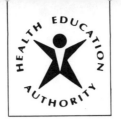

Every Woman's Health

Information and resources for group discussion

ISBN 1 85448 447 8

Contents

Acknowledgements

Thanks are especially due to the Project Coordinators and Project workers in the three WEA districts in which the book was developed – Melanie Pleaner, Linda Pepper, Jill Bedford, Hazel Millar and Norma Wilson.

A large part of the book has been written by Jill Bedford and Linda Pepper, who amended, updated and added to many of the ideas and activities in the previous book. They have also written substantial new chapters, on sexual health and older women's health.

We would also like to thank the following for their specific contributions: Kate Woodhouse for the section on Smoking; Victoria Fitch and Pam Naylor for the section on Drinking; Lesley Pattenson for Worksheet 9.4B, and, together with Leeds Lesbian Line, Worksheet 9.5; Justine Pepperell for Information Sheet 3.3 and Activity 3.3.

Among the other women, at national and local level, in paid and unpaid work who contributed to the book are:

- Melanie Pleaner, Mary Curran and Jane Black (WEA North Western District), who wrote the original book.

- The many women who participated in women's health events on which this book is based.

- The women who have shared their knowledge and experience, and whose ideas have been adapted.

- Mary Tidyman, as Project Officer, HEA, and for her work on drawing together material from the original book with the new material.

- The WEA Management Team, and administrative staff in the three WEA Districts.

- Kath Locke, WEA North Western District, who contributed to the original book and the development of this one, but who did not live to see its completion.

- Marie Goldsmith, HIV/AIDS Officer, Health Education Authority.

- Barbara James and Paula McDiamid for the Resources sections.

- Angela Martin for her cartoons.

Foreword

There are many opportunities for health education with women in different settings. Women meet together in a variety of groups with health as a prime focus, for example: women's health groups organised by health promotion officers, health visitors or well-women volunteers; antenatal education classes offered by midwives, health visitors or voluntary organisations such as the National Childbirth Trust; Look After Yourself sessions offered within workplace settings or in the community; and self-help groups concerned with a particular health issue, such as the menopause.

Other settings where women meet together may not be primarily concerned with health. For example, women's refuges, drop-in centres, play groups, youth, community and adult education settings offer many opportunities for health education because women use the chance to talk together about issues which affect their health and their lives. Such discussions may start very informally, and groups may then seek ways of structuring what they do around health. This book offers ideas and activities for health education with women in all these and many more situations.

The Health Education Authority (HEA) is a special health authority within the National Health Service, which has a remit 'to help the people of England to become more knowledgeable, better motivated and more able to acquire and maintain good health'.

In setting out to develop this book, the HEA has benefited greatly by its collaboration with the Workers' Educational Association (WEA). This is a national voluntary organisation which provides adult education in many towns and villages nationwide. Women's health has developed and become established as part of a growing area of work on women's education and women's studies within the WEA.

The HEA's Health Education for Women Training Project has been based in three WEA Districts to develop women's health education over the period October 1988 to March 1992. The Districts involved in the Project have been North Western District (with a base in Manchester); West Mercia District (with a base in Birmingham); and Western District (with a base in Bristol).

The Project has developed and built on the ideas in the previous Health Education Council/WEA *Women and Health: Activities and Materials for use in Women's Health Courses and Discussion Groups*, published in 1986. This new book, *Every Woman's Health* includes new ideas and activities, covers some additional health topics, and has updated information on health issues and about other resources on women's health.

A companion Handbook has been developed by the same Project: *Women Together: A Health Education Training Handbook for Ourselves and Others* (1992), available from the HEA price £12.95. It provides information and practical suggestions on how to plan, organise and facilitate women's health education as well as how to identify new opportunities for health promotion initiatives. The information will help women who are running health sessions themselves or are training others to do so.

1 Introduction

ABOUT THIS BOOK

How this book was developed

This book is a revised, updated and extended edition of the HEC/WEA *Women and Health: Activities and Materials for Use in Women's Health Courses and Discussion Groups*, first published in 1986. It has been developed alongside the HEA's *Women Together: A Health Education Training Handbook for Ourselves and Others* through HEA's Health Education for Women Training Project, 1988–1992, in collaboration with the Workers' Educational Association (WEA).

The project has developed the ideas and activities included in these two resources by working with a variety of women in different settings, including workers in:

- the National Health Service;
- community education;
- social services;
- youth and community services;
- probation services; and
- self-help and community groups.

Information has been updated, revisions made and the contents reorganised in response to women's experiences of using the original resource pack. A number of new topic areas are included, reflecting gaps in the original material identified by the project. This book includes new sections on:

- women and HIV and AIDS;
- contraception;
- sexually transmitted diseases;

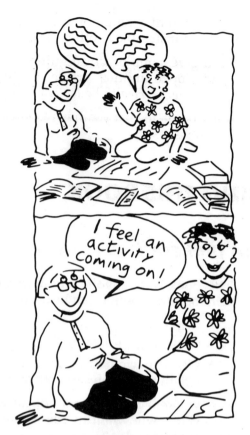

- older women's health;

- smoking;

- alcohol; and

- coronary heart disease.

This material has been developed and piloted through running women's health sessions and training events.

Material has been revised and extended to make it more relevant to the needs of Black women. The project has achieved this through:

- working with Black women at training events;

- discussions with Black women in each project locality to identify ways of meeting their health education needs;

- input from Black women in national organisations; and

- resourcing and supporting Black women to run women's health education sessions, to feed back good practice and write activities for the pack.

Aims of this book

1 To provide practical ideas and activities on a range of health topics to use in women's health sessions and courses.

2 To present a range of approaches for tackling health topics, which are also transferable to other topics.

3 To give some practical guidelines for working with groups. (These are developed in much greater depth in the companion publication *Women Together: A Health Education Training Handbook for Ourselves and Others*.)

4 To point to many other resources available on women's health topics and issues.

USING THIS BOOK

Who is it for?

This book is for anyone who wants to teach or learn about women's health with other women. It can be used in a variety of situations by:

- workers in statutory or voluntary organisations, involved with health education with women;
- self-help women's health groups who want to provide support or health education sessions for themselves; or
- workers in women's education who are familiar with group work skills, who want to use women's health as a useful tool to empower women.

It offers a starting point for those who may not otherwise have the confidence or skill to work in participatory ways on health issues, and an opportunity for those with experience of working with women in groups to extend their skills and cover new topics and issues.

How this book is organised

The book contains the following eleven chapters.

1 *Introduction*, giving the aims and background to the work which produced this book, and describing who the book is for, and how it is organised.

2 *Running women's health sessions*, considers why women and health should be an important subject focus, looks at opportunities for women's health education, and discusses differences between women, and health issues for Black women.

3 *The NHS and patients' rights*

4 *Mental health*, includes sections on emotional and mental health, stress, and relaxation and massage.

5 *Food and body image*, includes sections on food, diet and healthy eating, and self/body image.

6 *Female cycles*, includes sections on knowing our bodies, menstruation and menopause.

7 *Motherhood*

8 *Older women's health*

9 *Sexual health*, includes sections on sexuality, contraception, sexually transmitted diseases (STDs) and women and HIV and AIDS.

10 *Staying healthy*, includes sections on vaginal health, premenstrual syndrome, cancer prevention, complementary medicine, coronary heart disease prevention, smoking and drinking.

11 *General resources*, lists some general resources on women's health and provides details of distributors and organisations referred to throughout the book.

Chapters 3 to 10 each include:

- a contents page;
- background information;
- practical points;
- information and activities; and
- resources.

At the end of the book there is:

- an index of activities, worksheets, information sheets; and
- an evaluation sheet for the book.

Activities

All the activities detailed in this book include:

- aims;
- materials needed;
- methods;
- group size – groups are referred to as 'large', meaning the whole group, preferably up to 14 or 16, but no more than 20 women; or 'small', meaning sub-groups used in various learning methods, of around three to five women.

When using small groups, make sure someone in each group is noting comments and will report back, where necessary.
Stress that women should share what feels comfortable for them, and check they are happy about what is to be reported back to the large group.

● Discussion points, giving an idea about the possible issues or information that may arise from an activity, and suggesting points to raise with the group if they do not come up spontaneously.

Worksheets and information sheets

For some activities, there are corresponding worksheets and/or information sheets. You may photocopy these pages without obtaining permission.

● Worksheets can be used as they are, or adapted to suit your own needs.

● Information sheets can be used during the session or given out to take home for reference.

★ denotes an activity which needs particular care and experienced facilitation. It could provoke strong responses and emotions in some groups which could be damaging if not handled well. With experience you will have a better 'feel' for when a group is ready for this sort of activity. You could get support from a co-tutor in sessions where sensitive activities are being used.

Resources

● The resources suggested are by no means exhaustive, but suggest some useful and accessible material for each topic, and useful contacts.

● Inclusion of resources does not mean recommendation. All distributors are listed at the end of the book, in Chapter 11 *General resources*, rather than with individual listings.

DIFFERENT WAYS TO USE THE BOOK

Whilst the topics covered in this book are not exhaustive, they reflect those often requested by women. They therefore provide a good starting point for planning a women's health session or course. As you get going you will probably find that women will suggest other topics they also wish to cover.

You will need to decide which topics to include, and an order appropriate to your group. Whilst all women's health topics are potentially sensitive, some are more so than others. For example, it may be better to let group members get to know each other and you, and allow a certain level of trust to build up before introducing a topic such as sexual health.

The book is divided into different topic areas, but the boundaries between topics are not so clear cut. It's useful to take a "mix and match" approach, creating your own way of covering a topic by using activities from different chapters. For example, if you are working on *sexual health*, it may be relevant for your group to use activities from *female cycles* and *mental health* as well.

The activities offer ideas for ways of working with a group, but there is no one right way of doing things. You may find it is useful to adapt activities

- to suit different groups of women
- to give you ideas for covering different women's health topics.

With practice and experience you will find you can develop your own activities which work best for you and your groups.

2 Running women's health sessions

Why women's health?

Opportunities for women's health education

Differences between women

Health issues for Black women

Teaching and learning in groups

WHY WOMEN'S HEALTH?

Work with women is important and valuable for the following reasons.

Women have their own specific health concerns. They use the health services more than men – for themselves and for their families. They therefore need access to relevant information to feel confident in requesting the services they need.

Working with women on health offers the opportunity to question women's traditional roles, develop leadership skills, and promote and extend women's self-confidence.

Women's health sessions or courses can cover a wide range of aims, including to:

- find out about women's health issues generally;
- focus on a particular issue of interest or concern to group members (e.g. menopause, depression, older women's health);
- achieve a common goal (e.g. give up smoking, learn relaxation skills);
- campaign for, or organise, a particular service related to women's health (e.g. set up a well-women's centre); and

- provide the opportunity for women to develop knowledge and skills to enhance their health.

OPPORTUNITIES FOR WOMEN'S HEALTH EDUCATION

The following settings may provide opportunities for women's health education.

Within the Health Service, for example:

- health promotion units;
- well-women clinics/centres;
- GP health promotion clinics; and
- women's groups run by health workers in health centres or community venues.

Within local authorities, for example:

- youth and community work;
- women's refuges;
- community and adult education;
- social services;
- probation services; and
- health promotion units.

Within voluntary or community settings, for example:

- family planning agencies;
- well-women drop-in services;
- HIV and AIDS agencies; and
- community projects and groups.

Within workplaces, for example through:

- occupational health; and
- unions.

Below are some examples of how and why groups have started.

The mothers wanted to do something stimulating and challenging whilst their children attended the playgroup. They approached the local adult education centre about putting on a course at the centre. The group were all interested in women's health so I planned a course with the group to run for six weeks initially.

Community education worker

We met and discussed the isolation we experienced living on the estate, with young children, no transport and poor facilities in the area.

Mothers' support group

We started off as an exercise group but soon we were discussing other women's health topics. Women now come to the group to talk to each other, find out more about health and generally have time away from the kids.

Young women's health discussion group, meeting in a youth club

We wanted to attract women who would be unlikely to go to traditional adult education classes, who could not afford the fare to travel all the way from the estate to town and who could not attend daytime courses because they had young children at home. We tried to find a venue that was on the estate and where they would feel comfortable meeting. We were able to use the local primary school as the venue for a 10 week free women's health course with child care provided.

HEC/WEA Health Education for Women Training Project

We wanted to start a women's group, and looking at women's health issues seemed a good starting point to attract women.

Asian women's group in a community centre

We approached the WEA to run a women's health course as the first step in trying to establish a well-women centre.

Well-women group

Most of my patients who came to me because of menopausal/premenstrual problems seemed to want to talk and seek reassurance rather than actually wanting medication. I started a women's health discussion group once a week at the health centre.

Woman GP

We wanted to work with the parents of the children on changing diet and healthy eating. We advertised a talk on food for the parents and seven of the mothers attended. They were then keen to go on to other topics related to their own health. This became a regular forum and numbers gradually increased.

Health education worker

Many of the mothers I was working with seemed to be experiencing stress related problems. I started a women's stress and relaxation group at the health centre – the response has been overwhelming!

Health visitor

The group is intended for women who are going to have, or who have had hysterectomies. We share information, give support, give women the opportunity to ask questions and express anxieties and so on.

Hysterectomy self-help group

DIFFERENCES BETWEEN WOMEN

Differences between women in a group can be seen as a potential *problem*, because it may seem harder to find points of contact and communication and therefore conflicts may arise. Differences can also be seen as *enriching* because a variety of perspectives will be present within the group. Differences may include:

- class;
- race/culture/religion;
- sexual preference;
- age;
- ability (physical or emotional);
- marital status;
- the paid or unpaid work women do; and
- whether or not the women have children.

Differences between women within a group may well affect the group dynamics. While gender will be the common factor in the group, power will be distributed according to whether women are white or Black, working class or middle class, have disabilities or not, their sexual preference, ages and so on.

Some differences between women are more obvious than others (for example colour of skin, or the use of a wheelchair are obvious, while hearing problems, or sexual preference may not be). Often the norm is assumed to be white, middle-class, young, heterosexual, able-bodied women. Women who do not fit this stereotype may face discrimination. Women need to be aware of their own assumptions, attitudes and prejudices towards women who are different from themselves.

One Black woman, one lesbian, one woman with a disability in a group can provide a *perspective*, but not the views of all Black, lesbian or disabled women. It is important that their involvement in the group should not be limited to their experiences of race, sexuality or ability. Where a group does not have many differences among its members, the tutor may need to ensure that issues related to differences are considered.

Working individually or in small groups may encourage women to tackle sensitive areas relating to differences between themselves. Knowing that *issues*, rather than *specific personal information*, will be fed back to the large group can help group members feel 'safe'. Ground rules (see p. 18) are also important for this.

HEALTH ISSUES FOR BLACK WOMEN

The term 'Black' is used here to distinguish those groups of women who are discriminated against in Britain because their skin is not 'white'. This book has been developed specifically with African-Caribbean and Asian women to address some issues particularly relevant to them.

Health issues for Black women are similar to those for women in general. Yet the consequences of living with racism are that Black women face specific challenges in getting their health needs met. Discrimination and oppression faced by Black women as a result of both gender and race may have detrimental effects on their health. This 'double oppression' can often lead to a third type of oppression, that of poverty, which is known to be related to poor health.

Issues such as class, status, sexual preference, religion, ethnicity and ability, all serve to distinguish between Black women in the same way as they do for white women. Although culture has its place in exploring health issues, these other factors also need to be considered. Research has tended to focus on specific diseases which affect Black people, such as coronary heart disease, sickle cell or rickets, and offer either genetic or cultural explanations for their prevalence which are not always appropriate. For example, the high rate of rickets in Asian children was taken to be the result of inadequate diet and restrictive cultural practices limiting access to sunshine on skin. Yet in the past, there was widespread occurrence of rickets in the white working class population due to economic and social deprivation. Vitamin D was introduced into margarine to counteract this.

Black women face specific health challenges when health workers make assumptions about their lives which may be based on stereotyping and value judgements. For example, assumptions are made about family life: Asian women are seen as submissive within a rigid patriarchal family structure; African-Caribbean families may be viewed as lacking discipline. Such attitudes may affect both the way health workers relate to women, and also the options made available to Black women.

Access to health services may have an impact on the health of Black women. Language may be a barrier to health care, as may racist attitudes of staff, culturally insensitive practices, and the prevalence of male doctors.

Different lifestyles, diet and religion may be seen as a problem in relation to an inflexible organisation of services.

The day to day stress which Black women face may have an effect on their health. For example, Asian women show very high rates of coronary heart disease which have not been correlated with high incidence of accepted risk factors such as smoking, cholesterol or high blood-pressure. The Coronary Prevention Group (1986) put forward other possible causal factors needing research, including migration and discrimination.

TEACHING AND LEARNING IN GROUPS

Informal learning in groups can be effective because it enables:

- active involvement of group members in the planning and content of sessions;

- participatory learning methods, where learning takes place through enquiry, discovery and sharing of ideas;

- learning from each other by sharing experiences, enabling women to begin to see the more general patterns of health issues affecting their lives; and

- mutual support.

A wide variety of informal and participative methods can be used in women's health education. Some of those described below appear in

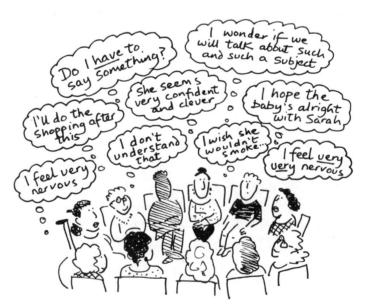

activities throughout this book; many activities use a combination of methods. It is important to be aware of factors such as the group's literacy, language and mobility when choosing methods.

Group discussion

is a very common method, and can be used with other methods. The skills of the facilitator are important to:

- draw out the group;
- encourage discussion between members;
- allow time for thought, rather than rushing in to fill silences; and
- encourage the group to look for links and connections, and to draw their own conclusions.

If the group is large, participation by all members can be increased by splitting into smaller groups where women may feel less daunted and more willing to contribute. (see below)

Pairs or small groups

can be valuable not only for discussion but also to work on a specific task, for example to fill in a questionnaire, play a game, do a role play or a practical activity. It also makes it easier to deal with sensitive or intimate issues, which could be difficult for some women in a larger group. Sometimes reporting back is not needed; in other situations it is valuable to feed back small-group discussions into the large group.

Round

involves asking a group of women in turn for a verbal response, which can then be written down on a flipchart for all to see.

Brainstorming

is putting a question or issue to the group for their immediate thoughts or ideas. It may be useful to set a time limit. Making a list of responses on the flipchart for everyone to see can be used:

- as a basis for more detailed discussion;
- for sorting ideas into different categories or in order of importance;
- to establish priorities for further action; and
- to refer to throughout the session.

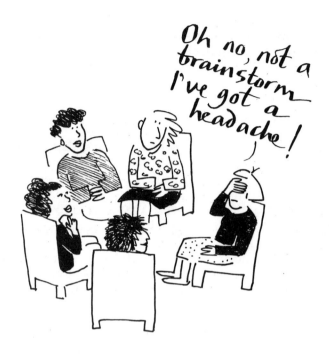

Questionnaires

can be used as a basis for group discussion, or to enable individuals to reflect on their own experiences, needs, or options. They are also useful for evaluation. Multiple-choice, true-false, or open-ended questions are some possible formats.

Sentence completion

is a method similar to questionnaires, but more open-ended. It can stimulate individuals or a group to express ideas or feelings about an issue verbally or in writing, with minimal prompting or guidance.

Case-studies

are a useful and non-threatening way of illustrating and bringing to life important issues. They can generate discussion on sensitive matters since they allow women to explore problems that might be close to their own, but in a more detached way. They also provide an opening for women to tell about their own situation if they want to.

Guided fantasy/visualisation

is a method whereby women are taken through a prepared fantasy, read out by the group leader, or developed in the session by women in the group. It can be a private method for individual women, or afterwards feedback can be shared with the group. Because some women in groups resist the letting-go aspect of a visualisation, it can sometimes be useful to do some simple relaxation techniques first.

Role play

involves acting out situations to bring issues alive, to explore attitudes, feelings and different points of view, and to develop insight. It can also be used to develop and practise skills, for example in being assertive in situations where women feel powerless. Role play can be a powerful teaching method and needs to be used carefully and sensitively when familiarity and trust have developed in the group. Some women will voice anxieties over this method, while at the same time acknowledging its benefit. In such instances, it can be useful for a more confident member of the group and the group leader to do a role play to begin with. Sometimes it is necessary to de-role afterwards, to bring women back to real life.

Debates

can be a useful approach to controversial issues. Whether formal or informal, they can develop confidence in critical thinking, arguing a point of view, assessing conflicting arguments and highlighting issues such as prejudice and objectivity. Careful preparation by the group leader can make this method particularly effective.

Course diary or scrapbook

gives women the opportunity to express their impressions and feelings about the group. Women can take turns recording each session in the diary, pasting in worksheets or activities, or even drawings. Course diaries are also useful for evaluation.

Group projects

are a valuable means of encouraging self-directed learning and co-operative activity. Projects can be done during a session or between sessions. Project work can be used in various ways, for example to find out more about local services and campaigns, or about a particular health topic.

Newspaper or magazine articles

can trigger discussion, introduce different ideas and opinions, or provide case-studies. 'Problem pages' from women's magazines can be used in the same way.

Videos

can stimulate discussion, especially on particular topics. They are especially useful when there are difficulties over literacy.

Creative work

such as collage and drawing can enhance discussion on many topics. Magazines, newspapers, felt-tips, crayons, scissors and glue can be used in many imaginative ways, providing a means of expression other than writing or talking.

Photographs

can trigger discussion and group cohesion. Asking women to bring in photographs of themselves when they were younger can stimulate discussion on issues such as self-image or different life-stages. Current photographs can promote discussion on different lifestyles, cultures and issues around the family.

Index cards

can have useful applications! You can ask women to write down things on one side of the card, stressing that what they write will be anonymous (though the information will be shared with the group). Place all the cards in a bin, box or bag, then let each woman take out a card (replacing it and taking another if they happen to pick their own) and read out what it says. This method can be used for a variety of topics and issues, for example to find out expectations and fears for the event, to find out women's concerns over HIV and AIDS, to elicit what is going wrong in the group, to evaluate a session, and so on. You are more likely to find out what women really feel with this method than if you had asked them to respond verbally in a round.

Games

have the advantage of getting women moving and can be a fun and lighthearted way of dealing with sensitive topics.

The role of tutor

- There is no absolute blueprint for a tutor.

- Some common difficulties tutors experience[1]:
    - the tutor being seen as an expert;
    - the group wanting information, not discussion;

[1] There are lots of guidelines and practical ideas for dealing with these issues in the companion book *Women Together: a Health Education Training Handbook for Ourselves and Others* (1992), HEA.

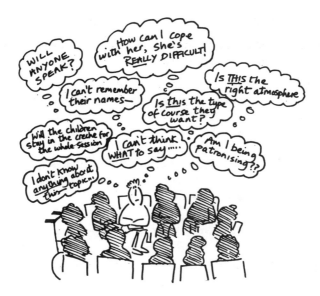

- working with people's emotions;
- dealing with dominant women;
- dealing with quiet women;
- the issue of self-disclosure;
- how to generate discussion; and
- resistance to some learning methods.

● Try to create an atmosphere of tolerance, respect and equality where learning can take place.

● Be clear about your own role, and its limitations – you don't have to be a social worker, an expert or a therapist. The group members need to know and accept this also.

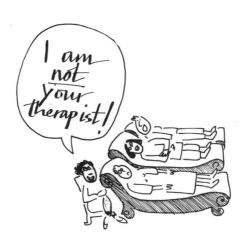

- Try to be aware of your own views, feelings, prejudices.
- It is useful to understand something about group dynamics and group processes, and the 'life' of a group.
- However experienced you are with leading groups, the unexpected can always happen! Try and use these instances for learning.

Ground rules

Groups are more likely to be effective if guidelines for working together – or 'ground rules' – have been agreed at the outset by all group members. Such ground rules might include:

- confidentiality;
- only one woman to talk at a time;
- listening as well as talking;
- respecting other women's opinions (even if you disagree with them);
- no one being forced to contribute;
- everyone taking responsibility for starting and finishing on time;
- giving equal time to everyone; and
- changing direction if appropriate.

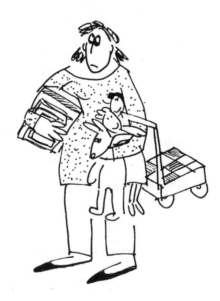

Practicalities

A women's health session or course is more likely to be successful if practical issues have been carefully considered. These will include:

- targeting the event;
- costing and funding;
- the venue;
- timing;
- providing creche facilities;
- publicity;
- structuring the event;
- running the event; and
- evaluation.

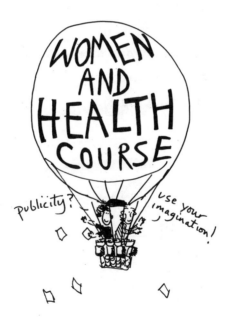

Evaluation

For group members, it is important to evaluate a women's health session or course, to:

- enable changes to be made to improve the relevance and quality;

- encourage them to have control over and participate in their learning process; and

- enable them to reflect on their learning and personal development.

For the tutor, evaluation is important to:

- clarify aims and objectives and check they are being met;

- measure the suitability of session/course content;

- assess adequacy of organisational arrangements;

- assess process and outcome;

- judge cost, time and effectiveness;

- assess whether original needs are being met;

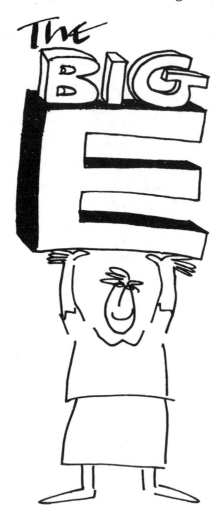

- generate change and improve ways of working;
- share experiences and models of good practice;
- demonstrate effectiveness in order to secure continued support and funding; and
- be accountable to ourselves, our colleagues, funders, employers and participants.

You may want to evaluate:

- the process – planning, running the event, the programme, learning methods, and venue, creche and refreshments;
- the outputs – any reports, articles or other publications produced as a result of the work; and
- the outcomes – effects of the session or course on women's health including changes in knowledge, attitudes or skills demonstrating other health behaviour.

Women Together (HEA, 1992) looks in much more detail at evaluation, what it is, what it is for, what, who, when and how to evaluate, including ways of evaluating what participants feel about a session or course and evaluating yourself as a tutor/trainer. It also includes suggestions for what to do with evaluation.

3 The NHS and patients' rights

BACKGROUND INFORMATION

- Women use the National Health Service (NHS) more than men (for both themselves and their families), they work in large numbers in the health services, and they tend to take on a carer's role in the community. It is important that women understand the organisation of health services, and how decisions are made and priorities set that will affect them.

- Recently there have been profound changes in the way the NHS is organised, and it is important for women to understand the implications for them, and the impact on local services. The activities *Understanding the NHS reforms, Contracting for women's health work I and II*, and *What kind of health services do we want?* address issues related to the new NHS, and are backed up with information sheets.

- Women's contact with the NHS may well be when we are at our most vulnerable. Sometimes we feel we are seen as a symptom, rather than as a whole person. We may feel nervous or intimidated when dealing with some health professionals, and we may not therefore make the best use of the consultation. The activities *Dealing with health professionals* and *Talking to your doctor* provide an opportunity to explore this area and develop communication and assertiveness skills.

- The greater our knowledge of our rights and responsibilities as patients, the more confidently and effectively we can work with health professionals. There are information sheets on *Patients' rights*, and *The Patients' Charter*. Information on making use of *Community Health Councils* is also included.

- The NHS and patients' rights is a large topic, and may be a theme running throughout a women's health course. The activity *Women's health Snakes and Ladders* can provide a fun and thought provoking introduction, raising issues such as social and economic factors which affect our health, availability of services, and positive action we can take to improve our health.

- Other issues that may be useful to cover include:

  - What is good health? What is good health care? Is the NHS a National Health Service or a National Illness Service?

  - To what extent does the NHS meet the needs of particular groups? Class and race can affect the way people are treated in the NHS. How can working class and Black women get their voices heard and their needs met in the NHS?

  - How can we as individuals and groups influence and gain more control over health care and health services?

    – What is the relationship between complementary medicine, private medicine and the NHS? What should it be?

PRACTICAL POINTS

Groups often request sessions about the NHS, but some tutors may feel intimidated by the topic because it is complex, and rapid changes are occurring. The information in this chapter will provide a good grounding, and there are useful ways to approach the topic without detailed knowledge:

- by focusing on the broad issues such as 'what is good health care'?
- by focusing on more personal issues such as relationships with health professionals; or
- by encouraging the group to do a 'project' over a number of weeks to find out about local health services.

It may be useful to invite someone to come and talk to the group about local health services; for example, someone from:

- the **Community Health Council** – they will have an overall grasp of the NHS reforms, and how they affect local services;
- the **Family Health Services Authority** (FHSA), who will be able to give information about GP services, including GP fund-holding and the new GP contract, and tell you about Health Promotion Clinics offered by GP practices; some FHSAs employ staff to link with the community, and they should be able to help you;
- your local **Hospital Trust** which may have a 'user forum' – you could ask a member to come and explain how the patient's voice is fed into decision-making processes; or
- a **health union** (e.g. NUPE or COHSE), who will have knowledge and experience of what is happening locally.

If you do invite someone to talk to the group, it is useful to find out beforehand what the group wants to know, and to let the speaker know this. Speakers are sometimes accustomed to 'lecturing' styles – it may be helpful to explain that women want to discuss issues as well as listen to information.

INFORMATION SHEET *3.1*

Organisation of the NHS in England

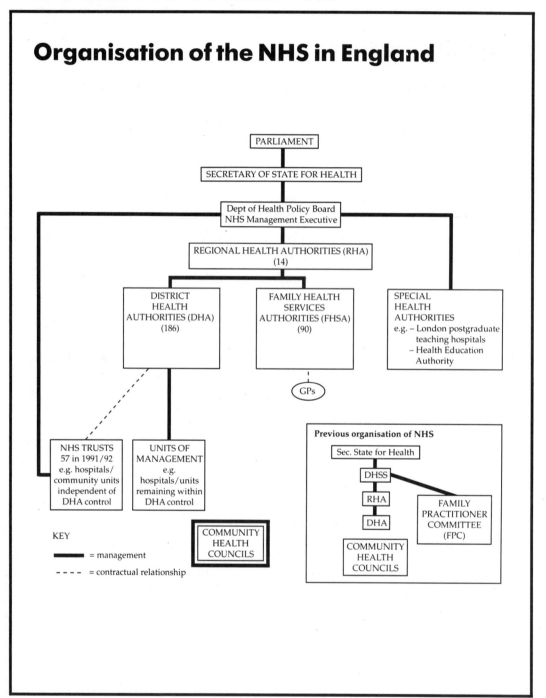

© Health Education Authority, 1993

INFORMATION SHEET *3.2*

Composition of NHS authorities

	Regional Health Authority	District Health Authority	Family Health Services Authority	NHS Trust
Chair appointed by	Secretary of State	Secretary of State	Secretary of State	Secretary of State
Non-executive members on the Authority	5 members appointed by Secretary of State (including FHSA chair and member from a university with a medical or dental school	5 members appointed by Regional Health Authority (teaching districts have to include a member from a university with a medical or dental school)	5 lay members and 4 professional members appointed by Regional Health Authority	Up to 5 members appointed from local community by Regional Health Authority; the rest appointed by the Secretary of State
Executive Members on the Authority	Up to 5 members including Chief Executive and Finance Director	Up to 5 members including Chief Executive and Finance Director – often the Director of Public Health	Chief Executive	Up to 5 members including Chief Executive, Finance Director, Medical Director, Senior Nurse

INFORMATION SHEET *3.3*

Contract culture

It is important to understand the way statutory agencies now work within a contract culture if you wish to influence or contribute to service provision in your area, and/or intend to fund-raise for work you are doing. Contracting involves statutory agencies (Health Authorities, Local Authorities, Family Health Service Authorities) buying services for their residents from other agencies (statutory, private, not-for-profit, or voluntary). A division has been created between the 'purchasing' and 'providing' of services. The philosophy applies to a range of services including health care, refuse collection, community care, and in some cases is enshrined in law e.g. the NHS and Community Care Act. The following terms are used.

Purchaser: the statutory authority responsible for buying services for its residents; holds a budget.

Provider: the agency providing the services to the purchaser, (directly managed unit, Trust, not-for-profit, voluntary, private).

Contract: the formal agreement between purchaser and provider about what services will be provided at what cost.

Contract specification: the details of the contract – who to; how much; where; what; when; quality assurance; monitoring.

Commissioning: creating new services and bringing new services into the purchasing process.

Contract culture: the philosophy of separating the purchasing and providing of services i.e. operating in a market place.

▷

▷ 3.3 cont.
There are opportunities for contracting services related to women's health with all three statutory agencies.

Possible contractual arrangements

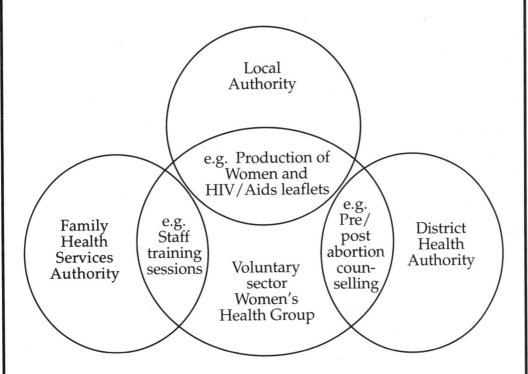

INFORMATION SHEET *3.4*

New GP contract

- GP practices must provide a practice leaflet (giving information about names and sex of doctors, kinds of clinics offered, out of hours cover, etc.).

- GPs must write an annual report and send it to the Family Health Services Authority (FHSA).

- The FHSA must produce and maintain a local directory of family doctors.

- GPs can claim reimbursement at a fixed rate from the FHSA for Health Promotion Clinics (provided the clinic has been run to an agreed standard, and covers one of the approved areas, such as smoking, diabetes, stress management). New arrangements are to be introduced.

- There are new target payments for immunisation and vaccination, and cervical smears.

- There is a special fee for doctors undertaking minor surgery, and child health surveillance (under five).

- Doctors accepting new patients must do a health promotion consultation, and obtain a medical history.

- Doctors must arrange to see patients not seen in the last three years, although this is being reviewed.

- Patients over 75 years old must receive at least one home visit from their GP per year for assessment purposes.

INFORMATION SHEET *3.5*

Budget-holding GPs

- Since 1 April 1991, General Practices with a large list of registered patients have been able to seek budget-holding status.

- They still remain in a contractual agreement with the Family Health Services Authority (FHSA) for the provision of general medical services.

- They are allocated a budget (by the Regional Health Authority in consultation with the FHSA) to cover the cost of:

  - a range of diagnostic tests;
  - outpatient/day patient/in-patient services;
  - prescribing drugs; and
  - staff and premises.

- Budget-holding GPs are free to negotiate contracts with directly managed hospitals/units or other providers (e.g. Trusts or private organisations) for services for their patients.

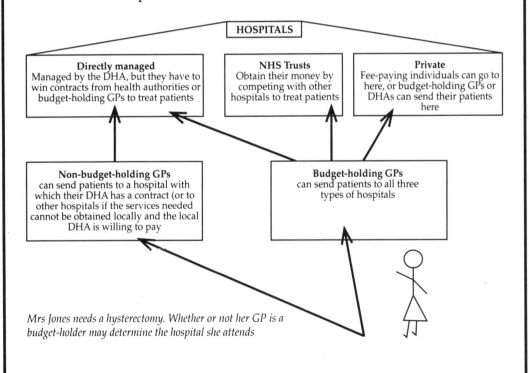

HOSPITALS

Directly managed
Managed by the DHA, but they have to win contracts from health authorities or budget-holding GPs to treat patients

NHS Trusts
Obtain their money by competing with other hospitals to treat patients

Private
Fee-paying individuals can go to here, or budget-holding GPs or DHAs can send their patients here

Non-budget-holding GPs
can send patients to a hospital with which their DHA has a contract (or to other hospitals if the services needed cannot be obtained locally and the local DHA is willing to pay

Budget-holding GPs
can send patients to all three types of hospitals

Mrs Jones needs a hysterectomy. Whether or not her GP is a budget-holder may determine the hospital she attends

INFORMATION SHEET *3.6*

Patients' rights

Getting treatment from a GP (family doctor)

Getting on a GP's list

Everyone living in this country has the right to be on a GP's list of patients. You can choose your GP, as long as the GP is willing to accept you. You'll find lists of GPs in main post offices and libraries, at the local Family Health Services Authority (FHSA), Community Health Council, Citizens' Advice Bureau, or general advice centre. If you can't find a GP to take you on, the FHSA will find you one. All GPs should produce a leaflet with details of the services they offer.

Seeing your GP
At the surgery

You have the right to see a GP (not necessarily your own) at your GP's surgery, at any time during surgery hours: these should be clearly displayed on a notice outside. The only exception is if there is an appointment system and you haven't made an appointment. In this case, you should be given an appointment at a later surgery, as long as the delay would not risk your health. Your GP's surgery should have a phone number at which you can leave messages, 24 hours a day, 365 days a year.

At home

You can ask your GP for a home visit but you have no right to one. You should speak to your doctor and explain what's wrong. The doctor is responsible for deciding whether to visit or not. If you are 75 or over you are entitled to at least one home visit each year.

Away from home

If you're away from home for up to three months, you can ask a GP to accept you as a temporary patient. A GP who won't accept you as a patient must give you any treatment that is immediately necessary. ▷

▷ 3.6 cont.

Emergencies

In an emergency, a hospital accident and emergency department will treat you.

Maternity and contraceptive services

You have to register separately for maternity and contraceptive services. If your GP does not provide these you can register with another GP just for maternity or contraceptive services while remaining on your first GP's list. The Family Health Services Authority (FHSA) will tell you which GPs offer these services.

Many areas have family planning clinics as well, where you can get free contraceptive advice. You can find out about them from FHSAs or Community Health Councils.

Changing GPs

If you move, you can apply to a GP in your new area. If you're unhappy with your GP you can change to another without giving a reason. Apply to another GP and send your medical card to the FHSA saying you want to change. If you change GPs, it may be up to 14 days before you can see the new one. You can also be removed from your GP's list without any reason being given. But the FHSA must make sure that you are not without a doctor.

Getting treatment from hospital doctors

You can't usually just walk into a hospital for treatment; you have to be sent by a GP or a clinic. But you don't need a doctor's letter to go to an accident and emergency department, or to a special clinic for treatment of sexually transmitted diseases. You have no absolute right to choose which hospital you're sent to, or which consultant you see. But if you have a preference, tell your GP.

Leaving hospital

Normally you can leave hospital (discharge yourself) at any time. If you do this against doctors' advice, they may ask you to sign a note recording your decision. This does not necessarily relieve them of legal liability. But you can be kept in hospital against your will if you are there by order of a Justice of the Peace because you have a longstanding or infectious disease, or if you are being detained under the Mental Health Act 1983.

▷ 3.6 cont.

Getting a second opinion

You have no absolute right to a second opinion. But doctors should take reasonable care to seek one if they are not sure what's wrong with you or how to treat you. So it's worth asking, if you want a second opinion.

Getting an abortion

Except in an emergency, you can get an abortion only if two doctors decide that:

- it would be a smaller risk to your life, your physical or mental health or the physical or mental health of your existing children than if your pregnancy continues; or

- the child, if born, would be seriously handicapped.

Giving your consent

In general, if you are examined or treated without your consent, it is a form of assault. Consent is only valid if you understand what your treatment involves and agree to it. You may be asked to sign a consent form showing that you accept treatment. However, if you go to see a GP or a hospital doctor, this is usually taken to mean that you are consenting to be examined and treated.

Refusing treatment

You are free to decide whether to accept treatment or not, and can stop treatment at any time even after signing the consent form. So make sure you tell your doctor if there's any sort of treatment you don't want. If doctors want you to have treatment that is unusual, or involves particular risks, they should discuss with you the consequences of any risk of injury (even in careful treatment) becoming a reality. You can stop treatment even if this could lead to your death.

Consent for abortion

For an abortion, only the woman's consent is needed, although doctors might want to consult your partner if you are willing. ▷

▷ 3.6 cont.

Consent for sterilisation

For sterilisation, doctors will normally want to consult your partner. But a partner's agreement is not legally necessary.

Not able to give consent

If you are unconscious or temporarily incapable of understanding and consenting to treatment, doctors should give you only essential treatment. If you are permanently incapable (through mental illness or confusion due to old age) it may be necessary for a court to decide whether treatment should go ahead. Usually relatives and doctors are asked to agree to the treatment although the consent of relatives is not legally binding (except in the case of parent and child).

Medical students

If you don't want to have medical students watching you being examined or treated, you can simply tell the doctor, who must go along with your wishes.

Finding out about your illness and treatment

In general, if you specifically ask about something to do with your illness or treatment, doctors should reply fully and truthfully. But doctors should take reasonable care to volunteer information even if you don't ask for it. In some cases, doctors may keep things back if they think the anxiety may injure your health.

Seeing medical records

From November 1991 doctors and hospitals have been obliged to let you see your written medical records (unless they consider that you could be harmed by seeing them) and to correct any mistakes, if you ask. If you have any difficulties getting hold of information, contact your local Community Health Council (CHC) who may be able to help.

If your doctor writes a report on you for your employer or an insurance company, you have the right to see it before it is passed on (unless the doctor decides that you could be harmed by seeing it). You can refuse to let your employer or insurance company see the report or you can add your own written comments. ▷

▷ 3.6 cont.

Confidentiality

In general, doctors must not pass on information about your case without your permission – except to other people involved in your treatment, or to close relatives. Doctors should not, for example, give information about you to employers without your permission. If there is something you don't want relatives to be told, tell the doctor what it is. If doctors suspect that a child is being deliberately injured, they may tell the local authority social services department or the NSPCC.

The law requires doctors to give information about you to health or other authorities if:

- ordered to by a court;
- you have certain infectious diseases or food poisoning;
- they suspect you're addicted to a hard drug (such as heroin);
- they arrange an abortion for you; or
- required by the police to help identify a driver who is suspected of motoring offences.

Children

- Everyone can reasonably expect to be able to consult a doctor confidentially. The older you are and the more you can understand the more 'reasonable' this expectation is. If you are 16 or over, you can give your own consent to examination and treatment. If you are under 16, the answer will depend on how mature you are and how much you can understand.

- The more serious or extensive the proposed treatment, the more likely the law is to expect the doctor to involve your parent(s) if you are under 16. But doctors may give advice and treatment to people under 16 without involving their parents, if there is sufficient need.

- If you are in hospital, your parents can visit at any time and should be able to stay overnight.

Charges

There is no charge for basic GP or hospital treatment (though people not living in

▷

▷ 3.6 cont.

this country do have to pay for most kinds of hospital treatment). There are the following exceptions:

Prescription charges

There is a charge for prescriptions. If you need a lot of prescriptions, you can get four-monthly and yearly 'season tickets'. Post offices, FHSAs and social security offices have the application form FP95.

But prescriptions are free automatically if you are:

- under 16 (or under 19 and still in full-time education);
- a woman 60 or over or a man 65 or over;
- pregnant or have a child under 12 months old;
- on income support or family credit (or if your partner is);
- suffering from certain medical conditions, including permanent physical disability which prevents you leaving home without the help of another person; or
- a war or service pensioner and you need prescriptions for your disability.

Post offices and social security offices have leaflets P11 and AB11 which explain about getting prescriptions free.

You may also be able to get free prescriptions if you or your partner are on a low income. Details are on form AG1 which you can get from any social security office.

GP charges

GPs can charge for services not normally provided by the NHS, including:

- certificates of sickness or injury other than those required for social security purposes;
- vaccinations or immunisations for travelling abroad if they are not recommended by the Department of Health; international certificates of vaccination; or
- check-ups needed by employers or insurance companies.

Hospital charges

Hospitals can charge for amenity beds (paying to get a bed with more privacy); and prescriptions for outpatients' drugs and appliances.   ▷

▷ 3.6 cont.

Road accident charges

GPs and hospitals can claim fees for emergency examination or treatment following road accidents. The patient is usually charged but this can often be reclaimed from the drivers of the vehicles involved or their insurance companies.

Making a complaint

GP services

Only if GPs fail to follow their terms of service (a sort of job description) can you make a formal complaint which is investigated by the Family Health Services Authority (FHSA). FHSAs also have informal ways of dealing with other complaints, for example about GPs' attitudes.

At present, if you can't sort out the problem with your GP you have to write to the FHSA, usually within 13 weeks of the incident. If you need advice on how to complain, or help in phrasing the letter, contact your local Community Health Council.

Hospitals

If you can't sort out a complaint with the person involved, or don't want to discuss it with them, the hospital should have a senior member of staff who will deal with your complaint. If your complaint is about the actual treatment you received, you can ask for the matter to be referred to the Regional Medical Officer (or, in Wales, the Medical Officer for Complaints).

Unethical or unprofessional behaviour

If a doctor behaves in a way which is unethical or unprofessional, you can complain to the General Medical Council (GMC), 44 Hallam Street, London W1; telephone 071 580 7642. Such behaviour includes neglecting patients, charging for free services, excessive drinking, or having a sexual or emotional relationship with a patient. You can also write to the GMC if a doctor appears to be incapable of doing the job because of a mental or physical illness. In the same way, if you believe that a nurse, midwife or health visitor has acted in an unprofessional way, you can complain to the UK Central Council for Nursing, Midwifery and Health Visiting, 23 Portland Place, London W1N 3AF; telephone 071 637 7181. ▷

▷ 3.6 cont.

Health service commissioner

If you are not satisfied with the way your complaint was dealt with, you can complain to the Health Service Commissioner for England, Church House, Great Smith Street, London SW1; telephone 071 276 3000. (For Wales: 4th floor, Pearl Assurance House, Greyfriars Road, Cardiff; telephone 0222 394621.) Normally you must do this within a year of realising you have something to complain about. The Health Service Commissioner cannot deal with doctors' decisions about diagnosis and treatment.

Legal action and compensation

Health authorities sometimes make voluntary payments to people who are injured by health care staff. But the only way to be sure of compensation or an award of damages is to sue and win. To win, you must normally prove negligence. You will therefore need legal advice from a solicitor or a law centre.

Source: The above information is based on a leaflet *Patients' Rights* published jointly by the Association of Community Health Councils for England and Wales, and the National Consumer Council and Welsh Consumer Council, November 1990. The leaflet is also available in the following languages: Welsh, Punjabi, Hindi, Bengali, Gujarati, Urdu, Cantonese, Vietnamese, Turkish, Greek and Armenian – please ask at your Community Health Council.

For legal reasons, the above information cannot be guaranteed as absolutely correct.

INFORMATION SHEET *3.7*

The Patients' Charter

The Patients' Charter sets out clearly for the first time your rights to care in the NHS. In addition to seven established rights, three new rights came into being on 1 April 1992. The Patients' Charter also identifies national charter standards which are not legal rights but specific standards for the NHS to achieve as circumstances and resources allow. In addition, Health Authorities will set and publicise local charter standards.

Established rights

Every citizen has the following NHS rights:

- to receive health care on the basis of clinical need, regardless of ability to pay;

- to be registered with a GP;

- to receive emergency medical care at any time (through GP, or emergency ambulance service and hospital accident and emergency services);

- to be referred to a consultant (acceptable to you) when your GP thinks it necessary, and to be referred for a second opinion if you and your GP agree this is desirable;

- to be given a clear explanation of any treatment proposed (including any risks and any alternatives) before you decide whether you will agree to the treatment;

- to have access to your health records, and to know that those working for the NHS are under a legal duty to keep their contents confidential; and

- to choose whether or not you wish to take part in medical research or medical student training.

New rights as from 1 April 1992

- to be given detailed information of local health services, including quality standards and maximum waiting times; this information is available from the District Health Authority, your GP, and your local Community Health Council;

- to be guaranteed admission for treatment by a specific date no later than two

▷

▷ 3.7 cont.
years from the day when your consultant places you on a waiting list; this is the responsibility of the District Health Authority, and your GP; and

- to have any complaint about NHS services (whoever provides them) investigated, and to receive a full and prompt reply from the chief executive or general manager. If you remain unhappy about your complaint you have the right to take the matter up with the Health Service Commissioner.

National charter standards (to be aimed for)

- Respect for privacy, dignity and religious and cultural beliefs.

- Arrangements to ensure everyone (including people with special needs) can use services.

- Information to relatives and friends.

- Waiting times for an ambulance service should be not more than 14 minutes in an urban area, and 19 minutes in a rural area.

- In an accident and emergency department, you should be seen immediately and your need for treatment assessed.

- In an outpatient clinic, you should be seen within 30 minutes of a specific appointment time.

- Your operation should not be cancelled on the day you are due to arrive in hospital (except because of emergencies or staff sickness).

- A qualified nurse, midwife or health visitor should be responsible for each patient.

- On discharge of patients from hospital, your hospital will agree arrangements for meeting decisions made regarding any continuing health or social care.

If you feel you are being denied one of the national charter rights, you should write to:
Duncan Nichol (Chief Executive of the NHS)
Department of Health, Richmond House
79 Whitehall, London SW1A 2NS   ▷

▷ 3.7 cont.

Local charter standards

In addition to national charter standards, health authorities will set and publicise local charter standards, including:

- waiting times for first outpatient appointments;

- waiting times in accident and emergency departments (after your need for treatment has been assessed);

- the waiting time for taking you home after you have been treated (where your doctor says you have a medical need for NHS transport);

- enabling you and your visitors to find your way around hospitals (through enquiry points and better signposting); and

- ensuring that the staff you meet face-to-face wear name badges.

Your Health Authority will publicise the name of the person you should contact if you want more information about the local charter standards they have set.

INFORMATION SHEET *3.8*

Community Health Councils

Community Health Councils (CHCs) are statutory NHS bodies which represent users of the NHS.

Membership and resources

- Membership of CHCs is drawn from the local community which they are set up to serve. Members are appointed for four-year periods of office, with half the membership being subject to re-appointment every two years. CHC membership is entirely voluntary.

- Total membership of each CHC may vary from 18-24 members, nominated or elected from: local authorities (half of the total membership) voluntary organisations (at least one-third membership); and the Regional Health Authority (RHA).

- Funding for CHCs is via the RHA, which determines the number of members as well as being responsible for premises and staffing.

- Members elect a Chair on an annual basis (the Chair is unpaid, unlike the Chair of all other health authorities).

Staffing

Each CHC has a Chief Officer, appointed by the CHC and employed by the RHA. Chief Officers are supported by at least one other member of staff, usually an Assistant.

Obligations

Health Authorities are obliged to:

- consult formally with CHCs on proposals for 'substantial' development or variation of services;

- provide information required by CHCs to carry out their public duties;

- permit CHCs access to NHS-owned premises, for purposes of visiting; and

▷

▷ 3.8 cont.
- arrange an annual statutory meeting between CHC and Health Authority.

CHCs are obliged to:

- maintain an interest in the health care status of their resident population;
- challenge plans for substantial development or variation in services if they feel they are not in the interests of their resident population;
- hold a council meeting at least every three months; and
- publish an annual report.

The role of Community Health Councils

CHCs act in the public interest by:

- monitoring the quality of existing services;
- responding to authorities' consultation exercises;
- promoting the interests of users of services;
- providing information and advice;
- assisting people with complaints over services; and
- campaigning for specific services.

Many CHCs have specific interests and they have 'working groups' on these, for example 'women and children', 'women's health', or 'cancer screening'.

With the NHS reforms, the role of the CHC is being developed. As District Health Authorities (DHAs) merge, so CHCs are also being merged. DHAs are less involved with managing units, and more involved with planning and purchasing of services. Patient satisfaction is a key feature of the NHS reforms; national and local charter standards are being developed through the Patients' Charter (see Information Sheet 3.7 *The Patients' Charter*) and there will be a role for the CHC to be involved in the monitoring of these.   ▷

▷ 3.8 cont.

The wider structure of Community Health Councils

- Many CHCs liaise with each other through a Regional Association of CHCs; the boundaries coincide with the boundaries of the Regional Health Authority.

- A national association – the Association of Community Health Councils for England and Wales (ACHCEW) – exists to protect the interests of CHCs. It is funded mainly through subscriptions from member CHCs. ACHCEW produces: an information service; the Community Health News newsletter; and briefing papers on current issues (for their address, see Chapter 11 *General resources*).

Your local Community Health Council

- CHCs may be found in Health Authority premises, in 'shop fronts' in the centre of towns or in other locations.

- Look in the telephone book for the address of your local CHC, or phone your District Health Authority (DHA) or Family Health Services Authority (FHSA).

- Contact your local CHC to find out if women's health issues are a feature of their work.

- Many CHCs are supportive of local health groups, self-help groups and campaigning groups. While they are unable – because of lack of resources – to fund such groups, they are often able to help with information, administrative back-up, use of premises, etc. CHCs will also have up-to-date information on 'who's who' in the Health Authorities, and useful contacts.

- Some may have well stocked libraries with facilities for borrowing books. CHCs will have copies of official documents on current concerns and issues for reference.

Make use of your local Community Health Council – it's *your* voice in the NHS!

INFORMATION SHEET *3.9*

Case study of a local self-help group

The following case study shows how one local self-help group, in Bristol, grew over a period of years, obtained funding and developed their services for women.

Well Women Information

Starting out

We started in 1978 as a small self-help group, the 'Bristol Women's Health Group', concerned about our own health problems such as contraception, fertility awareness, thrush and cystitis. We spent a lot of time learning about how our bodies worked, and about treatments provided by the medical profession. Working together, we gained skills which improved our own health and helped us challenge the one-dimensional approach of the medical model.

We built up a wealth of information relevant to women wanting to take a more active part in their health care, and we wanted to widen the scope of the process of information-sharing and support which went on in and around the group.

Going public

The opportunity came when we were offered the use of a room in the Health Authority's Health Education Department, based in a large clinic in the centre of Bristol. We launched a drop-in information service which was immensely popular, with women queuing outside on the first day we opened. Through this we recognised that women just wanted somewhere to talk about their health, with someone to listen and believe how much pain and distress they were in. They also welcomed the good quality health information we had accumulated – much of it from other women's groups – which could fill in the gaps in their knowledge.

The *Well Women Information* service was soon set up, run on a voluntary basis by a group of women who were unemployed or could adjust their schedules to work the rota. It continued on this basis for four years, during which time work expanded into community development work, helping to set up a women's health group in a town nearby, and responding to requests for an input into existing groups. New volunteers were drawn in, and two training courses were run.   ▷

▷ 3.9 cont.
Funding

In 1987 the formation of the Women's Committee of Bristol City Council brought hope of security to many women's organisations in Bristol. They visited and saw the strength of our commitment, and supported our work with a 'setting-up grant'. Avon County Council also provided some funding.

Receiving grant aid was controversial for us, with arguments on both sides (including the tension between self-help politics and having to account to funders). Funding meant we were providing a service for other women, not for ourselves; but we knew through our own health struggles how much this support and information was needed and valued. As a self-help group run by volunteers, it was hard to gain recognition and respect from some members of the medical profession and we often felt marginalised and dismissed. Funding helped increase our status and stability. Funding has changed some other aspects of our work, but we have tried to maintain the key principle of providing a 'user-led' service, responding to what women ask for in the way of help with health issues.

Mental health work

Our work demonstrated time and again that what women wanted was to talk, and that being heard and believed was more important than the leaflet that was the original reason for coming in. We started to explore issues around counselling and the complex issues involved in direct mental health work.

Some of us took training, and developed personal experience of one-to-one counselling and psychotherapy. Over time, we became better able to understand much more about the emotional content of the enquiries we got. The exhaustion and pain we were often left feeling after a busy drop-in morning became more tolerable. Gradually, we felt more able to focus on emotional health and to offer a small counselling service.

Community development and self-help work

Community development work focused on working with women's groups and running workshops and courses with different communities. Using our equal opportunities policy we were able to prioritise certain types of work, for example work with Asian women. Health groups, workshops, stalls, and consultations with Asian women's groups provided a crucial focus for the development work. We raised money to pay for some sessional work in mother tongue and both the sessional worker and the community development worker built up a network of contacts and information about what was needed.

Applications for funding of an Asian Women's Health Project were submitted and

▷

▷ 3.9 cont.

after three years one was successful. An Asian development worker is now in post, building on the work already done. She goes out to groups and networks with Asian women's organisations. Individual Asian women's health needs are becoming more articulated and both a women's health working group and a women's counselling group have recently been formed in the Asian Women's Network.

Alternative therapies

Our interest in supporting women in holding onto or regaining their health has also led us to look at some alternative approaches, in particular the use of herbs. Herbal treatments seem particularly useful for hormone problems such as premenstrual feelings and menopause. We have made creams and use herbal teas to treat thrush, nappy rash, period pains and tension. We work closely with the Clinic of Herbal Medicine and now buy a small consultancy service from them for three appointments per week for women on low incomes.

The future

It is fourteen years since we started meeting as a self-help group, and despite the economic and political climate we intend to be around for the next fourteen! If the inspiration, hard work and commitment of all the women involved is anything like that of the past, then we will see our hopes and plans come to reality. For many of us the involvement has been tremendously rewarding and for this we wish to thank all the women who have used our services.

At the moment we have three full-time workers – a community development worker, a women's health counsellor and a community development worker for Asian women. We hope to sustain and develop these areas of work. Future plans include developing our work with young Black women, and possibly creating a mobile service.

Source: Well Women Information, Bristol.

ACTIVITY *3.1*

Women's health Snakes and Ladders

Aims

- To provide a fun introduction to a complex topic.

- To introduce the wide range of factors which affect our health and the health care we get.

Materials

A copy of Worksheet 3.1 *Women's health Snakes and Ladders* for each woman; dice and counters (or improvise – see below).

Method

1 Introduce the activity and give out copies of the worksheet.

2 In small groups, play the game, using dice and counters to work round the sheet.

3 In large group, discuss what happened to the women in the game, relating it to the discussion points below.

Discussion points

- Do you think that what happened during the game was anything like real life?

- What things affect our health? Think of as wide a range as possible, including social and economic circumstances, local health care provision, and our own knowledge and assertiveness skills.

- What can we do to improve our health individually, and together with other people?

- How can we influence the provision and quality of health services in our area?

Note: To improvise, you can make a dice with blutack or plasticine, and use coins for counters.

ACTIVITY 3.2

Understanding the NHS reforms

Aims

- To help women understand the current changes in the NHS
- To find out the effects of NHS reforms on local health services

Materials

A flipchart, markers and copies of all the information sheets from this section for each woman.

Method

1 Brainstorm a list of issues that women have heard about to do with the NHS reforms (for example: purchaser/provider split; GP fundholding; GP contract; Trusts; contract culture).

   You may need to prompt – different groups will have different levels of knowledge.

2 Take each issue on the list and ask women to share what they know about each one.

3 Use appropriate information sheets to check out information.

4 Discuss how the NHS reforms have been implemented locally:

   - which hospitals/units have become Trusts?
   - have women experienced any differences as a result?
   - have women experienced any differences due to the new GP contract?
   - is their GP a budget-holder or not, and if so has it made any differences?

If women do not know how local services have been affected by the reforms, you could encourage them to find out for the next meeting, or plan to invite a speaker in (see Practical points, p. 25).

Discussion points

- What are the fundamental changes being introduced through the reforms?
- Does the contract culture/business analogy work for health care?
- If women are unsure as to how NHS reforms have affected local services, why might this be so?

- How can women find out about local services?

- How can women work together to get the kind of health services they want in the new NHS?

ACTIVITY *3.3*

Contracting for women's health work I

Aims
- To enable women to develop their understanding of the contract culture.

- To explore ways in which contracting may affect women's health work.

Materials
A copy of Worksheet 3.2 *Contracting for women's health work* and the Information Sheet 3.3 *Contract culture* for each woman; pens, a flipchart and markers.

Method
1 Give women copies of the information sheet and brainstorm information women have about the contract culture.

2 In pairs, women go through the worksheet and note their responses.

3 In the large group, feed back and flipchart key points under the headings 'advantages' and 'disadvantages'.

4 Discuss the issues raised.

Discussion points
- Are some issues on both lists? Why?

- Are there any similarities between issues raised by contracting and current funding arrangements for particular projects?

- Do some women/women's health groups face different possibilities/ difficulties from others? In what ways?

The points on the next page may be identified through this activity, or you could feed them in during the discussion.

Advantages	Disadvantages
Stability of funding – contracts could last 3–5 years.	The contract agreement could distort the aims or remit of the project.
Potentially new agencies and possible sources of funding for the work.	Negotiating a contract is time consuming and requires specific skills.
Opportunity to include and specify issues such as equal opportunities, user involvement.	Work will be more rigorously defined through contract specifications and it will be difficult to respond directly and quickly to new areas of work or newly identified needs.
Will change relationships with funder and may lead to more power and status.	Difficult for the group to carry out an advocacy or campaigning role and provide services due to conflict of interest.
Will lead to development of new skills, for example, negotiation.	Groups and agencies will be competing with each other, which will have an impact on collaborative work.
	The contracts might omit issues the group considers vital, e.g. equal opportunities.
	Smaller voluntary groups may go under as they might not have the resources and back-up to negotiate contracts.

ACTIVITY *3.4*

Contracting for women's health work II

Aims:

- To enable women to develop their understanding of the contract culture.

- To develop action plans for securing and developing women's health work within contracts.

Materials

A copy of Information Sheets 3.3 *Contract culture* and 3.9 *Case study of a local self-help group* for each woman; flipchart and markers.

Method

1 Check women's understanding of the contract culture, using the Information Sheet *Contract culture*. (You could also use Activity 3.3 *Contracting for women's health work I*.)

2 In small groups, women read through the case study, and discuss the prompt questions below.

Variation: women could choose to discuss their own project/work instead of the case study.

3 Still in small groups, draw up an action plan for securing and developing the work within contracts.

4 In the large group, feed back and flipchart key ideas, and discuss.

Discussion points

• What local and national networks are there for women to get advice, information and support about contracting?

• How can voluntary groups develop their links with statutory agencies?

• How can women develop their knowledge and expertise around contracting?

Prompt questions

• What are the implications of the contract culture for the development of the work of the project described.

• What opportunities might the contract culture offer? What threats?

ACTIVITY *3.5*

What kind of health services do we want?

Aims

• To consider our own health needs and the adequacy of the health services in providing for them.

• To consider ways in which we as consumers can generate improvements and changes in the health services.

Materials

A copy of Worksheet 3.3 *What kind of health services do we want?* for each woman; flipchart and markers.

Method

1 Introduce the activity and give out the worksheet.

2 Ask women to form three or four small groups based on the issue they are most interested in.

3 In small groups, discuss and write checklists.

4 Pool findings in the large group and discuss.

Discussion points

1 What experiences do the group have of trying to influence health services?

- what methods did women use?

- how successful were they?

2 In what ways can we make changes and improvements in health service provision? For example:

- working with the Community Health Council;

- making individual complaints if not satisfied with a service;

- using the Patients' Charter; and

- using the NHS reforms (which put the patient at the centre of the NHS) to make our voices heard.

*ACTIVITY 3.6

Dealing with health professionals

Aims

- To enable women to discuss their feelings and experience of dealing with health professionals in a constructive way.

- To identify what makes an encounter with a health professional a good or bad experience.

- To explore the ways we can improve our encounters with health professionals.

Materials

A copy of Worksheet 3.4 *Dealing with health professionals* for each woman; pens, a flipchart and markers.

Method

1 In small groups, go through the worksheet, each woman in turn describing a good and a bad experience she has had.

2 Still in small groups, draw together key factors that make experiences positive or negative, and list them.

3 In the large group, pool findings and discuss.

4 On the flipchart, develop a checklist of ways women can improve encounters with health professionals.

Discussion points

● Do women find it hard talking to authority figures in general?

● Do women find it particularly hard talking to doctors?

● How could health professionals improve our encounters with them?

● How can we influence them to make changes?

● What can we do to deal more confidently and effectively with health professionals? (For example by going armed with more information and a list of questions, taking a friend, or practising assertiveness.)

*ACTIVITY 3.7

Talking to your doctor

Aims

● To enable women to consider how they relate to doctors.

● To develop and practise skills which can help in future dealings with doctors.

Materials

Copies of Worksheets 3.5 *Talking to your doctor – checklist* and 3.6 *Talking to your doctor – role plays* for each woman; pens.

Method

Introduce the activity, with some initial discussion about why it can sometimes feel difficult to talk to doctors. Then follow one or other of the two sequences below.

1 Role play a doctor/patient consultation for the rest of the group to observe.

You will have to pre-arrange this with a co-tutor or willing member of the group.

- First, role play a good consultation, where the patient gets exactly what she wants from the consultation. Repeat, this time enacting a bad consultation in which the patient is obviously having difficulty with the doctor.

- The group all act as observers, using the checklists on the worksheet so they know what to look out for and can record what happens.

- Discuss the questions on the worksheet.

2 The group members all participate in role playing.

- Divide into groups of three. Each group chooses a situation from the Worksheet *Talking to your doctor – role plays*, or writes one that is more relevant to them.

- In turn, one woman plays patient, one plays doctor, and one observes, using the Worksheet *Talking to your doctor – checklist*.

- Swap roles, so that each woman has a turn at being patient, doctor and observer.

- Still in small groups, discuss the questions on the worksheet.

- In the large group, feed back and discuss.

Discussion points

- How might the 'patient' have encouraged a more positive consultation with the doctor?

- How can you best prepare for a visit to the doctor?

- What have you learned from the role play that you may use when you next visit the doctor?

WORKSHEET *3.1*

Women's health Snakes and Ladders

Finish!

35 Your local geriatric hospital is closed. You are left to look after your elderly and confused mother at home.

34 Using self-help remedies, you catch your cystitis early enough and prevent it developing into a severe attack.

33

Your family planning clinic isn't open at a time that is appropriate for you to attend. **29**

30 miss a turn

28 You take a friend with you to the doctors to insist you get a hospital appointment to get your stomach pains investigated.

15

14

1 Start here! – you must throw an odd number to start.

23

31

32

You take up your work place health issues with your trade union Health and Safety Representative. **26**

You attend your GP's Health Promotion Clinic for information on stopping smoking – move forward 2 squares. **16**

13

2

You are pregnant with your second child. The antenatal clinic has no facilities for children so it's difficult for you to attend. **22**

21

You keep getting severe pains in your stomach, but your doctor does not take it seriously. Stay here till you throw a 4 **24**

25

You get in touch with a tranquilliser self-help group. They give you support to come off them. **18**

A new kind of chemical is introduced at work. You develop a skin rash. If you threw an odd number, go back 1 square, if even, down the snake. **27**

17

You are in BUPA so you need not wait for an operation on your varicose veins. **12**

3

8

Your BUPA membership does not cover treatment for your chronic illness. Miss 2 turns. **20**

You manage to stop smoking! **19**

Move forward 5 squares. **10**

Your council flat is damp and you can't afford to keep the electric heating on. Your children get bronchitis. **11**

You are depressed and the doctor gives you tranquillisers. You now can't manage without them. Stay here till you get a 2. **27**

You have bad arthritis and need a hip replacement. The waiting list is 18 months. Miss three turns. **4**

9

6

A Well Woman Clinic has opened in your area – they give you advice about coping with the menopause. **7**

You join a Women and Health Course and gain in confidence, skills and knowledge so you can use the health service more effectively. **5**

WORKSHEET *3.2*

Contracting for women's health work

Think about what you know about the contract culture; your own experience of contracts in your life (e.g. contracts of employment, marriage, for purchasing or renting your home) and your knowledge about funding and fund-raising for women's health work (either your own group/project or an imaginary project).

Brainstorm the *advantages* and *disadvantages* related to contracting for women's health work, and write down your ideas below.

Advantages	Disadvantages
e.g. It will give me a more defined relationship with the funding body.	e.g. It is time consuming to negotiate a contract.

WORKSHEET *3.3*

What kind of health services do we want?

At a time of changes in health services provision, consumer health groups have often focused on resisting any cuts and defending the NHS. Yet some of us have criticisms of the NHS and feel that it does not always provide the type or quality of health care we would want.

As consumers in the NHS, we have a lot of valuable experience and knowledge – about our own health needs, about how health care and services could be improved, and the kind of health service provision we would like to have in an ideal world.

1 In your group, discuss and make a checklist of the kind of health service provision you would like to be available. Start with your own health needs, and those of your family.

2 You might then want to focus on one of these issues, or consider a different issue, for example:

- the health needs of particular groups in the community (e.g. Black people, people with a disability, or older people);

- well-women clinics (providing care for emotional as well as physical health);

- maternity services (e.g. antenatal care, birth options); or

- work-place health care (e.g. protection from work hazards, screening facilities).

3 How might you get the health service provision you want?

- as an individual;

- through working with others e.g. by lobbying/campaigning, in a self-help group, or otherwise.

WORKSHEET *3.4*

Dealing with health professionals

We all have many experiences of dealing with health professionals – our family doctor, hospital doctors and nurses, health visitors, community nurses and midwives. We may feel anxious or lacking in confidence when talking to them. We may be ill or worried about our health or speaking for someone close who is ill. Health professionals seem to know more than us and do not always explain things in words we can understand.

Think about experiences you have had with health professionals. Go round the group, and in turn describe a good experience you had – tell them what happened and how you felt about it. As a group you will probably find things in common. Make a list of what makes an encounter with a health professional a good experience for you. Do the same for a bad experience you had.

Key factors for good experiences with a health professional	Key factors for bad experiences with a health professional
For example, 'The doctor introduced herself and asked me about my feelings and needs'.	For example, 'The doctor only asked me questions when I was undressed on the examination couch'.

WORKSHEET *3.5*

Talking to your doctor – checklist

As an observer during the role play, watch out for the following points (if you want to record what happens, tick the boxes and add any other comments):

Physical arrangements   √ **for yes**

Is the doctor sitting behind a desk?   ☐

Are the chairs opposite each other?   ☐

or side by side?   ☐

Are they far apart?   ☐

or close together?   ☐

Body language

Doctor

To greet the patient, does the doctor:

get up?   ☐

look up?   ☐

Does the doctor sit back as if s/he has time to listen?   ☐

Is the doctor's hand hovering near the prescription pad?   ☐

Does the doctor keep looking at his/her watch?   ☐

Does the doctor look directly at the patient?   ☐

Patient

Does the patient greet the doctor?   ☐

Is the patient sitting in a relaxed way?   ☐

or on the edge of her seat?   ☐

Does the patient look at the doctor when she is speaking?   ☐

▷

© Health Education Authority, 1993

▷ 3.5 cont.

Does the patient appear distressed? ☐

Does the patient appear to be expecting the consultation to be a positive experience? ☐

Interaction

Doctor

Does the doctor speak to the patient by name? ☐

Does the doctor appear to listen? ☐

or keep interrupting? ☐

Does the doctor answer questions in a direct way? ☐

Does the doctor use language which the patient appears to understand? ☐

▷ 3.5 cont.

Patient

Does the patient allow the doctor to interrupt? ☐

Does the patient explain clearly what exactly is the problem? ☐

Does the patient give any additional information which may
help the doctor? ☐

Does the patient seem comfortable in disagreeing with the doctor? ☐

Does the patient ask many questions? ☐

Was the consultation ended by the doctor? ☐

or by the patient? ☐

Discussion points

- How did the physical arrangements of the surgery affect the consultation?
- What did the body language tell you about how the patient and doctor were relating?
- Did the patient ask what she wanted?
- Did she get what she wanted from the consultation?
- How could the consultation have been improved?

WORKSHEET *3.6*

Talking to your doctor – role plays

Role play 1

Patient

You are in your thirties and your marriage has recently broken up. You are tense, depressed and want to talk. You could break down and cry.

Doctor

You have had a hectic and stressful day and are nearing the end of a busy surgery. You are tired and want to get home to your family.

Role play 2

Patient

You are in your middle forties and your periods have been getting heavier. You feel there is something wrong and would like to be referred to a gynaecologist.

Doctor

You think the patient's problem is due to her age and that there is nothing abnormal. Tell her she has to put up with it, and it would be a waste of a consultant's valuable time to refer her.

▷ 3.6 cont.

Role play 3

Patient

You are in your early twenties with three children and you live in a council flat. You have been on the transfer list for a house for four years. Your middle child, age two, has never needed much sleep and has been difficult to cope with. You think she is hyperactive. You need practical help.

Doctor

You don't believe in hyperactivity; no one had even heard of it years ago. You think the woman is lucky to have such healthy, lively children. You are prepared to repeat a prescription for tranquillisers.

Role play 4

Patient

You are a young woman with a strict Muslim background. You are going for your routine internal examination after having your second baby. You feel tense at the thought of being examined but at least you know your doctor well. You do not want a student present.

Doctor

You have a student with you training to be a GP, who needs experience of all aspects of general practice. You are required to ask the patient if she minds the student being present but consider this to be a formality. You don't expect her to refuse.

RESOURCES

For contact details of distributors and organisations listed here, see Chapter 11 *General resources*.

Publications

Baxter, C, Poonia, K, Ward, L, and Nadirshaw, Z, *Double Discrimination: Issues and Services for People with Learning Difficulties from Black and Ethnic Minority Communities* (1990) King's Fund Centre/Commission for Racial Equality, £9.95, ISBN 0 903060 79 5. Available from Bailey Distribution Ltd.
A handbook which brings together suggestions on the improvement of services for people with learning difficulties from Black and minority ethnic communities. Well designed and clearly presented, with useful reading and resource lists.

Connah, B, and Pearson, R (eds), *NHS Handbook* 7th Edition (1991), Macmillan, £18.95. Available from bookshops (especially medical ones).
Produced by the National Association of Health Authorities and Trusts, this useful handbook is published annually and contains up-to-date information on new NHS structure, its management and funding, current issues in health, care in the community, partnerships with NHS.

Davies, Anne and Edwards, Ken, *Twelve Charity Contracts: Case Studies of Funding Contracts between Charities and Local Authorities and Other Bodies* (1990), Directory of Social Change, £7.95. Available from Directory of Social Change.

Farrell, Elaine, *Choices in Health Care* (1989), Optima, £5.99.
An assessment of the options available to people in Britain from home birth to health insurance and more.

Frain, J, *How to Know your Rights Patients* (1991), How to Books Ltd. £6.95.
This handbook for every health service user meets an important need for information on the rights of patients using the health services, about visiting doctors and hospitals, confidentiality, consent to treatment, right to information and records, complaints and compensation. Includes further reading, glossary and useful addresses.

Gabe, J, Calnan, M, and Bury, M (eds), *The Sociology of the Health Service* (1991), Routledge, £12.99.
A series of essays aiming to develop a sociological analysis of current health policy. Topics cover privatisation and health service management to health education and the politics of professional power. Also included is a historical view of sociology's contributions to health policy, and proposals for an agenda for sociological health research in the 1990s.

Gann, Robert, *The Health Care Consumer Guide* (1991), Faber and Faber, £7.99. ISBN 0 571 14298 2.

A valuable source of information for users and providers of health care. Highlights the needs for healthy communities as well as healthy individuals and covers: self-care; general practice and family health services; care in the community; going into hospital; making special choices such as having a baby; HIV, AIDS and cancer; using health services abroad, finding health information; and self-help resources.

Gutch, R, Kutz, C, and Spence, K, *Partners or Agents? Local Government and the Voluntary Sector: Changing Relationships in 1990s.* Available from the National Council for Voluntary Organisations.

Health Rights, *Information Pack on the National Health Service White Paper and Working Papers* (1989), £5. Available from Health Rights.
Sets out in detail the main White Paper proposals, and contains discussion documents on implications of the proposals. Sections on accountability, financial issues, choice, public expenditure, the role of markets in health care and primary care proposals.

HMSO, *Caring for People Implementation Document: Purchasing and Contracting.* Available from HMSO.

Hogg, Christine and Winkler, Fedelma (eds), *Community/Consumer Representation in the NHS with Specific Reference to Community Health Councils* (1989). Available from Greater London Association of Community Health Councils.
Papers on representation of the user and the community in the post-review NHS and a discussion paper on recognising the major contribution of CHCs in involving the community in health care.

Leathard, Audrey, *Health Care Provision Past, Present and Future,* (1990), Chapman and Hall, £10.95, ISBN 0 412 33190 X.
A valuable account of the development of the NHS and its place in the wider context of social policy. Looks at the 1989 review and discusses implications for the future. Interesting for anyone wishing to gain a wider perspective on the NHS and relate it to the 1990s.

McIver, S, *Obtaining the Views of Users of Health Services* (1991), King's Fund Centre, £7.50.
A practical guide on how to obtain the views of people using the NHS – the *who* you want views from, *why, how.* Offers a basic introduction to the subject, including discussion of the concept of patient satisfaction and describes an approach which avoids some of the pitfalls associated with this complex area.

McNaught, Allan, *Health Action and Ethnic Minorities* (1987), NCHR/Bedford Square Press, £4.45. Available from National Community Health Resource.
Looks at the response of the NHS to the needs of ethnic minorities and at how a number of community health initiatives have been established.

National Consumer Council and the Association of Community Health Councils for England and Wales, *Patients' Rights* (leaflet) – Armenian, Bengali, Cantonese, Greek, Gujarati, Hindi, Turkish, Punjabi, Vietnamese, Urdu, English. Price 10 copies £2 (plus postage and packing). Available from the National Consumer Council and the Association of Community Health Councils for England and Wales.

National Extension College, *Coming into Hospital: an Information Booklet for Patients* – Arabic, Bengali, Chinese, Greek, Gujarati, Punjabi, Turkish, Urdu, Vietnamese and English. Available from the National Extension College.

NCVO, *Changing the Balance: Power and People Who Use Services* (1991), £3. Available from National Council for Voluntary Organisations, Community Care Information Service.
People who use services write about their experience, the things that need to change and their own efforts at creating change. Contributions include 'Being Black with learning difficulties', 'User participation in Derbyshire', 'Mental health users' group', and 'Mid-Suffolk Rethink for Disabled People'. Publications and contacts list.

Contracting In or Out? Guidance Notes on Contracting for Voluntary Organizations. Available from National Council for Voluntary Organisations.
Set of papers covering different aspects of contracting eg: legal, management, organisational, from the voluntary sector perspective.

North East and North West Thames Regional Health Authorities, *Contracting for Ethnic Minority Health (a workshop report)*. Available from North East Thames RHA.

North East Thames RHA, *Health in any Language: A Guide to Producing Health Information for non-English Speaking People*, (booklet). Available from North East Thames RHA.

North East Thames RHA, *Health Services for People from Ethnic Minorities (a conference report)*. Available from North East Thames RHA.

North Manchester Health Promotion Unit, *A Strategy for Information: Health Promotion and Equal Opportunities*, £30.00. Available from North Manchester Health Promotion Unit.

Rodwell, Lee, *Women and Medical Care* (1988), Unwin, £3.50.
Practical guide to using the NHS.

Torkington, N P K, *Black Health: A Political Issue* (1991), Liverpool Institute of Higher Education, £7.95, ISBN 0 9515847 1 5. Available from National Community Health Resource or from the Liverpool Institute of Higher Education.
This study focuses on Black people and health and addresses issues of race and class inequalities in the provision of health services. It is based on the personal experiences of Black people from a number of ethnic backgrounds living in Liverpool.

Woolf, J, *Contracts and Small Voluntary Groups*. Available from London Voluntary Service Council.

Videos

Rights and Choices in Maternity Care, (Hindi, Bengali, Urdu, Gujarati, Punjabi, Cantonese all with English subtitles) 20 minutes. Available from Health Care Productions Ltd.

Working for Patients (Bengali, Gujarati, Hindi, Punjabi, Urdu, English) 23 minutes. £25 (including one booklet). Available from Lancashire FHSA.

Haringey Health Authority/Age Concern/Department of Health, *Looking After Your Health – Where To Go For Help*, £15.00 inc. VAT & £2.50 p&p. Available from SCEMSC (Standing Conference of Ethnic Minority Senior Citizens).

Organisations

Association of Community Health Councils for England & Wales
Represents consumers' views in the NHS. Publishes briefing papers on current health issues, leaflets (also in languages other than English), has library, can provide information and advice. Write/phone.

College of Health
Aims to give people the information they need to make effective use of the NHS, improve communication between doctors and their patients, and provide information about self-help groups.

Directory of Social Change
Directory of Social Change, in conjunction with NCVO, has developed training courses on the contract culture. The organisation specialises in voluntary organisation funding. They also produce good publications and a list is available from them on request.

London Voluntary Service Council (LVSC)
LVSC is developing a 'training the trainers' package; a series of seminars; a training pack for trainers; and various publications. All their work has an emphasis on the needs of Black and minority ethnic groups and smaller voluntary agencies.

National Association for Patient Participation (NAPP)
Aims to spread information about patient participation and offer encouragement and resources for the formation of new groups. Provides a national forum for the consideration of patient-centred issues.

National Council for Voluntary Organisations (NCVO)
NCVO has a team working specifically on the impact of the contract culture on the voluntary sector, and produces various publications including a newsletter available on subscription.

4 Mental health

INTRODUCTION

This chapter consists of three sections: *Emotional and mental health*, *Stress*, and *Relaxation and massage*.

However, there is no clear dividing line between the three units, and much overlap.

- It is important to include mental health in any discussion of women's health, and indeed it is hard to separate physical and mental health issues because they impact on each other so closely.

- Women patients outnumber men by roughly 2 to 1 at all levels of the mental health services. Although various explanations have been put forward (e.g. women are more likely to ask for help, men express distress in different ways) it is generally accepted that women's mental health *is* poorer than men's.

- It is useful to start thinking about what mental health is, and what needs women have in order to be mentally and emotionally healthy. By working together on this issue, women are able to validate each other's experiences, and express feelings within a positive and supportive environment.

- This chapter tries to focus on a positive approach to mental health, including understanding feelings and dealing with them in appropriate ways, and developing skills for dealing with stress, and for relaxation and massage.

Emotional and mental health

BACKGROUND INFORMATION

- Emotional and mental health is about how we feel about ourselves, and our ability to express feelings. Self-esteem and self-confidence are key factors. Increasingly, links are being made between a woman's mental health and the extent to which her needs are met in society – access to a comfortable lifestyle, and the freedom she has to make positive choices about her life.

- Black women have been active in voicing their concern about their experience of higher rates of poverty, unemployment, poor housing, as well as racial harassment, racism and the impact of immigration laws, and the effect of all these on their physical and mental health.

- The definition of mental health and what is acceptable and normal changes over time. It was not so long ago that some unmarried women who had children were put into mental hospitals, and homosexuals were given aversion therapy. Definitions are closely bound up with dominant cultural values in society, and those who do not fit easily may be labelled mentally ill or deviant.

- Different views about what are normal and appropriate feelings and behaviours occur between cultures, classes, and between men and women. A lack of awareness about different ways of life and different beliefs and values on the part of health professionals may be the product of institutional racism. It may lead to people being viewed as having a mental health problem. This is recognised by many Black people in this country as having a large impact on their lives.

- Women's mental health is related to how valued they feel – within personal relationships and within society as a whole. At its most extreme, women subjected to emotional or physical violence by those they live with are likely to experience a crisis of confidence, and feelings of depression and fear. This may be most severe when domestic violence is not openly acknowledged and an image of normality is presented to the outside world.

PRACTICAL POINTS

- Exploring the issue of emotional and mental health may raise many issues for the tutor. It is important that you are clear about your own aims, and limitations – what you are and are not – and that the group is also clear about this. Avoid falling into the role of therapist.

- You cannot be responsible for:

  - personal counselling;
  - giving medical advice; or
  - women who might not want to take steps that you or the group feel they ought to take.

- Try to balance the activities you use, so that if a session has been at all 'heavy' you end on a positive note.

ACTIVITY *4.1*

What is mental health?

Aims

- To promote an awareness of mental health as opposed to mental illness.
- To relate this awareness to the needs of the women in the group, and of women in general.

Materials

Copies of Worksheet 4.1 *What is mental health?* for each woman; pens.

Method

1 Introduce the key issues in this area, some of which are outlined above in the Background information section.

2 In pairs, work through the worksheet.

3 In the large group, pool findings, and discuss.

Discussion points

- Is it helpful to look at mental *health* in this way?
- How would you now define mental *illness*?
- How common are the responses from different pairs?
- Can women think of some strategies to get their needs met?
- See Activity 4.2 *Images of mental health*.

ACTIVITY *4.2*

Images of mental health

Aims

- To explore creatively the feelings associated with feeling low.
- To examine what women need to feel emotional and mental well being.

Materials

Scissors, glue, magazines, coloured pens, a large sheet of paper for each small group, blutack; tactile items such as wire, nails, tacks; coloured wool, fabric bits, foam scraps, glitter, balsa wood bits, etc.

Method

1 In small groups, use the available materials to produce a collage or picture which expresses feelings associated with feeling low.

2 Display the pictures on the walls or floor. Encourage women to explain/ interpret their own and others' work.

3 Discuss what women feel they need to encourage emotional and mental well being.

Discussion points

- What types of feelings did women identify?

- How common are women's experiences of feeling low?

- What do women feel they need in order to be emotionally and mentally well?

- How are/can these needs be met?

ACTIVITY 4.3

Identifying and expressing feelings

Aim

- To develop a greater understanding of feelings

Materials

Copies of Worksheet 4.2 *Identifying and expressing feelings* for each woman; pens, flipchart and markers.

Method

1 Introduce the activity, talking about the value to our mental health of identifying and acknowledging both positive and negative feelings and emotions.

2 Ask women to fill in the worksheet in pairs, and then discuss the talking points.

3 In the large group, feed back what women want to share, and flipchart the main points.

Discussion points

- Are some feelings easier to deal with than others? Which ones?

- Does the pressure to 'carry on as normal' make it harder to express feelings at the time?

ACTIVITY 4.4

Looking at anger

Aims

- To stimulate discussion about anger.

- To identify some strategies for dealing with anger.

Materials

Copies of Worksheet 4.3 *Looking at anger – case study* for each woman; pens.

Method

1 In small groups, women discuss the case study on the worksheet, and share situations where they have felt angry.

2 In the large group, feed back and discuss strategies for dealing with anger.

Discussion points

- Is anger an acceptable emotion for women? How easy is it for women to express anger?

- Can anger be a positive emotion? In what way?

- It may be useful to look at Activity 7.10 *Coping with feeling angry* in Chapter 7 *Motherhood*.

ACTIVITY *4.5*

Being positive

Aims

- To encourage discussion about self-esteem.

- To validate times when women have felt positive and valued.

Materials

Copies of Worksheet 4.4 *Being positive* for each woman; pens, flipchart, paper, markers.

Method

1 In pairs, women go through the worksheet.

2 Pairs join to make fours, and share responses. Each group chooses their six most relevant experiences, with at least one from each woman.

3 In the large group, feed back and flipchart six situations from each group of four and discuss.

Discussion points

- How difficult is this activity? Why?

- What is the range of experiences? Can they be grouped at all? For example, achieving, being valued, and so on.

- What can women do to learn from these past experiences?

ACTIVITY *4.6*

Depression – finding the words

Aims

- To introduce the issue of depression.

- To encourage the group itself to define the terms of discussion.

- To look at links between physical and mental feelings associated with depression.

Materials

Copies of Worksheet 4.5 *Depression – finding the words* for each woman; pens, flipchart paper and markers.

Method

1 Emphasise the value of starting with our own experiences, rather than with medical definitions.

2 In small groups, ask women to work together to list words on the worksheet.

Variation: Ask some groups to list physical feelings; other groups to list mental feelings.

3 In the large group, feed back and flipchart words, and discuss.

Discussion points

- Is it easy to separate physical and mental feelings?

- Is there overlap between the two lists?

- Does this help us to begin to understand more about depression?

- There are many meanings attached to the word 'depression': it can mean 'feeling low' in everyday terms, but in medical terms it can mean a serious and debilitating illness.

- It can be linked to specific events such as the upheaval associated with the birth of a baby or a bereavement. Sometimes it can seem as if it is not tied to anything and this can be hard for people to accept.

ACTIVITY *4.7*

Why do women get depressed?

Aims

- To examine depression in relation to women in particular.

- To explore the connections between life situations and depression.

Materials

A copy of Worksheet 4.6 *Why do women get depressed?* for each woman.

Method

1 Ask women to form small groups, read through the worksheet and share their ideas about the statements.

2 In the large group, feed back and discuss.

Discussion points

- Are women more prone to depression than men, or are there particular factors in their lives which make them more vulnerable? If so, what might these be?

- Are there cultural differences, and if so, why might this be so?

ACTIVITY 4.8

Families

Aims

- To help women understand their own position in their family.

- To consider strategies for dealing with difficulties which arise out of family relationships.

Materials

Flipchart paper for each woman; different coloured markers.

Method

1 Give each woman a sheet of flipchart paper, and have different coloured markers available.

2 Ask women to draw a diagram which shows themselves and their family (e.g. relationships with spouse/partner, parents, siblings, children, in-laws).

Note: Some women may find it easier to draw the family as a train, or a tree, or whatever. Encourage creativity!

3 With different coloured markers, ask women to:

- Indicate the nature of different relationships, for example: who supports them financially, whom they support financially, who supports them in other ways, whom they support in other ways, whom they are responsible to, and whom they have responsibility for.

- Put an asterisk next to family members who live in the same household.

- Highlight relationships within the family which they find difficult.

4 In small groups, discuss each woman's sheet.

5 In the large group, feed back what women wish to share, and flipchart any difficulties in relationships.

6 Discuss strategies for overcoming difficulties within the family.

Discussion points

- Are there common difficulties that arise between family members?

- Are there difficulties affected by living in the same household?

- Are there differences between cultures regarding family relationships?

(Thanks to Nigar Sadique and Ghazala Hussain.)

WORKSHEET *4.1*

What is mental health?

1 How would you define mental health? Jot down any ideas that come to mind.

2 List as many things as you can think of that women need in order to be mentally healthy.

3 Is it easy for women to get what they need? What can they do to help this?

WORKSHEET *4.2*

Identifying and expressing feelings

Can you think of any instances in the last couple of weeks when you have felt any of the following feelings? Note the situation/s when they occurred, and think about how you expressed the feelings.

Feelings	*Situation*
Anger	_____
Anxiety	_____
Contentment	_____
Guilt	_____
Insecurity	_____
Warmth/Affection	_____
Frustration	_____
Lack of confidence	_____
Confidence	_____

Talking points

- Choose one or two feelings you would like to look at more closely. Think back to when you felt this way, looking at the situation more closely. Can you see why you had this feeling? Was it OK to feel this way? Was it easy to express the feeling?

- Are there any feelings you would prefer to respond to differently from the way you tend to? How do you think you could do this:
  – by yourself?
  – with support from others?
  – by trying to change your situation?

WORKSHEET *4.3*

Looking at anger – case study

One of the strongest conflicts I have is when I get this immense desire to express the pain and outrage I feel about it, which wells up in quite an overwhelming way, and what happens is that a part of me says 'no, you can't do that. You've got to keep a stiff upper lip, you mustn't give in to that, you mustn't feel distressed.' But a very strong part of me is saying: 'You've every right to feel outraged and you must express it.'[1]

1 Can you identify with what the woman is saying?

2 Think back to the last time you felt really angry. Were you able to let this anger out? How did you cope with the situation?

3 What could you do in future in this sort of situation?

[1] From Naire, K, and Smith, G, *Dealing with Depression* (1984), Women's Press. (Reprinted with permission of the publisher.)

WORKSHEET *4.4*

Being positive

Think back to times when you have felt good about yourself. They may be recent occasions, or some time in the past, and may be happy, serious or even sad occasions.

Examples from women have included:

- 'When I asked for a refund and got it';
- 'When I achieved what I set out to do';
- 'When X really listened to what I had to say';
- 'When I was asked for my opinion';
- 'Doing my best in difficult circumstances'.

Make your own list.
I felt good about myself when:

WORKSHEET *4.5*

Depression – finding the words

What words do we use to describe how we feel when we are depressed?

Physical Feelings	Mental Feelings

WORKSHEET *4.6*

Why do women get depressed?

- There are many meanings attached to the word 'depression': it can mean 'feeling low' in everyday terms but in medical terms it can mean a serious and debilitating illness.

- It may be linked to specific events such as the upheaval associated with the birth of a baby, moving to a new country, or bereavement.

- Sometimes it can seem as if it is not tied to anything and this can be hard for people to accept.

Below are the conclusions of some research studies.[1]

1 Women are twice as likely as men to be diagnosed as depressed.

2 In one study in London, 40% of mothers with children under 5 were suffering from depression.

3 1 in 6 women and 1 in 12 men spend some time in their life in a mental hospital.

4 There are more tranquillisers and anti-depressants prescribed in the UK than any other drugs, and these are mostly prescribed to women.

5 Married women are more prone to depression than single women, while single men are more prone to depression than married men.

- What explanations do you think there are for these findings?

- Do you think these findings will have changed since their publication in 1978?

[1] Brown, D W, and Harris, T, *Social Origins of Depression* (1978), Tavistock.

RESOURCES

For contact details of distributors and organisations listed here, see Chapter 11 *General resources*.

Publications

Birchwood, Max and Smith, Jo, *Understanding Schizophrenia* (1990), West Birmingham Health Education Unit, 6 page booklet. Available in Bengali, English, Gujarati, Hindi, Punjabi, or Urdu from West Birmingham Health Education Unit.

Brown, George and Harris, Tirrill, *The Social Origins of Depression: a Study of Psychiatric Disorder in Women* (1990), Routledge, £12.99.
The classic study of women from a sociological point of view.

Burningham, Sally, *Not on Your Own: the Mind Guide to Mental Health* (1989), Penguin, £3.99.
Explanation of the different types of mental health problems, with both professional and self-help suggestions.

Community Education Training Unit, *Assertion and How to Train Ourselves* (1990), £4.65. Available from Community Education Development Centre.
These materials cover setting up and running assertion training courses and are easy to use and adapt. They are aimed at community groups, voluntary organisations and local authorities.

Corob, Alison, *Working with Depressed Women* (1987), Gower, £5.95.
A feminist perspective. Useful for social workers and others in caring professions. Includes interviews with women.

Confederation of Indian Organisations (UK), *A Cry for Change: An Asian Perspective on Developing Quality Mental Health Care*, £7.50 + £1.15 for p&p. Available from Confederation of Indian Organisations

Cox, G, and Dainow, S, *Making the Most of Yourself* (1990), Sheldon Press, £4.99.
A self-help book which encourages everyone to take responsibility for themselves in becoming more self-aware, more successful at personal problem-solving and more confident. Uses exercises and action planning methods. Case histories are included.

Dickson, Anne, *A Woman in Your Own Right: Assertiveness and You* (1982), Quartet, £5.95.
A useful guide to assertiveness aimed particularly at women.

Ehrenreich, B, and English, D, *For Her Own Good: 150 Years of the Expert's Advice to Women* (1979), Pluto Press, £5.95.
Reassesses 150 years of advice on subjects from childcare to gynaecology, showing how a male-dominated body of 'expert' scientific opinion undermines women's age-old skills.

Ernst, Sheila and Goodison, Lucy, *In Our Own Hands – a Book About Self Help Therapy* (1992), Women's Press, £7.95.
A practical book on how to set up a women's self-help therapy group.

Ernst, Sheila and Maguire, Marie, *Living with the Sphinx: Papers from the Women's Therapy Centre* (1987), Women's Press, £5.95.
A selection of papers covering topics such as racism, abortion and envy.

Fensterheim, Herbert and Baer, Jean, *Don't Say 'Yes' When You Want to Say 'No'* (1989), Futura, £2.99.
A guide to assertiveness in a number of situations.

Hare, Beverley, *Be Assertive* (1990), Optima, £5.99.
A practical guide to assertiveness with lots of exercises.

Hite, S, *The Hite Report of Love and Passion and Emotional Violence* (1991), Optima, £11.99.
Questions the belief that insecure women seek out destructive relationships; rather it documents a hidden, socially acceptable pattern of behaviour in relationships which puts women's needs last.

Horley, Sandra, *Love and Pain: A Survival Handbook for Women* (1988), Bedford Square Press, £5.95, ISBN 0 7199 1214 8. Available from booksellers or by post from Plymbridge Distributors Ltd.
Written by an experienced counsellor and campaigner for the rights of abused women, this handbook provides advice and information on different types of abuse and aims to help women take control of their lives.

King's Fund Centre, *Is Race on your Agenda: Improving Mental Health Services for People from Black and Minority Groups*, £2.95. Available from King's Fund Centre.

King's Fund Centre, *A Question of Race: Report of a Conference on the Future of Mental Health Services for the Black Community*, £3. Available from King's Fund Centre.

Leicester Black Mental Health Group, *Sadness in My Heart: Racism and Mental Health* (1989), University of Leicester. Available from The Mental Health Shop.
Report of a research project which surveyed a group of Black patients diagnosed as schizophrenic, their parents and siblings and a group of Asian women suffering from depression. Contains lengthy interviews and analysis of NHS structures and provision.

Litvinoff, S, *The Relate Guide to Better Relationships* (1991), Ebury Press, London, £6.99.
Practical ways to help sustain a relationship, by understanding your partner, testing your compatibility, learning how to listen and hear, improving your sex life, and tackling problems together.

McKeon, Patrick, *Coping with Depression and Elation* (1990), Sheldon, £4.99.
How to recognise and deal with mood swings.

MIND, *Women and Mental Health*, Information leaflet available from MIND.

Nairne, Kathy and Smith, Gerrilyn, *Dealing with Depression* (1984), Women's Press, £3.95.
Women talk about their own experiences of depression and how they have learned to cope with it. Also looks at the causes of depression and ways to deal with it.

Rowe, Dorothy, *Depression, the Way Out of Your Prison* (1989), Routledge, £6.99.
A detailed, practical guide.

Sanford, Linda, Tschirhart and Donovan, Mary Ellen, *Women and Self Esteem: Understanding and Improving the Way we Thrive and Feel About Ourselves* (1989), Penguin, £7.99.
Looks at how women's attitudes are formed and offers suggestions for help including step-by-step exercises.

Survivors Speak Out, *Self-Advocacy Action Pack: Empowering Mental Health Service Users*, £5 (£1 for "survivors"). Available from Survivors Speak Out.
Designed to give practical information and advice to people involved in mental health self-advocacy. Contains sheets on setting up a group, fund-raising, resources, publicity, role of mental health workers, contact list and overview of mental health self-advocacy.

White, E C, *Chain Chain Change: for Black Women Dealing with Physical and Emotional Abuse* (1986), Seal Press, USA, £4.95. Available from women's or radical bookshops.
This book explores the cultural and institutional barriers Black women face, and offers Black abused women an understanding of the role of emotional abuse and violence in their lives. It discusses stereotypes and cultural assumptions and offers positive suggestions on getting support from statutory and voluntary bodies.

Wilson, Amrit, *Finding a voice: Asian Women in Britain* (1978). Virago, £4.99.
Describes old and new attitudes, tells of love, marriage and drastic changes imposed on family relationships and friendships of Asian women in the UK.

Videos and audio tapes

Asian Women in Their Own Words (video), £43.85 (including VAT and p&p). Produced by Berkshire Education Department. Available from Dramatic Distribution.
Describing ourselves; overcoming struggle, influences, histories, frustrations, happiness and aspirations.

Breakdown, 40 minutes, £3.50. Available from MIND.
An audio documentary to share the experience of a 'breakdown' through first-hand accounts.

Depression in Ethnic Minorities (video), £35.50 inclusive. Produced by N Films for NAFSIYAT. Available from CFL Vision.

Mistaken for Mad, (video), 40 minutes. Available from Healthcare Productions Ltd. Two-part video looking at the problems experienced by Afro-Caribbean and Asian communities in Britain with regard to mental illness.

Post-Natal Depression (1986), (video) 20 minute, £22.47 (including VAT and p&p). Produced by the Royal Society of Medicine Film and TV Unit for the Asian Mother and Baby Campaign. Available in Bengali, English or Hindi from Healthcare Productions.
Attempts to explain and promote debate about post-natal depression using interviews with health professionals. Aimed at health care providers and the Asian Community. Includes trainer leaflets.

Sharing Power, (video) 40 minutes, £48. Available from MIND.
Looks at efforts to involve users of mental health services in decision-making and provision of services.

We're Not Mad, We're Angry (video) 64 minutes, £20. Available from MIND.
For trainers and teachers this powerful documentary has users offering an explicit and wide-ranging critique of their experiences in hospital and making positive statements about the mental health care they want.

Organisations

British Association of Counselling
Represents counsellors in Britain. Provides information to the public on available counselling. Publishes information.

Concord Video and Film Council
Concord lists a number of videos under the heading mental illness in their catalogue. See Chapter 11 *General resources* for distributors.

Good Practices in Mental Health
Provides information, an enquiry service, publications and rural networking.

London Black Women's Health Action Project
Produces information on Black women's health issues with emphasis on mental health. Aims to provide a national network.

London Rape Crisis
Support for women who have been sexually assaulted.

Mental Health Media Council
Provides information to link the media and the consumer, with a database of over 4,000 film and video titles relating to mental health and well-being. Will also organise activities and discussion groups to complement programmes. Produces *Mediawise* on women and mental health.

MIND (National Association for Mental Health)
Newsletter and numerous publications. Acts as a focus of information and expertise on mental health issues. Has regional centres.

Survivors Speak Out
A facilitating organisation which provides information and a news sheet for its membership and can provide speakers and workshop leaders.

Women's Aid
Information on refuge for women in violent relationships.

Women's Therapy Centre
Offers workshops in many areas of women's concerns and group psychotherapy.

Stress

BACKGROUND INFORMATION

- Stress is a normal part of human experience and can be a positive response to changing conditions. However, when it becomes a long-term habitual response to situations which don't become any easier, stress may be a problem.

- The 'flight or fight' response to dangerous situations involves the production of hormones to prepare the body for increased awareness and activity – to run or fight. In modern life, our responses may be internalised as anger, frustration or anxiety, and this may affect both physical and emotional health.

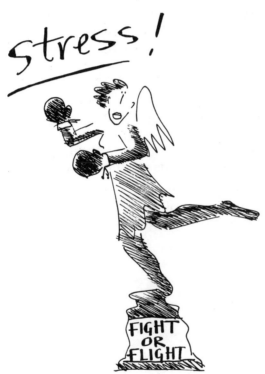

- People have different tolerance levels for stress. What is stimulating for one person, may induce headaches and insomnia in another. In general, women are subject to stressful lives. Experiences may be viewed as stressful or not depending on past experiences, or different material circumstances.

- There are many different causes of stress for women, including:

  – working at home looking after dependants;
  – working at home and in paid employment;

– living within a violent relationship;
– coping on little money, in poor housing conditions; and
– being the target of racism.

- Racism is a real cause of stress for Black women, affecting them in different ways through:

  – limited opportunities for employment;
  – tokenistic employment;
  – racist remarks; and
  – assumptions, for example, about their lifestyle, attitudes and education.

- People respond to stress in different ways:

  – positive ways include identifying the causes; taking time for yourself and learning how to relax; learning skills such as assertiveness or communication skills, which help you to alter a situation which is causing stress; and
  – negative ways include using 'props' such as smoking, drinking or tranquillisers.

- Women from different cultures and social classes may view stress and the capacity for change in very different ways. Assertiveness and confidence building needs to be dealt with in a way which is sensitive and appropriate to the needs of different women.

- Where the underlying causes of stress appear to be insurmountable for individual women to deal with, it is important to seek the support of others. Campaigning may be used as one tool for change.

INFORMATION SHEET *4.1*

Stress and health

In the flight or fight response to stress, the pituitary glands secrete the alarm hormone ACTH. ACTH causes the adrenal glands to secrete adrenaline, noradrenaline and cortisone hormones.

This causes:

- increased heart rate;
- increased respiration;
- the liver to release sugars and fatty acids into the blood;
- pupils to dilate;
- sweating to increase;
- bowels and bladder to empty; and
- muscles to tense.

Yet, modern living does not allow for us to run away from our stress, and we tend to internalise anger, anxiety and frustrations. This may contribute to:

- high blood-pressure;
- ulcers;
- intestinal inflammation;
- migraine;
- asthma;
- constipation;
- back pain and hunched posture;
- shallow breathing;
- heart disease;
- skin complaints; and
- reduced immune system effectiveness.

▷

▷ 4.1 cont.

Other signs of stress include:

- insomnia and poor sleep;
- irritability;
- nail biting and teeth grinding;
- using sedatives;
- increased use of alcohol;
- being obsessive;
- being wound up;
- general dissatisfaction;
- shouting and slamming doors;
- stomach ache;
- eye strain and headaches;
- tightness in chest and chest pains; and
- increased smoking.

INFORMATION SHEET *4.2*

Stress and women's lives

Stress occurs at numerous points all through life. The diagram below shows many key points which may be particularly stressful for women. Additional factors such as racism, poverty, sexual violence and ageism may also affect the amount of stress experienced by individual women.

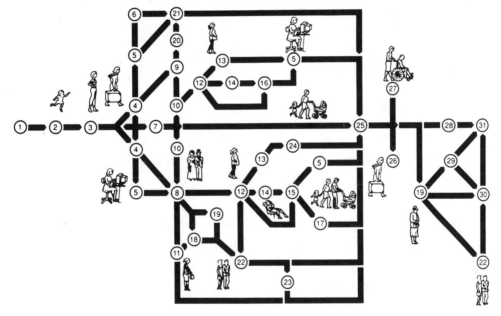

1 Infancy	17 Leave marriage
2 Childhood	18 Divorce
3 Puberty	19 Widow
4 Leaving home	20 Loss of partner
5 Job/Career	21 Living alone·
6 Loss of job	22 Remarriage
7 Fertility/infertility	23 Extra-marital affair
8 Marriage, cohabitation	24 Mature student
9 Cohabitation	25 Menopause
10 Conceive	26 Child leaves home
11 Housewife, childfree	27 Looking after elderly
12 Pregnancy	parents
13 Abortion	28 Old age
14 New baby/Adoption	29 Living with children
15 Parenthood	30 Institutionalised
16 Single parent family	31 Approach of death

Source: The Modern Women's Body (1990), Diagram Visual Information.

INFORMATION SHEET *4.3*

What is assertiveness?

Many women have difficulty in being assertive. Because we are brought up to look after other people and consider their needs, we are often out of touch with our own needs. Even if we know what our needs are, we may feel we do not have the right to pursue them, particularly if they appear to conflict with the needs of others.

Assertiveness is often confused with selfishness or aggression, with pursuing our own needs regardless of the effect on others. This is not assertiveness. Let's look at what assertiveness really is and compare it to other ways of relating to people – aggressiveness, passivity and being manipulative.

Assertiveness

- Recognising our needs and asking openly and directly for what we want.
- Recognising and respecting the rights and needs of other people.
- Relating to people in personal and working situations in an open and honest way.
- Feeling responsible for and in control of our own actions.
- Not seeing situations in terms of win or lose, but being prepared to compromise.
- Being able to resolve difficulties and disputes in a way that feels comfortable and fair to those involved.

Aggressiveness

- Expressing feelings and opinions in a way that punishes, threatens or puts the other person down.
- Disregarding the rights and needs of others.
- Aiming to get our own way no matter what.
- If we 'win' and get what we want aggressively it probably leaves someone else with bad feelings, making it difficult to relate to them in future.

▷

$\triangleright$ 4.3 cont.

Passivity

- Not standing up for our rights. Allowing others to take advantage of us.

- Avoiding responsibility for making choices – leaving others to make decisions for us.

- Not being in control of our lives. Seeing ourselves as helpless victims of unfairness and injustice.

Being manipulative

- Unable to ask directly for what we want.

- Trying to get what we want indirectly, by playing games or trying to make people feel guilty.

ACTIVITY *4.9*

How stress affects me

Aims

- To open up discussion about stress.
- To explore the physical and emotional effects of stress.

Materials

Prompt questions A and B (below) written on a flipchart, paper, pens, flipchart paper and markers.

Method

1 Divide into two small groups, giving prompt questions A to one group, and prompt questions B to the other.

2 Each group discusses the questions, and notes responses.

3 Both groups report back, flipchart and discuss. Add any further points to the lists.

Discussion points

- Are there overlaps between responses from both groups?
- How serious are these symptoms, and how should we deal with them?
- It may be useful to follow this with activities on how to deal with stress.

Prompt questions A

- From your own experience, list some of the physical signs and symptoms of being stressed.
- Are there others you know of?

Prompt questions B

- From your own experience, list some of the mental and emotional signs and symptoms of being stressed.
- Are there others you know of?

ACTIVITY 4.10

Sources of stress for women

Aim

- To explore and acknowledge causes of stress in women's lives.

Materials

Small cards, flipchart paper, markers, a bag.

Method

1 Each woman chooses a stress factor which she experiences, and writes it on a small card. Emphasise that these will be shared with the group anonymously.

2 Place cards in a bag and women each pick one at random.

3 Read out stress factors in turn, and flipchart.

4 Discuss.

Discussion points

- Is it possible to group the different factors, for example into feelings about home/relationships, money worries, juggling home and work?

- Are the stress factors more common to women's experiences than men's, and why?

- Racism may be identified as a major cause of stress by Black women.

ACTIVITY *4.11*

Women and stress

Aims

- To acknowledge stress in women's lives.

- To share common experiences of stress.

Materials

A copy of Worksheet 4.7 *Women and stress* for each woman; pens, flipchart paper, markers.

Method

1 Women fill in the worksheet individually, and then share in pairs.

2 Pairs join to make foursomes and compile a list of common areas of stress in women's lives.

3 In the large group, feed back, flipchart responses and discuss.

Discussion points

- Did some areas of stress come up for most women?

- Are there differences between older, younger, white and Black women? What other factors may affect responses?

- If men were to do this activity, what would the differences be?

ACTIVITY *4.12*

Time for yourself

Aims

- To explore what women already do and what else they would like to do to try to deal with stress.

- To look at what stops them from doing these things.

Materials

A copy of Worksheet 4.10 *Time for yourself* for each woman; pens, flipchart paper, markers.

Method

1 In small groups, ask women to go through the worksheet, noting their responses.

2 In the large group, report back and flipchart responses.

3 Discuss.

Discussion points

- How can women change situations to gain more time for themselves?

- Is it useful to acknowledge situations which are beyond the individuals' control?

- What other ways of dealing with stress are there, apart from finding time for yourself?

- How difficult is it to explore this issue?

ACTIVITY *4.13*

Stress – making changes

Aim

- To develop a personal action plan for making changes to reduce stress levels.

Materials

A copy of Worksheets 4.8 *Stress-making changes 1* and 4.9 *Stress-making changes 2* for each woman; pens.

Method

1 Give women Worksheet 4.8 and ask them to fill it in individually.

2 In pairs or small groups, ask women to fill in Worksheet 4.9, giving each other support and ideas.

3 In the large group, share ideas and compare first steps which women are going to take.

Discussion points

- How helpful is it to plan in this way?

- In what ways can the group support the plans each member makes?

ACTIVITY *4.14*

Seven-point plan for a calmer life

Aims

- To consider a range of options for reducing stress.

- To acknowledge the reality of women's lives.

Materials

A copy of Worksheet 4.11 *Seven-point plan for a calmer life* for each woman; pens, paper, flipchart paper, markers, post-its, blutack.

Method

1 In small groups, consider the seven points on the worksheet and discuss the questions, noting down responses.

2 In the large group, feed back and flipchart responses and discuss.

3 Ask each woman to write on a post-it one suggestion for how she could reduce stress for herself. (If women have difficulty on their own, they may pair up with someone.)

4 Stick post-its on a piece of flipchart paper to create the group's own plan for a calmer life, and display it on a wall.

Discussion points

- Is it helpful to think about taking time for yourself? It can be very threatening to start to think about making changes, especially if other people benefit from the way you currently organise your time.

- If it feels difficult to organise this, why might this be so?

ACTIVITY *4.15*

Responding to stress

Aim

- To explore both positive and negative responses to stress.

Materials

Flipchart paper and markers.

Method

1 In a large group, brainstorm both positive and negative ways in which women respond to stress, and flipchart them in two columns for example:

negative	*positive*
smoking	sitting still
being moody	long walk
alcohol	talking about it

negative	*positive*
not sleeping	soaking in the bath
tranquillisers	

2 Discuss the lists you have produced.

Discussion points

- How balanced are the two lists?

- What else can be done to foster a more positive approach to dealing with stress?

- Women may need prompting about positive responses they could adopt for themselves, such as massage, getting out for walks, and talking to others more often.

ACTIVITY *4.16*

What is assertiveness?

Aim

- To understand the difference between assertive behaviour and other types of behaviour.

Materials

A copy of Information Sheet 4.3 *What is assertiveness?* for each woman; prompt questions (below) written on a flipchart, flipchart paper, markers.

Method

1 Divide into four groups, and ask each group to use a different style of behaviour to deal with situations – aggressive, assertive, passive or manipulative.

2 Each group responds to prompt questions in the style allocated.

3 In the large group, feed back and flipchart responses. Encourage general approaches rather than specific ways of dealing with the case studies. Use separate sheets for the four approaches.

4 Compare flipchart lists with the information sheet and discuss.

Discussion points

- Does each group deal with the situations differently?

- How close is the fit between group responses and those on the information sheet?

- Are there any surprises for the group?

- How easy is it for women to identify their own behaviour (past or current) as being assertive or not?

Prompt questions
- 'Rita needs someone to babysit next week. She rings her friend to ask her . . .'

- 'Dee is the Health and Safety rep and has been meaning to talk to the manager for some time about dangerous working practices. A colleague sustains a minor injury at work and now she feels this is the time to broach the subject. She is feeling very anxious . . .'

ACTIVITY *4.17*

How assertive are you?

Aims
- To explore how assertive we are in a range of situations.

- To identify the situations in which we find it easiest, and hardest, to be assertive and to look at the reasons for this.

Materials
A copy of Worksheet 4.12 *How assertive are you?* for each woman; pens.

Method
1 Ask women to think about the questions on the worksheet, and fill it in.

2 Discuss the questions and answers, trying to identify any patterns.

Discussion points
- Did any clear patterns emerge from the questionnaire about your assertiveness in different situations:

  – with your partner?
  – with family?
  – with friends?
  – at work?

– dealing with those you pay for goods or services?
– dealing with authority figures?

● In which situations do you find it easiest to be assertive? Why?

● In which situations do you find it hardest to be assertive? Why is it so difficult?

● What can we do to become more assertive?

● Is assertiveness a help when dealing with stressful situations or relationships? If so, how?

ACTIVITY *4.18*

Making and refusing requests

Aims

● To explore feelings and difficulties about asking for something, and about refusing a request.

● To practise assertiveness skills in making and refusing a request.

Materials

A copy of Worksheet 4.13 *Making and refusing requests* for each woman; pens.

Method

1 Ask women to think of something they find it hard to ask for. Explain that they are going to ask the woman sitting on their right for this, and that when they are asked for something they must refuse.

2 Choose someone to start, who asks the woman on her right for something. She refuses the request, and then asks the woman on her right for something. Continue around the circle until everyone has asked for something and has also refused a request.

3 In small groups, go through the worksheet and share ideas.

4 In the large group, feed back and discuss.

Discussion points

● Are there any patterns about difficulties women have in making or refusing requests?

- How can women come to feel they have the right to make or refuse a request?

- What have women learnt from this exercise that could help them in making or refusing requests in future?

ACTIVITY *4.19*

Giving and receiving criticism

Aims

- To explore feelings and difficulties about giving and receiving criticism.

- To practise assertiveness skills in giving and receiving criticism.

Materials

A copy of Worksheet 4.14 *Giving and receiving criticism* for each woman; pens.

Method

1 You could do this activity in the whole group or in smaller groups. Ask each woman to think of a criticism she has avoided making, or made but felt she handled badly. Make it clear that you are not asking them to make real criticisms of the women in the room, but of other people in their lives.

2 Each woman in turn makes her criticism to the woman on her right, first identifying who she is criticising, e.g. 'You are my work colleague – I don't think you have really been pulling your weight recently. I seem to end up with all the difficult jobs'.

3 The woman on her right must respond to this criticism in any way which she feels natural to her. She may respond with a single statement which ends the dialogue, or provoke further discussion (or argument) for several minutes. Hopefully there will be a range of different responses which will provide much to talk about afterwards.

4 In the large group, use the worksheet to structure a discussion on how women handle criticism in this exercise, and in their lives.

Discussion points

- Why is criticism hard to deal with in an assertive way?

- How can we improve our handling of criticism?

ACTIVITY *4.20*

Rehearsing situations

Aims

- To provide an opportunity to rehearse difficult situations in a safe setting.

- To explore the concept of effective communication.

- To encourage self-confidence.

Materials

A copy of Worksheet 4.15 *Rehearsing situations* for each woman.

Method

1 Individually, women decide upon a situation that they would like to rehearse in pairs.

2 Using the worksheet prompts, women work in pairs, sharing time equally.

3 In the large group, feed back and discuss, allowing time for women to discuss how they felt about doing this activity.

Discussion points

- How useful can it be to rehearse situations?

- How difficult is it?

- Does the whole thing feel artificial? Could this be a problem for some women?

Note for tutor

This activity works best after some time has been spent with the group exploring areas of stress in their lives. It requires a level of trust and confidence within the group.

WORKSHEET *4.7*

Women and stress

Complete the following sentence with as many factors as you can.

As a woman I feel stressed when . . .

WORKSHEET *4.8*

Stress – making changes 1

1 Make a list of the main causes of stress in your life. They can be major and minor ones.

2 Now place a tick next to those causes which you would like to do something about or change. Put an x next to those which you feel may be hard to change. Put a ? for those you are unsure about.

Main causes of stress	*Would like to do something about*	*May be hard to change*	*Unsure*

3 Choose one of the stress factors that you have ticked, to work on with Worksheet 4.9. (Sometimes it is easier to start with a minor, fairly manageable example.)

WORKSHEET *4.9*

Stress – making changes 2

Using the stress factors you have identified through Worksheet 4.8, look at the Stress Action Wheel below and see if you can begin to make your own action plan.

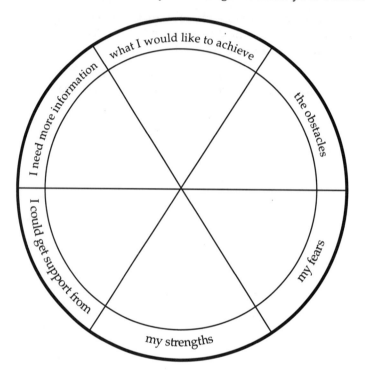

My first step will be:

WORKSHEET *4.10*

Time for yourself

Time for yourself means the time you take to do things for yourself – to enrich your life or to relax. It is the things you choose to do rather than the things you have to do. It may include things you do with others or by yourself.

- How much time do you have for yourself in a week?

- What sort of things do you do for yourself?

- What else would you like to do?

- What stops you from doing any of these?

WORKSHEET *4.11*

Seven-point plan for a calmer life

Read through the following suggestions and say which of these would be easiest to implement and which would be hardest.

1 Do one thing at a time.

2 Listen without interrupting.

3 Escape into tasks that demand concentration.

4 Eat slowly and savour the food.

5 Find a private retreat in the home.

6 Plan some idleness every day.

7 Avoid hurry by every conceivable measure.

WORKSHEET *4.12*

How assertive are you?

1. When a friend or neighbour asks you a favour you do not want to do, can you refuse?

2. Can you accept criticism?

3. If you do not understand what your doctor is telling you, can you insist she or he explains?

4. Do you feel able to ask your husband/partner for what you want from the relationship?

5. When you need help, is it easy for you to ask others to give it to you?

6. If you are paying for a job or service to be done and you are not satisfied with the result, can you insist it is completed to your standards?

7. Do you feel confident about dealing with authorities, e.g. employers, social security staff, housing officers, landlords?

8. If you are treated unfairly at work, do you try to do something about it?

9. Do you readily admit your mistakes and apologise?

10. If you are sold faulty goods, do you take them back?

11. If you feel hurt by something a friend has said or done, do you tell them how you feel?

12. Do you find it easy to talk to your child's teacher?

WORKSHEET *4.13*

Making and refusing requests

Making a request

- How many women prefaced their request with an apologetic phrase, such as: 'I don't like to bother you but . . .' or 'Do say if it's inconvenient, but perhaps you wouldn't mind . . .'?

- Why did you feel the need to apologise?

- Did you find it hard to ask for something?

- How did it feel to be refused?

- In your own life, what requests do you find it hardest to make?

- What are the worries about asking?

- How do you feel if you are refused?

- If you are refused do you feel able to make a similar request again?

Refusing a request

- How many women justified their refusal with a reason, such as: 'I'm going out on Tuesday, so I can't babysit'?

- Would you find it hard simply to say no, or that you just don't want to?

- Did you leave a loophole in your excuse, making it hard to refuse a second request: 'Well it doesn't really have to be Tuesday, the film is on all week – any night would do'?

- Did your reason make clear whether your refusal was for this particular occasion or for all time: 'I can't babysit this week, but do ask me another time with more notice, I may be freer', or 'No I don't feel able to do any babysitting'?

- In your own life what kind of requests do you find it hard to refuse?

- What are your fears about refusing?

WORKSHEET *4.14*

Giving and receiving criticism

Giving criticism

- Was the criticism of the person's behaviour or of the person themselves, for example: 'Your work is disorganised', or 'You are a disorganised person'?

- Was anything positive said along with the criticism: 'We've generally worked well together, but recently . . .'?

- When criticising, did you acknowledge your own feelings rather than assuming you were stating objective facts, for example: 'I can't stand the mess in your room any more', rather than 'Your room is an absolute disgrace'.

- If the person you are criticising rejects the criticism, do you back down, or even sometimes end up apologising and taking the blame yourself?

- Generally, do you make criticisms in the heat of the moment, or when you are feeling calm?

- In your own life, in what situations have you avoided giving criticism which you felt was justified?

- In what situations do you feel you have handled giving criticism badly?

Receiving criticism

- In the responses to criticism were there some you could identify as largely aggressive, passive, manipulative or assertive?

- Do you tend to have an automatic response to criticism – either rejecting it out of hand, or accepting it even when it's not justified?

- Do you often regret your initial response later when you've had time to think about the criticism?

- Do you ever reject criticism by going on the attack, for example: 'It's not me who isn't pulling her weight, you're the one who doesn't . . .'?

- Does being criticised remind you of other situations when you have been criticised in the past, by your parents or school teachers for instance?

WORKSHEET *4.15*

Rehearsing situations

Working in pairs, decide who will speak first and who will listen.

If you are doing the talking make sure your partner knows what you expect from her. This could be listening silently while you talk at her, or it could involve her answering you back in a way you have specified.

If you are doing the listening be clear about what you need to be doing. If you are to listen, then focus upon what your partner is saying and don't think about what you would be saying or doing in the same situation. It can be helpful to give an indication that you are hearing what is being said to you, by nodding and making eye contact.

RESOURCES

For contact details of distributors and organisations listed here, see Chapter 11 *General resources*.

Publications

Patel, Chandra, *The Complete Guide to Stress Management* (1989), Optima, £8.99.
Looks at factors causing stress and how to cope with stress through fitness, diet, mental relaxation, etc.

Saunders, Charmaine, *Women and Stress: how to Manage Stress and Take Control of Your Life* (1990), £4.99.
Covers types of stress, life roles, and how to deal with stress.

Videos

Shanti – Asian Women and Stress, in Bengali, Gujarati, Hindi, Punjabi, Urdu (all with English subtitles), or English. Available from the SHANTI Project.
Aims to give Asian women culturally appropriate information and skills to manage stress, working with groups and individual women in the community to develop suitable programmes in stress management skills; to train volunteers and other workers in skills of stress management; and to improve access for Asian women to information and services which promote mental health.

Stress at Work (undated), 24 minutes. Available from Concord Video and Film Council.
Looks at different jobs and the stresses associated with them.

Relaxation and massage

The views expressed in this section are those of the authors and do not necessarily reflect the views and policies of the Health Education Authority

BACKGROUND INFORMATION

- Relaxation plays an important role in promoting good health. It is one approach to the relief of a range of mental and physical conditions including stress, tension, high blood-pressure, hot flushes in menopause, and pain, for example during childbirth or during periods.

- Techniques and exercises for relaxing can easily be learned, but they need to be incorporated into daily life in order to be really effective. Relaxation is also about saying no to others and yes to yourself.

- Relaxation may be harder for women than men, because of the variety of responsibilities that women juggle. It may be more acceptable for men to relax at the end of a working day, while many women, especially those with young children, are always 'on duty'. It is worth taking time for positive relaxation rather than collapsing with exhaustion on a regular basis.

- Relaxation is an approach which is free, requires no equipment, and has no adverse side effects. It can make us feel good in a short time.

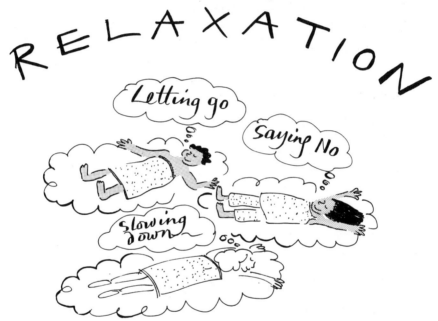

- Relaxation can be useful as an aid to giving up smoking and other dependent habits such as drinking and tranquilliser use.

- Massage can bring immediate beneficial effects from headaches and muscle tension, and is an important aid to relaxation. Combining it with the use of aromatic oils can make it even more beneficial (see Information Sheet 10.3 *Aromatherapy* in the complementary medicine section in Chapter 10).

- Attitudes to massage are affected:
  - by the public image of 'massage parlours'; and
  - because touching others usually happens within sexual relationships.

- Massage can be used as therapy for physical and emotional problems, such as depression and premenstrual syndrome.

PRACTICAL POINTS

- Both massage and relaxation are easily incorporated into women's health sessions – although it is useful to discuss the feelings of the group beforehand. Activity 4.27 *Attitudes to massage* may help the group explore feelings.

- Tutors do not have to be experts in yoga, physiotherapy or massage. The group can do activities at a fairly simple level to start with. If the group is keen to do more, you could invite in a woman yoga teacher, a masseuse, or use a book as a group learning exercise.

- There is no need for removal of clothes if the group is not happy with this. Feet, head and neck massages are usually acceptable. Women in the group may have different ideas about what they are comfortable with.

- It is possible to devote whole sessions to relaxation and massage or integrate them into each session – as a wind-down at the end, or to balance discussion activities.

- Guided fantasies are not suited to everyone as some women find it hard to relax and visualise in a group setting, or have fears relating to the scene of the fantasy – so check with the group.

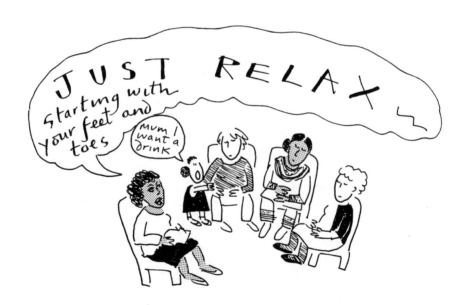

- Massage works well in groups where there is a degree of trust established already. It can leave a warm and open feeling within a group and enable women to communicate at a more personal level. Leave time for discussion and a balanced close.

- When doing massage sessions it is vital to have a warm room to work in as draughts will produce tension in the muscles.

- Some activities can be done sitting in a chair. For any activity requiring women to lie on the floor ask them to bring a towel or mat to lie on, depending on the type of room being used.

- Quiet rooms enable women to relax more easily. If there is a creche, try to ensure the noise of children cannot be heard. Sometimes a quiet piece of music helps.

INFORMATION SHEET *4.4*

Helpful hints for massage

- Make sure the room is warm.

- Apply pressure when you massage – this will vary, but some pressure is always necessary. People first learning massage are often nervous about hurting someone, so tend to apply almost no pressure. Don't worry. Pressure feels good, as you'll see yourself. You can always check this out by asking the person.

- Use your weight rather than your muscles to apply pressure.

- Relax your hands. It's harder to relax a limb while you're using it than to relax it while it's lying still. But try to keep your hands as loose and flexible as possible, when you are moving them. Giving a good massage, as well as helping the other person, will also help you get rid of the tension in your hands. A lot of women experience this.

- Mould your hands to fit the contours over which they are passing.

- Keep a gentle pressure most of the time, but if you need to use more pressure, or to massage faster, especially in the shoulder area, then do so.

- Try to 'listen' to the body you are massaging, e.g. feel the tension in the neck and work on it.

- It is important not to break contact with the skin of the person you are massaging until you have finished. This will benefit the person you are massaging and help them keep the continuity of feeling.

- Massage with your entire body, not just your hands, i.e. make your hands an extension of your whole body.

- Feel centred and relaxed about the way you are standing, sitting or kneeling.

- You can use oil if you want to. Coconut oil and almond oil are available cheaply from the chemist. They are non-greasy and smell good. Talcum powder is an alternative.

ACTIVITY *4.21*

Learning to unwind

Aims

- To encourage women to consider their own needs for relaxation.

- To begin to see time for relaxation as a positive choice.

Materials

Flipchart paper, markers.

Method

1 Going round the group, ask everyone to think of at least one situation in which they would like to relax, but find it hard to. List these on the flipchart.

2 Going round the group again, ask everyone to think of their favourite ways of unwinding, or relaxing. Make another list of these.

3 Now try to 'match' the two lists. Ask each woman to see if there is a way of relaxing which could be helpful for her stressful situation.

Discussion points

- Which list was easier to make?

- How easy is it for us to find time to unwind?

- Is it harder for women than for men? If so, in what ways?

- How many of us feel guilty if we take time to relax? What can we do about this?

ACTIVITY *4.22*

Warm-up exercises

Aims

- To warm up the body before doing relaxation.

- To lighten the mood and make the group feel at ease.

Materials

A copy of Worksheet 4.16 *Warm-up exercises* for each woman.

Method

1 In the large group, talk through points 1–8 on the worksheet, and discuss opportunities for women to use them in everyday life as well as before an exercise and relaxation activity.

2 Follow with a practical relaxation activity.

Discussion points

• In everyday life, it may not be possible to work through all of these exercises at one time. They can be used individually for different tension spots.

• Points 4, 6 and 7 can help reduce tension in the shoulders and neck during the day as soon as one becomes aware of it, or to prevent the build-up of tension in those areas. These may be particularly useful for women involved in activities such as typing, computer operations, sewing, or knitting.

ACTIVITY *4.23*

Five-minute relaxation in a chair

Aim

• To demonstrate one quick, accessible and adaptable relaxation activity.

Materials

A copy of Worksheet 4.17 *Five-minute relaxation in a chair* for the tutor.

Method

1 Introduce some basic principles of relaxation (see Background information p. 120) and discuss.

2 Make sure women are sitting comfortably and ready for the activity.

3 Take the group slowly through the relaxation activity by reading out from the worksheet.

4 Get women to feed back how it felt, and discuss.

Discussion points
- How easy is it for women to find the space and time to relax at home?

- How easy is it to relax our minds as well as our bodies?

- This is one way of relaxing – there are other methods. In time, relaxation is something that can be used almost anywhere in everyday life. (For example, see Activity 4.26 *Quick release of tension*.) Have women found their own ways of relaxing during everyday life?

ACTIVITY *4.24*

Relaxing the mind

Aim
- To relax the mind after a period of muscle relaxation.

Materials
A copy of Worksheet 4.18 *Relaxing the mind* for each woman.

Method
1 Explain the activity to the group, and why it is useful.

2 Choose *one* of the images from the worksheet, and ask the women to let their minds focus on it, imagining every detail. (Start off doing the activity for one minute, building up to five minutes, as they get more used to it.)

3 Slowly, ask the women to return to reality.

4 Get the group to feed back how it felt, and discuss.

Discussion points
- Was it possible to relax the mind and shut out everyday thoughts and the environment around you? This takes practice, so don't be put off if you don't succeed initially. In time it will become easier.

- This activity can be repeated at other sessions, with each group member focusing on their own chosen image, either from the worksheet or of their own choice.

- Women may choose to take the worksheet home to try out the activity for themselves.

ACTIVITY *4.25*

Guided fantasy

Aim

- To take the group on a fantasy trip away from reality and day-to-day worries.

Materials

A copy of Worksheet 4.19 *Guided fantasy* for the tutor.

Method

1 Explain the activity to the group, and check that the women feel happy about doing it. Make sure women are sitting or lying comfortably.

2 Slowly read out the *Guided fantasy* worksheet.

3 Carefully bring the group back to where they started from, and let them slowly come to.

Discussion points

- These types of activities are often used in yoga to help people switch off for a few minutes from worries and responsibilities.

- This fantasy was written for use in a situation where there was some

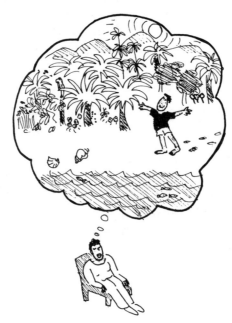

sound from the nearby creche – in the fantasy the sounds are monkeys and parrots! The group could also create other fantasy worlds for use in this way.

- How easy did women find it to get carried away? What might help?

Note to tutor: This activity is useful after a practical relaxation activity, and/or Activity 4.24 *Relaxing the mind*.

ACTIVITY *4.26*

Quick release of tension

Aim
- To enable women to deal with everyday tension quickly and at the time.

Materials
A copy of Worksheet 4.20 *Quick release of tension* for each woman.

Method
1 Go through the worksheet together, and practise.
2 Discuss situations in which this technique could be used.

*ACTIVITY *4.27*

Attitudes to massage

Aim
- To examine the range of attitudes held towards massage.

Materials
Flipchart paper, markers.

Method
1 Ask the whole group to think about what comes into their head when they hear the word 'massage', and list responses on the flipchart.

2 Discuss the issues raised.

Discussion points

- What kind of dominant image do we have of massage?

- How does this affect how we feel about giving or getting a massage?

- Have any women in the group had a massage? Does the image of massage fit with their own experiences?

ACTIVITY *4.28*

Ideas for massage

Aim

- To help women develop skills for massage.

Materials

Copies of Information sheet 4.4 *Helpful hints for massage* and Worksheet 4.21 *Ideas for massage* for each woman.

Method

1 Give women the information sheet, read it through and share ideas and experiences women may have.

2 Using the worksheet, let women choose to work individually, trying ideas for self-massage, or in pairs, massaging each other. Allow plenty of time.

3 In the large group, discuss how women found the activity.

Discussion points

- Did women find the self-massage beneficial – in what situations might they want to use this in future?

- How comfortable were women about massaging each other? How did it feel to give a massage? And to receive one?

Notes for tutor

- This activity may work best in a group where some trust is already established.

- If women are not comfortable with doing the activity in the session they could have the worksheet to try out ideas in other situations.

WORKSHEET *4.16*

Warm-up exercises

It is a good idea to do a few exercises to warm up the body before doing relaxation. Warm muscles relax more readily.

1. *Stretch.* Raise one arm as far as you can, gently reaching upwards, then let it relax and drop. Do the same with the other arm, then lift both arms, stretch and let them go.

2. *Shake arms loosely by your side.* Shake one then the other in a rotary movement. Do the same with your legs – hold on to something if you are wobbly.

3. *Sway.* With feet apart, lean forward a little. Sway a little, let your arms move, don't control them, let them stop on their own.

4. *Circle shoulders.* Circle shoulders backwards, first one then the other.

5. *Slapping.* Slap yourself all over, especially thighs and tummy.

6. *Head roll.* Allow your head to flop to the left. Let it roll across your chest and up to the right. Then let it go back to the starting position. Next roll your head slowly in a circle – then back again.

7. *Hands.* Shake hands loosely as if they were wet, then clench and stretch several times. Rest them in the cradle position in your lap.

8. *Face.* Frown, then let it go; raise eyebrows, then let go; do both together; now smooth your forehead – use your hands to help if you wish.

WORKSHEET *4.17*

Five-minute relaxation in a chair

This technique is for when you have only a short time to spare. It is better to have a chair with arms, but ideally, you should be able to learn to relax anywhere you find yourself. Use a cushion in the small of the back if it helps. Make sure you are warm.

1 Sit upright and well back in the chair so that your thighs and back are supported, and rest your hands in the cradle position on your lap, or lightly on top of your thighs. If you like, take off your shoes, and let your feet rest on the ground (if they don't touch the floor, try to find a book or similar object to rest them on). If you want to, close your eyes.

2 Begin by breathing out first. Then breathe in easily, just as much as you need. Now breathe out slowly, with a slight sigh, like a balloon slowly deflating. Do this once more, slowly . . . breathe in . . . breathe out . . . as you breathe out, feel the tension begin to drain away. Then go back to your ordinary breathing: even, quiet, steady.

3 Now direct your thoughts to each part of your body in turn, to the muscles and joints.

- Think first about your left foot. Your toes are still. Your foot feels heavy on the floor. Let your foot and toes start to feel completely relaxed.

- Now think about your right foot . . . toes . . . ankles . . . they are resting heavily on the floor. Let both your feet, your toes, ankles start to relax.

- Now think about your legs. Let your legs feel completely relaxed and heavy on the chair. Your thighs, your knees roll downwards when they relax, so let them go.

- Think now about your back, and your spine. Let the tension drain away from your back, and from your spine. Follow your breathing, and each time you breathe out, relax your back and spine a little more.

- Let your abdominal muscles become soft and loose. There's no need to hold your stomach in tight, it rises and falls as you breathe quietly – feel that your stomach is completely relaxed.

- No tension in your chest. Let your breathing be slow and easy, and each time you breathe out, let go a little more.

- Think now about the fingers of your left hand – they are curved, limp and

▷

▷ 4.17 cont.
quite still. Now the fingers of your right hand . . . relaxed . . . soft and still. Let this feeling of relaxation spread – up your arms . . . feel the heaviness in your arms up to your shoulders. Let your shoulders relax, let them drop easily . . . and then let them drop even further than you thought they could.

- Think about your neck. Feel the tension melt away from your neck and shoulders. Each time you breathe out, relax your neck a little more.

- Now before we move on, just check to see if all these parts of your body are still relaxed – your feet, legs, back and spine, tummy, hands, arms, neck and shoulders. Keep your breathing gentle and easy. Every time you breathe out, relax a little more, and let all the tensions ease away from your body. No tensions . . . just enjoy this feeling of relaxation.

- Now think about your face. Let the expression come off your face. Smooth out your brow and let your forehead feel wide, and relaxed. Let your eyebrows drop gently. There's no tension round your eyes . . . your eyelids slightly closed, your eyes are still. Let your jaw unwind . . . teeth slightly apart as your jaw unwinds more and more. Feel the relief of letting go.

- Now think about your tongue, and throat. Let your tongue drop down to the bottom of your mouth and relax completely. Relax your tongue and throat. And your lips . . . lips lightly together, no pressure between them.

- Let all the muscles in your face unwind and let go – there's no tension in your face – just let it relax more and more.

4 Now, instead of thinking about yourself in parts, feel the all-over sensation of letting go, of quiet and of rest. Check to see if you are still relaxed. Stay like this for a few moments, and listen to your breathing . . . in . . . and out . . . let your body become looser, heavier, each time you breathe out.

5 Now continue for a little longer, and enjoy this time for relaxation.

6 Coming back – slowly, wriggle your hands a little, and your feet. When you are ready, open your eyes and sit quiet for a while. Stretch, if you want to, or yawn, and *slowly* start to move again.

Variation: this activity could be followed by Activity 4.25 *Guided fantasy* for a longer session.

WORKSHEET *4.18*

Relaxing the mind

- When your body is relaxed and heavy, it is useful to focus your mind so that it is prevented from thinking about everyday things which worry us.

- Try thinking of one of these, perhaps just for one minute to start with, building up to about five minutes over a period of time. Imagine every little detail – the sights, sounds, scents, colours:
  - a vase of flowers;
  - a picture or a painting;
  - a room in your house;
  - going for a walk in your mind;
  - looking around a garden you know well;
  - a field of corn or trees blowing in the wind;
  - a harbour with little boats bobbing in the breeze;
  - just use your ears and listen to the sounds around you; or
  - say 'one' mentally every time you breathe out.

- If everyday thoughts come into your mind to disturb you – just note them mentally and then let them pass – don't hang on to them – bring your attention back to your mind discipline.

- To come back to reality, slowly wriggle your hands a little, and your feet. When you are ready, open your eyes and sit quietly for a while. Stretch if you want to, or yawn, and slowly start to move again.

WORKSHEET *4.19*

Guided fantasy

Read the text below slowly, in a calm, soothing voice.

Image yourself walking out of this building and seeing a magic carpet outside. You get onto the carpet and make yourself comfortable. You are going to fly right away from here to somewhere much warmer. You are flying above towns and villages, fields and farms. The houses and cars look unreal, like match-box toys. Now you are over a beach and now the sea. At first the sea is grey but as we get to a warmer climate it gets bluer and bluer. You can feel the sun beating down on you, warming you up.

Ahead you see a lush island with palm trees, white sands and clear blue sea. You land on the beach and look around for a minute or two breathing in the richly scented warm air. You take a stroll on the beach barefooted and feel the warmth of the sand on the soles of your feet. Dip your toes into the sea, it feels warm but refreshing.

Now walk into the jungle. There are beautiful exotic flowers everywhere – they smell wonderful and are clear bright colours – pinks, yellow, turquoise. High above you are monkeys jumping from tree to tree chattering to each other, and parrots flying around. Ahead you see a clearing in the jungle and walk towards it. There is a sleepy green lagoon bathed in green light from the sun passing through the tallest palm trees. On the lagoon is a little dinghy and you get into it and lie down.

You are bobbing gently in the lagoon in a pool of green light. You can hear the monkeys and birds screeching in the jungle but they sound a long way away. You can smell the musky fragrance of the exotic flowers and fruit on the trees. Just enough sun can get through the trees to warm your body as you lie on the dinghy. Let yourself completely unwind as you relax breathing in the warmth, smells and sounds of the jungle.

When you are ready to come back, get up from the dinghy, walk slowly back through the jungle to your magic carpet. Make yourself comfortable on the carpet again for your journey home. You are flying over the sea, then over land and now you can see your home town. You land back where you started from and walk back into the room.

WORKSHEET *4.20*

Quick release of tension

Whenever you feel anxious, panicky or uptight . . .

1 Let your breath go (don't breathe in first).

2 Take in a slow, gentle breath; hold it for a second.

3 Let it go, with a leisurely sigh of relief.

4 Drop your shoulders at the same time and relax your hands.

5 Make sure your teeth are not clenched together.

6 If you have to speak, speak more slowly and in a lower tone of voice.

WORKSHEET *4.21*

Ideas for massage

Self-massage – face, head and neck

This can help relieve obstinate muscle tension or pain. It can also be done before loosening exercises or relaxation. Think of it as 'oiling' the joints and muscles to ease them into movement and stimulate the blood supply. Massage should be rhythmical and the pressure varied according to your needs. Some of these techniques can be done with a partner.

- Shoulders – hand on opposite shoulder, roll the back muscle up and forward.

- Neck – thumbs along edge of skull from ears towards spine; change to fingers and continue down spine; then push the back neck muscles up towards head.

- Forehead – for 'vertical wrinkles' – start at centre of forehead, stroke rhythmically out and down to ears. For 'horizontal wrinkles' – stroke from eyebrows to hairline, each hand in turn.

- Eyes – 'palming' – close your eyes and place the palms of your hands – one over each eye socket. Let your fingers cross over your forehead. The resulting darkness is very restful.

- Lips – with finger tips massage lips over teeth.

- For sinus pain – with finger tips massage over site of pain – gently.

- Scalp – 'hair washing' – move scalp over skull with finger tips.

With a partner

Forehead massage

This is very useful for relieving headaches and tension.

- Hold palms against the forehead for a few moments. Cover the forehead with the hands, let the fingers spread. Apply no pressure. Pause as long as it seems OK – let your partner grow used to your touch. Centre yourself and make sure you feel relaxed – focus on your breathing if this helps.

- Now begin to massage the forehead with the balls of your thumbs. First, mentally divide the forehead into strips about half an inch wide. Start with your thumbs at the centre of the forehead just below the hairline – glide both thumbs

▷

▷ 4.21 cont.
at once in either direction outwards along the top-most strip. Continue towards the temples, and end there by moving your thumbs in a circle about half an inch wide.

- Then, without taking your hands off the forehead, return to the centre of the forehead and begin again – the next strip down.

- Work progressively down – ending with a circle on the temples – to the last strip just above your friend's eyebrows. This is the first stage of complete face massage.

Variation: Two hands on the forehead, smooth one back from eyebrows over scalp and then the other.

Neck and shoulders

Stand behind your partner, put your hands on her shoulders and centre yourself.

- Place your hands on your partner's shoulders with your thumbs at the back. Use your thumbs in small circular movements – work up from the top of the spine to the hairline – slowly. With each circular motion you make, try to feel aware of the tension and try to work it away. Hold your whole hand in contact with her shoulders, and although you're concentrating on the neck, be aware of tension in the shoulders too, and try to work that away.

- Then try in any way that feels right to you, to smooth away tension in her neck and shoulders.

- To end, press down with the hands on top of the shoulders and then let the hands travel down the upper arms as far as the elbows. Repeat a few times.

Foot massage

This is wonderfully soothing! We often neglect our feet, hate them, think they are too ugly or smelly! It's good to give them a treat. Your partner can lie down, or sit with her foot on a stool.

- Massage the sole of the foot with the tips of your thumbs. Press hard, as if you were putting a drawing pin into a piece of wood. Press everywhere. Work slowly over the sole.

- Then lift the foot slightly and work the sides of the heel all the way to the ankle bone. Try to feel as if you are pushing away all the tension. Stop if it hurts, and change position.

- You can then work on the toes, and the top of the foot in the same way.

RESOURCES

For contact details of distributors and organisations listed here, see Chapter 11 *General Resources*.

Publications

Downing, George, *The Massage Book* (1990), Penguin, £5.99.
Shows how to do massage for relaxation.

Hewitt, James, *The Complete Relaxation Book* (1989), Rider, £7.99.
Second revised edition of the guide to a wide range of relaxation techniques.

Kirsta, Alix, *The Book of Stress Survival: How to Relax and Live Positively* (1986), Thorsons, £8.99.
Covers causes and ways to deal with stress including exercise, massage, meditation and diet.

Mitchell, Laura, *Simple Relaxation: Physiological Methods for Easing Tension* (1987), J Murray, £5.95.

Nagarathna, R, Nagendra, H R, and Monro, Robin, *Yoga for Common Ailments* (1990), Gaia, £6.99.
Illustrated guide which includes many women's stresses and problems.

O'Brien, Paddy, *A Gentler Strength: the Yoga Book for Women* (1991), Thorsons, £6.99.
A guide to the uses of yoga for women.

Phillips, Alison, *Relax* (1989), Outset Publishing, £4.00 (for more than 25 copies, £3.50 each). ISBN 0 95031 627 X.
Exercises to develop relaxation skills for use by individuals or groups, by professionals and non-professionals.

Tobias, Maxine and Steward, Mary, *The Yoga Book* (1986), Pan, £5.95.

Trimmer, Eric, *The 10 Day Relaxation Plan* (1985), Sphere, £1.95.

Organisations

Institute of Complementary Medicine
Send an SAE for details of a wide range of therapies for relaxation and healing, such as massage, spiritual healing and others.

International Stress and Tension Control Society
Information for professionals and the general public on stress management.

Relaxation for Living
Produce publications and run classes. For information, send a large SAE.

5 Food and body image

INTRODUCTION

This chapter is divided into two sections: *Food and healthy eating*, and *Self-image and body image*.

Women play a key role in relation to food, both as consumers, and with the main responsibility for buying and preparing food, and educating others about healthy eating. While women themselves may be actively changing this stereotypical view, the dominant picture presented through schools, the media and advertising is that food is a woman's domain.

For many women, trying to attain an 'ideal' figure leads them to focus constantly on what they eat, and provokes a diet of 'slimming' foods and excessive calorie watching. Eating disorders are often the presenting symptoms of much deeper needs for self-esteem, self-respect and tolerance and affection of ourselves. These two sections have been put together in this chapter because of the value of considering the way our image of ourselves affects our nutrition.

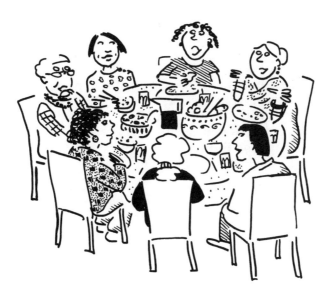

Food and healthy eating

BACKGROUND INFORMATION

- Food is a central issue for women:
  - as providers, they are seen as responsible for the health of the whole family, which brings pressures to bear upon women; and
  - as consumers there are complicated relationships between women and food – the following section on self-image and body image, looks at this in more detail.

- There can be a great deal of confusion about what is good for us. On one hand there are the claims of the 'healthy eating' lobby and on the other, claims by individual manufacturers. These can often seem to have conflicting messages.

- Women whose traditional diet is different from the typical English diet, such as Asian and African-Caribbean women, may have to spend much more buying basics as these are often classed as 'exotic' in supermarkets and so are expensive.

- Low income also brings a different attitude to food from women who can afford to experiment with different styles of cooking or different ingredients. Often women providing food on very low incomes have to choose filling, energy-giving foods which may lack the protein and vitamins available in more expensive foods and be high in fat and sugar. There is little opportunity to experiment with 'new' foods.

- Women as either consumers or providers are one part of the story. The other part is the organisation of the food industry itself, involving issues of food safety, labelling and food production. It is interesting to consider the amount of choice we have in using foods.

PRACTICAL POINTS

- This is a wide-ranging topic, difficult to contain in just one session. The final selection will need to be made by the tutor and the group, depending on the interests of the group and the areas women want to look at in more depth.

- Tutors will need to develop a basic level of information on the current opinions and debates about healthy eating, for example the eight guidelines for a healthier diet (see Information Sheet 5.2 *Healthy eating 1*). The Resources section provides a guide for further reading.

- Avoid the temptation to be judgemental or prescriptive, as this will only make women feel guilty or defensive. These sessions can raise awareness of the issues and facts, and encourage women to look at how changes can be integrated into their lives. Looking at attitudes, and economic and social constraints is as important as discussing what is or is not the perfect healthy diet.

- Present information carefully. Some information, for example about additives, can sound very alarmist. If you present figures or statistics, do this sensitively.

- This is one of the sessions where there is potential for a lot of enjoyable practical activities, for example: bringing in samples of wholefoods, foods with hidden 'unhealthy' ingredients (e.g. added salt, sugar); the group choosing to prepare some healthy snacks; exchanging recipes or compiling a recipe book. Another idea is to hold a family event to encourage other members of the family to come along and taste 'new' food.

INFORMATION SHEET *5.1*

How food affects our health

Today's diseases

Research has shown links between what we eat and many modern diseases. For example:

- heart disease may be linked with too much fat, especially saturated fat;
- tooth decay may be linked with too much sugar;
- high blood-pressure and strokes may be linked with too much salt in certain people;
- bowel cancer, constipation, and diverticulosis (a common bowel problem) may be linked with too little fibre;
- obesity is linked with too many calories. Diabetes, high blood-pressure, strokes, heart disease and cancer are all associated with obesity too.

Of course, what you eat is not the only factor in ill health. Smoking, lack of exercise and drinking too much alcohol also increase the chances of illness and early death.

Tomorrow's health?

The trouble is, the rewards of eating are immediate. It tastes good, it's comforting, it's sociable, it's convenient. The 'punishment' of ill health from a major disease may seem a long way away and not important to you now.

If you need encouragement to change what you eat, think about the benefits you might gain soon. For example, do you suffer from:

- being constipated? ☐
- having piles? ☐
- being overweight? ☐
- boredom with what you eat? ☐
- having high blood-pressure? ☐
- tooth decay? ☐

The more ticks you have, the more you stand to gain from making changes.

Yes, but . . .

▷

© Health Education Authority, 1993

▷ 5.1 cont.

Making changes raises doubts.

- Will I get enough protein?

- What about vitamins and minerals?

- I couldn't live without sugar...

- It'll take the pleasure out of food . . .

If you eat a varied diet with plenty of fruit and vegetables (fresh, frozen or tinned) you will get all the vitamins and minerals you need. And there's useful protein in bread, peas, beans, and nuts.

You don't need to give up anything entirely. There's no point in chomping away miserably on food you don't like. It's a question of finding the new patterns of shopping, cooking and eating that are best for you.

INFORMATION SHEET *5.2*

Healthy eating 1

Enjoying what you eat is important especially if you are changing to a healthier diet. The **eight guidelines** for a healthier diet are:

1 enjoy your food;

2 eat a variety of foods;

3 eat plenty of foods rich in starch and fibre;

4 don't eat too much fat;

5 don't eat sugary foods too often;

6 look after the vitamins and minerals in your food;

7 if you drink, keep within sensible limits; and

8 eat the right amount to be a healthy weight.

No single food contains all the nutrients which we need in order to remain healthy. It is important to eat a mixture of different foods. This can be done by eating a range of foods from the **four main food** groups each day. These groups are:

- starchy foods – bread, chapattis, rice, sweet potatoes;

- dairy produce – cheese, milk, yoghurt;

- meat, poultry and alternatives – fish, eggs, nuts, beans;

- vegetables and fruit e.g. cabbage, leeks, okra, peppers, mangoes, apples.

Starch and fibre

Starchy foods are filling without providing too many calories. They are also a good source of nutrients. So we should try to base our meals around these foods. The wholegrain varieties of starchy foods are a particularly good choice because they are high in fibre.

Fibre is what is sometimes called roughage. It is only found in foods that come from plants. Animal products contain no fibre. Fibre helps to prevent constipation and may help to reduce the amount of cholesterol in the blood.

▷

© Health Education Authority, 1993

▷ 5.2 cont.

Fat

The fat we eat comes mainly from:

- meat and meat products;
- spreading fats (butter and margarine);
- milk and milk products such as cheese;
- cooking fats; and
- biscuits, cakes, puddings and chocolate.

There are two problems with eating too much fat. Fat is loaded with calories so eating too much can lead to becoming overweight. For example, an ounce of butter has almost ten times as many calories as an ounce of boiled potatoes. Eating too much fat, especially saturated fat, can also push up the cholesterol level in the blood. The cholesterol builds up on the inside of the arteries, especially in the heart and can eventually lead to a heart attack (see Information Sheet 5.4 *Fats and heart disease*). One in four of all women in the UK are killed by heart disease.

Overall we eat more fat than the experts recommend, so we could benefit from trying to cut down, especially on the amount of saturated fat we eat. The main sources of saturated fat are dairy products, fatty meat, hard and soft margarine other than that labelled 'high in polyunsaturates', cakes, biscuits, and chocolate.

Sugar

- In Britain we use an average of 88lb (39kg) of refined sugar per person each year – and that does not include glucose sugar or honey. Less than half of this is bought as bags of sugar. The rest is found mostly in sweets, sweet foods and soft drinks.

- Sucrose, dextrose, fructose, glucose, maltose, honey, molasses and brown sugar are all sugars.

- There are good reasons for cutting back on sugar intake. Sugar contains no useful nutrients apart from energy – and we can get all the energy we need from healthier sources. It is unnecessary for health, and is a major factor in dental decay. Currently 30% of adult women have no natural teeth, and 36% are overweight.

Salt

- On average we eat about ½ an ounce (12g) a day. That's two whole tea-spoonfuls.

- Too much salt may lead to high blood-pressure in some people – and high blood-pressure is an important risk factor for heart disease and strokes. Other

▷

▷ 5.2 cont.

things are involved too – fat, smoking, stress, lack of activity. Cutting down on salt alone won't guarantee to reduce the risks. But it would certainly do you no harm.

- You can control the amount of salt you add in cooking and at the table. But much of the salt we eat is added to processed food by the makers. So you might also decide to look for products which are labelled 'low salt' or 'no salt added'.

INFORMATION SHEET *5.3*

Healthy eating 2

What you can do

Tick off the things you do already on this list. Then put an H or E against the rest, according to how hard or easy it would be for you to make each change:

	Hard (H)
Tick	*or Easy (E)*

To eat more starch and fibre

Eat more bread or chapattis

Eat more potatoes

Eat more sweet potatoes, cassava or plantain

Eat more rice

Eat more pasta

Eat more breakfast cereals

To further increase fibre

Eat more fruit and vegetables

Choose wholemeal bread instead of white bread

Use brown rice or wholemeal pasta

Eat more peas, beans or lentils

To cut down on fat:

Choose a low fat spread instead of butter
or margarine, or spread these more thinly

Buy skimmed or semi-skimmed milk

Use plain low fat yoghurt or low fat fromage frais

Buy lower fat cheeses such as cottage cheese
and half fat hard cheeses

Cut down on crisps, chocolate, cakes and biscuits   ▷

▷ 5.3 cont.

| | Tick | *Hard (H) or Easy (E)* |

Buy the leanest cuts of meat you can afford
or trim the fat off meat

Eat chicken or turkey without the skin

Eat more fish

Grill, microwave, casserole or poach rather than frying

Use as little oil as possible for cooking and choose
one that is high in unsaturates such as
sunflower, soya, corn or rapeseed oil

To cut down on sugar

Use less sugar in tea or coffee

Choose fresh fruit sometimes for pudding

Buy fruit tinned in natural juice

Halve the sugar in recipes – it works for most
things except jam, meringues and ice-cream

Cut down on sweets, chocolate and cereal bars

Cut down on cakes, biscuits and sweet pastries

Cut down on jam, marmalade, syrup, treacle and honey

Buy breakfast cereals which are not sugar- or honey-coated

To cut down on salt

Reduce cooking salt

Don't put salt on the table

Use more herbs and spices for flavour

Choose tinned vegetables with a
'no added salt' label

Cut down on salted meats such as bacon, gammon
and salt beef

Cut down on convenience foods with a high salt content

Cut down on salty snacks such as crisps, salted nuts
and other salty nibbles

INFORMATION SHEET *5.4*

Fats and heart disease

Heart disease is the leading cause of death in England, with one in three men and one in four women dying from the disease. These rates are among the highest in the world. Heart disease is caused by a combination of factors. Some of these cannot be altered, such as family history of heart disease. Others which can be influenced are smoking, high blood cholesterol levels and high blood-pressure.

A small amount of fat in the diet is essential to provide certain vitamins and to make foods more pleasant to eat. However, we often eat more fat than is needed. Eating too much fat is linked with a higher risk of heart disease.

There are two types of fat – saturated fats (or saturates) and unsaturated fats (or unsaturates). The unsaturated group includes two types – polyunsaturated fats and monounsaturated fats. The difference between these types of fat is in their chemical make-up. Saturates are found in dairy products and meat as well as in some vegetable oils, in hard and some soft margarines and cooking fats, and in cakes, biscuits, puddings, savoury snacks and chocolate. If hydrogenated vegetable fat/oil is included in an ingredients list this means that the food contains saturates. Unsaturates are found in vegetable oils such as sunflower, corn, soya, rapeseed and olive oils, in soft margarine labelled 'high in polyunsaturates', in nuts and in oily fish such as herring, mackerel, tuna, pilchards, sardines and trout.

All foods with fat in them contain a mixture of saturates and unsaturates, it is just that the balance is different in different foods. Some of the unsaturates are necessary in small quantities for good health. The saturates, however, are best kept to a minimum because these increase the level of cholesterol in the blood which increases the risk of developing heart disease.

Cholesterol found in the body is often called 'blood cholesterol'. Cholesterol is also found in some foods (dietary cholesterol) but this cholesterol does not have a major effect on the overall amount of cholesterol in the blood in most people. The amount of saturates eaten is the main influence on blood cholesterol levels. So try to cut down on the total amount of fat you eat, and when you do eat foods containing fat, choose ones high in unsaturates.

Some fats are easy to spot like cream, butter, margarine and fat on the outside of meat. These are known as visible fats. There are also hidden fats in cakes, chocolate, biscuits, crisps, and pastry. To help cut down on fat choose fish, chicken or turkey without the skin, lean cuts of meat and lower fat dairy products, and choose cooking methods that don't involve adding fat or oil.

© Health Education Authority, 1993

INFORMATION SHEET *5.5*

Labelling, additives and food safety

Labelling

By law most prepackaged foods must give:

- the name of the food;
- a list of ingredients in decreasing order of weight;
- the weight of the food;
- how long it can be kept and how to store it;
- how to cook or prepare it;
- the name and address of the maker, packer or seller of the food; and
- sometimes, the place of origin.

Nutrition labelling

More food labels now give nutritional information and some may make claims that the food has particular benefits. Specific claims like 'low in calories' or 'rich in vitamin C' have to meet legal conditions. Vaguer claims like 'all natural' are meaningless from a health point of view.

Many manufacturers and food stores are using labels or symbols to identify foods which are 'low fat', 'low sugar', or 'high fibre'. These can be useful as a quick guide but may mean something different on each food and there is no legislation to control their use. For example, a low fat spread is lower in fat than butter or margarine but still contains about 40% fat. A low fat yoghurt on the other hand contains less fat than an ordinary yoghurt and contains less than 1% fat.

Cream of
TOMATO
SOUP

INGREDIENTS: Water, Tomato Purée, Sugar, Thickeners (Modified Starch, Starch), Vegetable Oil, Salt, Double Cream, Butter, Citric Acid, Spices.

NUTRITION INFORMATION

Typical Values	per 100g	approx. per ½ can serving
Energy	284 kJ (68 kcal)	605 kJ (145 kcal)
Protein	0.5g	1.1g
Carbohydrate	8.9g	19.0g
(of which sugars	5.5g)	
Fat	3.6g	7.7g
(of which saturates	0.5g)	
Sodium	0.4g	0.9g
Fibre	0.5g	1.1g

Acceptable for gluten free and vegetarian diets.

Low fat black cherry yoghurt
NUTRITION INFORMATION

TYPICAL VALUES	Per 100g	Approx per pot
ENERGY	434 kJ (102 kcal)	650 kJ (155 kcal)
PROTEIN	5.7g	8.6g
CARBOHYDRATE	19.0g	29.0g
(of which sugars	19.0g	29.0g)
FAT	0.9g	1.4g
(of which saturates	0.6g	0.9g)
SODIUM	less than 0.1g	less than 0.1g
FIBRE	TRACE	TRACE
CALCIUM	160mg	240mg (48% RDA)

RDA = RECOMMENDED DAILY AMOUNT

ACCEPTABLE FOR GLUTEN FREE AND VEGETARIAN DIETS

Added Ingredients: Sugar, Black Cherry, Flavouring, Stabilisers (Pectin, Carob Gum)

▷ 5.5 cont.

A standard format for voluntary nutrition labelling is being introduced in the European Community. However, at present it is not compulsory to label nutrients. Where available, use these labels to compare similar foods to choose the lower fat, lower sugar varieties.

Additives

Additives are listed along with the ingredients on most packaged foods. Many additives are now shown by their European Community (EC) number (the E number). All of the additives with E numbers have been tested for safety, and passed for use in the EC. Numbers without an E in front are allowed in the UK, but may not have been passed for use in all EC countries.

A few people suffer from allergic reactions to some additives, whether natural or synthetic. The E numbers are helpful to these people because they can easily see whether the food contains an additive to which they are allergic. However, many more individuals are allergic to ordinary foods such as milk, strawberries, and shellfish.

Additives are sometimes used when there is no real need for them, for example artificial colours, but other additives may have a useful role. For example, preservatives help to prevent spoilage of food so that foods can be stored safely for longer.

It does seem wise to limit additives to essential uses but this is a consumer issue rather than a health issue. Many manufacturers and food chains are cutting down on the additives in their foods, because their customers are unhappy about additive use. By following a healthy, varied diet there is little need to be concerned about additives. It is when people are dependent upon highly processed foods that additives may become more of a concern.

Food safety

As well as choosing foods that help us to remain healthy over many years, we want foods that are safe and will not make us ill from food poisoning. There are controls to prevent food poisoning at all stages from production to sale of foods. The consumer is the last link in the chain. Whatever food you choose to eat:

- take chilled or frozen food home as quickly as possible, preferably in an insulated bag;

- keep your fridge or freezer at the correct temperature (below 5°C for fridges) – buy a fridge thermometer.

▷

▷ 5.5 cont.

- cook food thoroughly;

- do not eat raw eggs or products containing them;

- observe microwave standing times;

- store raw and cooked foods separately;

- check the dates on goods, and use food within the recommended period;

- where possible, do not reheat food – if you do have to reheat food then do not do so more than once;

- keep pets out of the kitchen, and wash your hands after handling them;

- keep your kitchen clean and dry – wash and dry utensils between preparation stages; and

- always wash your hands with hot soapy water before and after preparing food.

Foods that can go off within a few days carry a 'Use by' date. These foods should be eaten, cooked or frozen before that date or thrown away. Foods that keep longer carry a 'Best before' date which indicates when a food is no longer at its best, but should still be safe to eat.

INFORMATION SHEET *5.6*

Culture, religion and food

Many religions prescribe certain eating habits as acceptable, and prohibit others. Individuals will vary widely in how strictly they keep to these laws, which is a matter of personal values.

Hindu dietary restrictions

Many Hindus are vegetarians and do not eat meat, fish, eggs or anything made with them, as it is seen as wrong to take life to sustain your own. Cows are sacred to Hindus and beef is strictly forbidden. Alcohol is prohibited as it reduces self-control.

Some Hindus fast one or two days a week and this usually involves restricting food rather than eating nothing. It is considered physically and spiritually beneficial. Women in particular are likely to follow strict dietary principles as they are considered to be custodians of moral and religious values.

Sikh dietary restrictions

A similar code to that of Hinduism, where beef and alcohol are restricted.

Muslim dietary restrictions

Muslims may not eat pork or pork products. All other meat must be halal (the name of Allah must be said over the animal and its throat quickly cut and blood allowed to drain). Alcohol is not allowed.

Healthy adults must fast during the 30 days of Ramadan. This involves eating and drinking nothing between dawn and sunset. Pregnant, breastfeeding, and men-struating women are exempt from fasting, as are people who are travelling, old or ill. Everyone except old or ill people must make up days missed, fasting as soon as possible after Ramadan. Fasting is highly valued as having spiritual benefits and in understanding the suffering of those who never have enough to eat.

Jewish dietary restrictions

Jews may not eat pork or pork products, shellfish and fish without fins or scales. All other meat must be kosher – the throat of the animal is cut quickly and blood

▷

▷ 5.6 cont.

allowed to drain, then the meat is salted and steeped in water to remove any remaining blood.

For more orthodox Jews, milk and meat must not be used together. Jews fast for 25 hours at the feast of Yom Kippur. In Passover they may not eat food containing yeast.

Seventh-day Adventist dietary restrictions

Seventh-day Adventists may not eat pork or pork products.

Each culture has ideas about what constitutes a balanced diet. These will depend upon what is available in the area, what is known to be beneficial and what tastes good.

Aspects of some diets

	British	N India	Chinese	Caribbean	W African
STAPLES	potatoes bread	rice chapattis	rice noodles	rice yams plantain	yams & cassava (gari) plantain
MAIN PROTEIN	meat fish dairy products	meat fish cereals pulses dairy products	cereals pulses meat fish	fish chicken goat meat pulses	meat stews chicken goat fish
MAIN FATS	butter margarine lard veg oils	ghee veg oils	veg oils lard	veg oils especially coconut oil	veg oils especially palm oil

Most diets rely on a combination of vegetable and animal protein, although Western diets include more animal protein. Less affluent societies rely more upon vegetable protein such as pulses and grains being eaten together to enrich protein intake. Examples are rice and dahl, tacos and beans, peanuts with noodles and beans on toast.

Many Western countries have issued guidelines for healthy eating because of an increase in diet-related diseases. Recommendations involve a shift in diet which

▷

▷ 5.6 cont.

would bring Western diets closer to those of less affluent societies, i.e. less fats, sugar and meat, and more fibre-rich and starchy foods including fruit, vegetables, pulses and grains. Diet-related diseases in less affluent societies are linked to lack of food available rather than to bad diets.

A balanced diet may also include cultural ideas about 'hot' and 'cold' food. This is related to the principle of yin and yang. 'Hot' or yin foods are believed to raise body temperature, excite emotions and increase activity. They include spicy foods and animal based products. 'Cold' or yang foods are believed to cool the body, calm emotions and make a person cheerful and strong. They include bland food, mainly vegetable in origin.

The precise definition will vary from family to family and community to community. However, there is a common belief that too much of one type of food will unbalance the body and the emotions. There may be ideas of what foods to eat at certain times, especially when ill or when a woman is pregnant or breastfeeding.

Source: Adapted from Mares, P, Henley, A, and Baxter, C, *Health Care in Multi-Racial Britain* (1985), NEC/HEC.

*ACTIVITY 5.1

A typical day

Aim
- To raise awareness about how much of our daily routine is affected by food.

Materials
A copy of Worksheet 5.1 *A typical day* for each woman.

Method
1 Women work in pairs and interview each other using the worksheet as a guide.

2 In the large group, feed back responses.

Discussion points
- What is the average time spent on food in the group – in a typical day and a typical week?

- Which aspects of food do women spend most time on – and least time on?

- Which aspects of food do women in the group like best and least?

- How does this kind of profile differ depending on the kind of life a woman leads, e.g. whether she is single, a mother, or an elderly woman living alone.

- It may be useful to link this activity with Activity 5.6 *Family eating habits*.

*ACTIVITY 5.2

Feelings about food

Aim
- To explore the importance of food in women's lives.

Materials
A copy of Worksheet 5.2 *Feelings about food* for each woman; pens and flipchart paper.

Method

1 Ask women to look at the worksheet individually.

2 In small groups, women discuss the statements.

3 Back in the large group, discuss, using the points below as a trigger for further discussion.

Discussion points

Statements 1, 3 and 5 are concerned with women's role as head household cook:

- do women feel the constant pressure to be responsible for food?

- are there pressures (e.g. from children, the media, partners) to prepare certain types of food?

- how do we feel if our food isn't appreciated?

Statements 2, 4, 6 and 8 look at women's own feelings about and needs for food:

- are we concerned to eat well when we feed ourselves?

- why do we feel greedy or guilty if we eat too much?

- some women eat more when feeling low, others lose interest in food. Why do you think this is?

Statement 7 looks at the relationship between food and teenage rebellion:

- did this affect you in any way?

- if you have children, is this a helpful statement for you?

Food seems to be bound up with so many of our emotions – why do you think this is?

ACTIVITY *5.3*

Food choices checklist

Aim

- To explore the factors influencing food choices.

Materials

A copy of Worksheet 5.3 *Food choices checklist* for each woman.

Method

1 Ask women to work through the checklist individually.

2 Discuss their findings.

Discussion points

- Which are the most important factors influencing the group?

- How much influence do a woman's own likes or dislikes have over the food she chooses?

- It may be useful to link this with Activity 5.6 *Family eating habits*.

ACTIVITY *5.4*

Changing what you eat

Aims

- To get women to look at their current eating patterns.

- To encourage changing to a healthier diet.

- To discuss what is a healthy diet.

Materials

Copies of Worksheets 5.4 *What did you eat yesterday?* and 5.5 *Changing what you eat* for each woman. Copies of Information Sheets 5.2 and 5.3 *Healthy eating 1* and *2* for each small group. Pens and flipchart paper.

Method

1 In pairs, women work through Worksheet 5.4 *What did you eat yesterday?*.

2 They share findings in groups of four.

3 In the large group, discuss what differences and similarities there are.

4 Back in small groups, work through Worksheet 5.5 *Changing what you eat*.

5 In the large group, feed back and flipchart obstacles and practical steps, and discuss.

Discussion points

- Do you need to change your diet, and if so, how?

- How easy or difficult would it be to change your own diet? What are the obstacles? How could you make a start?

ACTIVITY 5.5

A healthy food industry?

Aims

- To explore what choices the food industry gives us.
- To find out any connections between consumer activism and what is available in shops.

Materials

Flipchart paper and pens; copies of Worksheet 5.6 *A healthy food industry?* for each woman.

Method

1 In small groups, women go through worksheet.

2 In the large group, flipchart responses from each question. Allow time for discussion, raising some of the issues below.

This activity could be used as the basis for a group project extending over several weeks requiring research outside the group sessions.

Discussion points

- In the late 1980s, 75% of food purchased came from just seven major food store chains in England.
- How far does advertising affect the food we buy?
- Do campaigns change what manufacturers supply?
- The government subsidises the production of sugar while the NHS spends money treating complaints stemming from too much sugar in our diet.
- Choice is only available to those with the money to buy. The link between poverty and poor diet has been established (see the Food Commission report in the Resources section).
- The London Food Commission (1988) stated that 'two thirds of 8 million people below poverty line are women, with British Asian *women* being the worst hit'.

- The London Food Commission (1988) also stated that: 'households on low incomes . . . tend to provide concentrated cheap energy sources containing few other useful nutrients such as proteins, vitamins and minerals . . . and at the same time are eating more potatoes, canned vegetables (in particular baked beans) and white bread. These are relatively cheap filling foods'.

- Are food choices a reality for only specific groups of the population, i.e. middle class people with the ability to buy and time and energy to campaign for more choice, e.g. organic foods?

ACTIVITY 5.6

Family eating habits

Aim

- To explore the family pressures for certain foods.

Materials

Flipchart paper and pens.

Method

1 Brainstorm food products and ways of preparing foods that women feel under pressure to provide and eat.

2 Brainstorm where the pressures come from, and discuss.

Discussion points

- What are the risk factors associated with any of these types of eating habits or ways of preparing foods?

- Where are these pressures coming from – children, partners, wider family, religion, tradition?

- How similar are the group members' experiences?

- How can the situation be improved?

ACTIVITY 5.7

Culture, religion and food

Aims

- To look at approaches to food within different cultural and religious groups.

- To extend knowledge about these differing communities.

Materials

Copies of Information Sheet 5.6 *Culture, religion and food*; flipchart and pens.

Method

1 Before looking at the information sheet, use the headings: Hindu, Sikh, Muslim, Jew, Seventh-day Adventist, and Christian, to brainstorm the known dietary restrictions for each religion.

2 Using the information sheet, find any others new to the group.

3 Discuss, raising some of the issues below.

Discussion points

- This may be a richer group experience if it is used in a multi-cultural group.

- Some religions have more dietary needs than others and some relate to only parts of the year.

- What problems could arise from these specific needs, such as availability, severe restrictions, costs.

- In many cases, traditional ways of preparing food are the healthiest.

- The activity can lead onto looking at wider cultural differences between communities.

- It may be useful to extend this activity over a few weeks so that women can do their own research.

ACTIVITY *5.8*

Seeing is believing

Aims

- To learn more about food labelling and additives.

- To understand more about food safety.

Materials

Food labels brought in by the tutor and/or the group; copies of Information Sheet 5.5 *Labelling, additives and food safety* and Worksheet 5.7 *Seeing is believing* for each woman.

Method

1 Use the labels and the information sheet as basis for small group work with the worksheet.

2 Share information in the large group, and discuss.

Discussion points

- What information is given on labels and what is missed out?

- How do different brands of the same food compare with each other?

- Do any additives have side-effects?

- Do you feel that the manufacturers are on the whole honest and open with information?

- Whose responsibility is food hygiene/safety – the manufacturers, retailers or the person who cooks/prepares the food?

WORKSHEET *5.1*

A typical day

Interview your partner, using the questions below.

1 Can you estimate how much of your time is taken up each day with:

Time
taken

planning meals

shopping

cooking

eating

in other ways related to food

TOTAL _____

_____

2 Can you estimate how much time you would spend on food in a typical week?

3 What are the occasions when you spend more time on food than on a typical day?

WORKSHEET *5.2*

Feelings about food

Discuss each of these statements. Are any of them close to your own views?

1 'My whole life seems to revolve around food. As soon as I've cooked one meal I have to think about the next.'

2 'Now there's just me, I don't bother with a proper meal – it doesn't seem worth the trouble.'

3 'I feel like a proper mother when I make a hot, traditional dinner for the children.'

4 'If I've eaten too much I feel guilty and bad about myself.'

5 'The more effort I put into cooking a meal, the more upset I get if my family don't eat it.'

6 'I enjoy food, but often when I am eating a big meal people will make comments. It seems that women are not supposed to have a healthy appetite.'

7 'My mum used to ply me with food. Not eating it was a way of rejecting her values and establishing my independence.'

8 'I eat more if I'm feeling low.'

WORKSHEET *5.3*

Food choices checklist

When we choose our food, we are influenced by many factors. Some of these are listed below. You may be able to think of others.

See if you can number the factors: 1 = very important
2 = quite important
3 = unimportant

Low price

Quick to prepare

No need for an oven

You've tried it before and it tastes good

It's good for you/them

It's not fattening

It can be bought locally

It looks good

The family likes it

I like it

It is fresh

Others:

WORKSHEET *5.4*

What did you eat yesterday?

Write down everything you can remember that you ate yesterday, including drinks, sugar, snacks and so on.

Breakfast

Mid-morning

Lunch

Mid-afternoon

Evening meal

Supper

Anything else (e.g. snacks, alcohol)

WORKSHEET *5.5*

Changing what you eat

Current nutritional knowledge recommends the following eight guidelines for a healthy diet.

1 Enjoy your food.

2 Eat a variety of different foods.

3 Eat the right amount to be a healthy weight.

4 Eat plenty of foods rich in starch or fibre.

5 Don't eat too much fat.

6 Don't eat sugary foods too often.

7 Look after the vitamins and minerals in your food.

8 If you drink, keep within sensible limits.

(For more information on this and practical suggestions for changing to a healthier diet see Information Sheets 5.2 and 5.3 *Healthy eating 1* and *2*.)

Make a list of any obstacles you may have to changing to a healthier diet.

What practical steps can you make to move towards a healthier diet?

WORKSHEET *5.6*

A healthy food industry?

1 Does the food industry provide us with a range of choices and the information to choose a healthy diet?

2 What is the relationship between the food industry and government policies?

3 How can consumers affect what the food industry offers for sale?

4 How much choice do people really have in what food they can buy?

WORKSHEET *5.7*

Seeing is believing

Using the labels try to answer the following questions.

1 What information are you given?

2 Does it tell you how much of the carbohydrates are sugars? Does this surprise you?

3 Does it separate saturated and unsaturated fats?

4 Does any label try to sell based upon 'low fat' or 'healthy'? Does this claim bear close inspection?

5 Is there anything which puzzles you and which you need to find out about? What is it?

RESOURCES

For contact details of distributors and organisations listed here, see Chapter 11 *General resources*.

Publications

Canon, Geoffrey and Einzig, Hetty, *Dieting Makes You Fat* (1984), Sphere, £1.95.
Revised edition of why dieting often does not work, and when it can, with guides to practical eating.

Department of Health, *While you are Pregnant: Safe Eating and How to Avoid Infection from Food and Animals*, Free booklet. Available from the Welsh Office.

Elliott, Rose, *Your Very Good Health: Recipes for Healthy Eating* (1981), Fontana, £3.99.
Easy recipes with an emphasis on nutrition.

Food Commission, *The Nutrition of Women on Low Incomes* (1991), £3.00. Available from the Food Commission.

Forbes, Alison, *Healthy Eating: Cooking with Vitamins and Minerals* (1990), Penguin, £4.99.
A guide to vitamins and minerals, toxicity and deficiencies, with recipes for each.

Hanssen, Maurice and Marsden, Jill, *New E for Additives* (1986), Thorsons, £4.50.
A comprehensive guide to additives with a commentary as to what they are, their uses and potential effects.

Health Education Authority, *Nutrition in Minority Ethnic Groups: Asians and Afro-Caribbeans in the United Kingdom* (Briefing Paper). Available from the Health Education Authority.

Hunt, Paula, Heritage, Zoe, and Haste, Frances, *Access to Healthy Food: Some Women's Views on How Primary Health Care Workers Could Help* (1991). Available from the Health Education Authority Primary Health Care Unit.
Report of a study asking women for their views on food, healthy eating and access to healthy and affordable food, and what role they felt primary health care workers could play. Contains recommendations to primary health care workers, family health service authorities, district health authorities and the Health Education Authority.

Lacey, Richard, *Unfit for Human Consumption: Food in Crisis – the Consequence of Putting Profit before Safety* (1992), Paladin, £5.99.
New edition of this book which analyses the food industry.

Lobstein, Tim, *Children's Food: the Good, the Bad and the Useless* (1988), Unwin, £3.95.
Excellent Food Commission guide.

NCHR, *Community Health Initiatives and Food: an Information Pack* (1991), National Community Health Resource, £4.00. Available from National Community Health Resource.
Brings together the issues of food and community development in health. The pack contains guidelines for a healthy diet and information to help women work on food in a community-based way. Aimed at a wide range of workers it explains community health initiatives, gives ideas for action, and provides lists of contacts and references.

NCHR, *Food and Health: Community Health Action Issue 22* (Winter 91/92), National Community Health Resource, £2.50 (voluntary groups) £3.50 (statutory bodies). Available from National Community Health Resource.
Articles on new approaches to nutrition education, healthy eating initiatives with women's groups, tackling food poverty, food co-ops, nutrition and child development, plus resources and contacts. Useful for ideas and contacts.

Paterson, Barbara, *The Allergy Connection* (1985), Thorsons, £5.99.
Looks at allergies and their links with food and chemicals. Includes self-help suggestions.

Taylor, Joan and Taylor, Derek (eds), *Parents for Safe Food: Safe Food Handbook*, London Food Commission/Geoffrey Cannon, Ebury Press, £6.99.
Aimed at concerned parents and the green consumer. Provides a wealth of information about the food we eat and its safety.

Webb, Tony and Lang, Tim, *Food Irradiation: the Myth and the Reality* (1990), Thorsons, £5.99.
A Food Commission guide to the issues surrounding irradiation.

Videos

Apni Sehth: Our Health, (1991) (Punjabi), 12 minutes, £40 (plus VAT; including 40 leaflets in English, Urdu and Punjabi). Available from Derbyshire FHSA.
Addresses the issue of obesity, aimed at the Punjabi community, and is sensitive to Punjabi cultural attitudes and dietary practices.

Diets for Asian Diabetics (1990) (in English, Hindu, Gujarati), Leicestershire Health Authority, Health Education Video Unit.
Information for diabetics on foods which are culturally acceptable, and guidelines on ways of cooking and modifying food to suit diabetics.

Academy Television, *Food: Fad or Fact* (undated), 6 programmes of 26 minutes.
Titles: *A Little of what you Fancy does you Good; Are Fats Harmful?; The Battle of the Fats; Salt; Sugar; Fibre.* Available from Academy Television.
Attempts to sort out fact from fiction in the Western diet.

Thames TV, *Good Enough to Eat? (Additives)*, (1985). 52 minutes. Available from Concord Film.
Looks at the additives put in food and what is being done to stop the trend.

A Taste of Health (1986) (English and Hindi), DHSS Asian Mother and Baby Campaign. Available from the Department of Health, London.
Outlines basic nutrition messages for all the family. Through Asian families going shopping, it illustrates the importance of a low sugar, salt and fat, and high fibre diet with traditional Asian foods and English junk foods as examples.

Organisations

Family Health and Nutrition Information Group
Publishes newsletter. Provides information; some emphasis on candidiasis.

The Food Commission
National organisation for both the public and professionals, independent of government and industry, which aims to provide information on the food we eat. Magazine: *The Food Magazine*, quarterly, covers a wide range of issues.

National Society for Research into Allergy
Offers diet sheets and advice for allergy sufferers. Membership scheme. Send s.a.e.

Parents for Safe Food
Provide information. For free information pack, send 60 pence in stamps.

Vegetarian Society
Produces a magazine, *The Vegetarian*. Membership scheme. Send large s.a.e. for information about vegetarian diet.

Self-image and body image

BACKGROUND INFORMATION

- Both self-image and body image are closely related to questions of emotional and mental health.

- Women are often defined in terms of their relationships to other

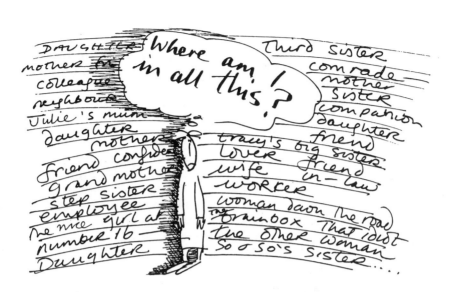

people . . . as someone's wife, daughter, or mother for example. This happens whether or not they have paid employment. Acceptable roles for women seem to be connected with providing for other's needs first and foremost.

- It can be difficult for a woman to move beyond this to develop an alternative image for herself based upon valuing her skills and strengths. This may seem indulgent and a waste of time.

- Many skills traditionally associated with women are undervalued and taken for granted. Women's work is often low or unpaid. Women still say of themselves – 'I'm just a housewife'. It's not difficult to see why women undervalue themselves.

- The images that we see in the media are usually of white women – often slim and beautifully dressed. There are very few images of Black women within mainstream media and this can isolate and lower esteem for Black women. It also serves to reinforce racist stereotypes as the few Black women who are portrayed usually conform to specific types such as exotic or sexual, or happy-go-lucky.

- Self-image is very closely linked to body image as women are often judged or valued by their appearance. As a result women judge their own appearance harshly.

- In many cultures women are encouraged to believe that there is an ideal body shape. The media usually present women as conforming to these ideals and these are used to advertise and to sell products.

- Many women feel that some part of their body does not look right. Even when rationally we can dismiss pressures to look a certain way, there can still be feelings associated with our body image. These feelings may be connected to size or age or to an ideal image of what is beautiful. There are few positive images of older women and Black women. Many Black women have spent pounds upon skin bleaching agents and creams and have had their hair straightened to conform to the 'ideal' image of long silky hair. These have had detrimental effects upon women's skin and hair.

● This section contains information sheets about the eating disorders anorexia and bulimia. Low self-esteem, visual appearance and sense of body image are closely linked to them both. Eating disorders stem from the individual's need to use food in a certain way as a response to how they feel about themselves. It is important to recognise that such disorders will not respond to simple information and activities about healthy eating, and individuals may need further help.

PRACTICAL POINTS

● This is a potentially emotive section as women have strong feelings about themselves and body image. These are usually negative feelings.

● Emphasise that if women are drawing, then the finished product is not going to be judged for artistic talent.

● If women feel they have a tendency to an eating disorder it would be useful to put them in touch with sources of further help, for example a local eating disorder group (see the Resources section for organisations to contact).

INFORMATION SHEET *5.7*

Eating disorders

Eating disorders are many and varied and are related to how a woman feels about herself. Living in a society which prescribes strict guidelines about what is attractive and healthy in terms of size, leads many women to feel an intense pressure to diet and 'lose weight'.

Women who have very low self-esteem, and possibly histories of sexual abuse or pressure to achieve academically, may feel they are overweight, even though others do not see them as such. This can lead to extreme forms of eating disorders such as anorexia nervosa or bulimia. Women with such problems seem to be acting out the classic feminine stereotype:

- extreme self-denial;
- repression of anger and conflict;
- desire to remain childlike in body shape; and
- conformity to the idea of a thin woman.

Anorexia nervosa takes the form of severe and deliberate self-starvation and can lead to death. Women who have anorexia see their body as bigger than it actually is.

Bulimia involves bingeing on many different types of food and then purging through either vomiting or taking laxatives. Women who have bulimia risk their health by:

- injury to intestines and oesophagus;
- severe tooth decay from regurgitated stomach acids;
- upsetting their electrolyte balance.

It can endanger long term health or can be immediately fatal.

In the past, remedial treatment for eating disorders has included wiring together of jaws, and forcing anorexic women to stay in bed until they have gained weight through forced eating. Currently, it is thought that building up self-esteem, developing a sense of control over one's life and receiving support from others are the key factors for recovery.

Women who do not fit into current ideas about what is a desirable size and shape may believe that they are overweight and use 'dieting' as a tool to remove the

▷

© Health Education Authority, 1993

▷ 5.7 cont.

'extra pounds'. Women who feel that they are fat come under considerable discrimination because of their size and the resulting stress can lead to reduced self-esteem, a sense of shame and feelings of guilt. A vicious circle comes into effect:

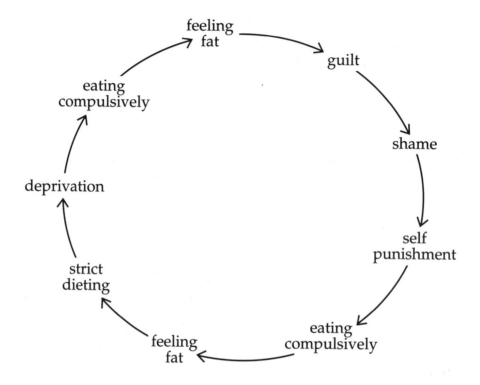

Slimming diets often recommend a daily intake of 700–1000 calories. With low levels of calorie intake you can easily miss out on necessary nutrients. Physical effects include the following:

- apathy;
- strain on kidneys;
- headaches;
- lethargy;
- dizziness, feeling high or light headed;
- irritability due to unbalanced blood sugar;
- depression;

▷

▷ 5.7 cont.

- using quick energy food like sugary snacks;

- losing lean body tissue instead of fat; and

- permanent tissue damage.

When dieting stops, weight may be regained, which may lead on to a series of diets. Hunger pains from strict dieting can lead to bingeing on food and this may lead on to bulimia.

Compulsive eating is a common issue for women: a woman may eat to relieve feelings caused by loneliness, boredom, isolation, frustration and dissatisfaction. Women may use food as a comfort for guilt or depression. A vicious circle forms: feeling guilty; eating for comfort; feeling fat; and feeling guilty.

Positive information about healthy eating is useful for women, but for those with severe eating disorders the focus needs to be on dealing with the source of negative feelings about themselves and learning to trust, respect, accept and love themselves.

It bears repeating time and time again that we cannot make any changes without loving and caring for ourselves. If we feel bad about our bodies, we neglect them. Such neglect underpins our own negative feelings about ourselves but if we begin to break this down and take care of our bodies, then the body responds and we feel better – not thinner or larger, but fitter, more supple, more accepted, more loved, and good enough to be loved. The emphasis has shifted: rather than trying to reduce our size, we can take very positive steps to feel good about our own bodies, whatever their size.[1]

[1] Greaves, M, *Big and Beautiful* (1990), Grafton Books.

INFORMATION SHEET *5.8*

Height and weight chart

Are you the right weight for your height? Use the chart below to find out. Children, expectant and nursing mothers and those with health problems or who are heavily overweight may have special needs.

Take a straight line across from your height (without shoes) and a line up from your weight (without clothes). Put a mark where the two lines meet.

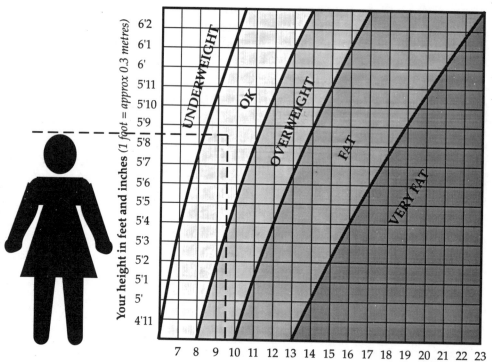

▷ 5.8 cont.

Underweight

Maybe you need to eat a bit more. But go for well-balanced nutritious foods and don't just fill up on fatty and sugary foods. If you are very underweight, see your doctor about it.

OK

Your weight is in the desirable range for health. You're eating the right quantity of food but you need to be sure that you're getting a healthy balance in your diet.

Overweight

Your health could suffer. You should try to lose weight.

Fat

It is really important to lose weight.

Very fat

Being this overweight is very serious. You urgently need to lose weight. Talk to your doctor or practice nurse. You may be referred to a dietician.

If you're trying to lose weight

- Be realistic – a weight loss of 1–2lb (½–1kg) per week is ideal and easier to maintain.

- Don't weigh yourself too often – once every two weeks is enough.

- Don't be discouraged if your weight loss slows down – everyone is different.

- Ask your family and friends for encouragement.

- Join a slimming group if you need extra support.

- Don't panic and resort to periods of starvation or crash diets or expensive slimming foods. You'll be more successful in controlling your weight if you change your long-term eating habits.

ACTIVITY *5.9*

Images of women in the media 1

Aims

- To explore the way images of women are represented in the media.

- To consider how this affects our images of ourselves and other women.

Materials

Large sheets of paper, scissors, pens, glue or sellotape. Magazines or newspapers. (Preparation: ask women to bring some to the group.)

Method

1 Divide into groups of 4 or 5, each taking some magazines and newspapers, glue, scissors etc. Each group makes a collage of images and words which represents the way they feel women are portrayed in the media, choosing and discussing what they want to use and using headlines, pictures, etc. grouped in any way they wish.

2 If the group members wish, they can then go on to do another collage of images of men.

3 Each group should then describe its collage to the other groups.

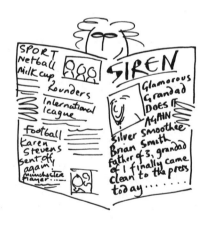

Discussion points

- What are the dominant images that come across?

- What kind of women make media headlines?

- Are there any images of women you found which surprised you?

- How many older women or Black women do you see?

- Are these generally positive or negative?

- Do these images affect us? If so, how?

ACTIVITY *5.10*

Images of women in the media 2

Aims

- To look critically at the images of women in the media.

- To discuss which are the predominant images portrayed.

- To consider the implications of this.

Materials

A copy of Worksheet 5.8 *Images of women in the media* for each woman; blutack, flipchart paper, pens.

Method

1 Divide into pairs and work through the worksheet.

2 All pairs pool their findings onto a large set of lists stuck on the wall.

3 Discuss findings in the large group.

Discussion points

- Are there general agreements and similarities between the lists? Do any aspects of them surprise you?

- Do any categories of women appear on more than one column? What do you think this might say about them?

- Which column(s) contain the largest number of images or references?

- Does this exercise have anything to do with us? How do we feel if we fit into the 'positive' column? Or if we fit into one of the other two columns?

- There can also be more detailed discussion about particular categories e.g. working women, Black women.

*ACTIVITY *5.11*

Positive and negative me

Aim

- To encourage women to think about how they see themselves, as opposed to how others see them.

Materials

Flipchart paper, pens, blutack.

Method

1 In small groups, each woman writes on a large flipchart sheet two positive and one negative word to describe herself.

2 Put sheets on the wall and look at them all.

3 In the large group, go round and each woman thinks of one aspect of her body she either appreciates or likes and shares this with the group.

4 Discuss.

Discussion points

- Which was the easiest to think of – positive or negative aspects?
- How did it feel to say a positive aspect out loud to the group?
- Is it easier in a small group or a larger group? Why?
- Which was easiest to focus upon – your body or your whole self?
- Were you surprised at what you came up with? Why?

*ACTIVITY *5.12*

Draw your body image

Aims

- To encourage women to think about how they see themselves.
- To explore the links between self-image and body image.

Materials

Paper, pens, crayons.

Method

1 Ask each woman to have a go at drawing herself – any way she wants to.

2 When this has been done, put the pictures together in a pile, and see if the group can guess who is who.

Discussion points

- Can you all recognise each other's drawings?

- What do you think your drawing says about you?

- Do other people in the group agree with you?

- Are there common points or anxieties from different women in the group?

ACTIVITY *5.13*

Our old photos

Aim

- To explore how images of ourselves may change over time.

Materials

Old and recent photographs of group members.

Preparation

Ask the group to look for any old photographs of themselves, either as girls or as younger women, and bring these in. You could also ask them to bring their favourite recent photo of themselves.

Method

Put the photographs together in a pile, and see if the group can guess who is who.

Discussion points

- Body image – how do we feel we have changed over the years?

- Clothes/fashion – how has this affected our image of ourselves over the years?

- Ageing – how do we feel about seeing our younger selves in the photos? What have we lost and what have we gained, as the years have gone by?

Note to tutor

If there is one woman in the group who is different from the majority, for example in a wheelchair, or a Black woman in a predominantly white group, *this activity can serve to marginalise them and may not be appropriate.*

ACTIVITY *5.14*

Food and body image

Aim

- To explore the relationship between food and body image.

Materials

A copy of Worksheet 5.9 *Food and body image* for each woman; pens.

Method

1 Individually, each member of the group completes the worksheet.

2 As a whole group, look at each question in turn, and see what the opinions within the group are. Use the group's responses to each statement as a basis for the discussion.

Discussion points

It may be interesting to reflect upon statements 4, 5 and 6 – how many women in the group do, for example, feel very comfortable about their body? Also question 12 – why are feelings of success and failure so closely bound up with dieting and slimming?

ACTIVITY *5.15*

Sizing up clothes

Aim

To examine the pressures on women to look and dress fashionably.

Materials

A copy of Worksheet 5.10 *Sizing up clothes* for each woman; flipchart paper and pens.

Method

1 In small groups ask women to go through the worksheet.

2 In a large group compare responses and flipchart if needed.

3 Discuss.

Discussion points

- There seem to be many examples of women who suffer to be beautiful – why do women do this?

- What are the advantages and disadvantages in doing this?

- Are there equivalent pressures for men?

*ACTIVITY *5.16*

Body reflections

Aims

- To explore feelings and attitudes about our bodies.

- To increase confidence in body image.

- To look at factors which increase social acceptance.

Materials

A large mirror; flipchart paper and pens.

Method

1 Ask each woman to stand before the mirror and state one thing she appreciates or likes about her body.

2 In small groups, discuss the prompt questions written up on the flipchart.

3 In the large group, report back and flipchart responses.

Discussion points

- How many women found it hard to look in the mirror and find something positive to say?

- How important are make-up, clothes, and jewellery to women's self-image?

- Would this alter with different groups of women from different cultures?

- How much care do women take of their appearance and their bodies?

Prompt questions

- How did you feel looking at your reflection?

- Was it hard or easy to make a positive statement about your body?

- Why should this be so?

*ACTIVITY *5.17*

Fat and thin

Aim

- To explore images of fat and thin women.

Materials

A copy of Worksheet 5.11 *Fat and thin* for each woman; pens, flipchart paper, Information Sheet 5.8 *Height and weight chart*.

Method

1 In small groups read the worksheet and make two lists of words associated with fat and thin women.

2 In the large group, compare lists and transfer all the words onto a flipchart.

Discussion points

- What kinds of images are conveyed by the word associations, for example, in terms of looks, personality and health?

- How much truth do you think there is in these images?

- What other factors affect the way we see fat and thin women?

- Do these kinds of images affect the way you see yourself?

- What pressures are there on women to be slim in our society?

- Refer to the information sheet for women to assess their own weight.

- How do the weight limits on the chart compare with what is socially acceptable?

WORKSHEET *5.8*

Images of women in the media

There are many images of women portrayed in the media – in advertisements, television programmes, newspapers, magazines and films. Are these images we can identify with? Do they present positive or negative statements?

Below is a list of some different kinds of women:

Slim women	Lesbians
Old women	Fat women
Black women	Rich women
Mothers	Poor women
Glamorous women	Working women
Women with a disability	Single parents
	Others

Working in pairs, take each of the above examples, and put them into one (or more) of the columns below to show how these women are portrayed in the media.

Positive images   Negative images   Few or no images

WORKSHEET *5.9*

Food and body image

Do you agree or disagree with the following statements?

1 People don't pay much attention to fat women.

2 If a woman is fat she only has herself to blame.

3 There isn't the same pressure on men to be slim.

4 I'd like to put on weight.

5 I'd like to lose weight.

6 I feel very comfortable about my body.

7 Thin people are healthier than fat people.

8 Thin people are more successful than fat people.

9 I want to be slim to be more attractive.

10 I feel less confident when I feel overweight.

11 I think more about food and eating when I'm dieting than when I'm not dieting.

12 I feel a failure and weak willed when I lose interest in a diet.

© Health Education Authority, 1993

WORKSHEET *5.10*

Sizing up clothes

In Victorian times women were supposed to look frail, with petite waists, so they wore corsets.

> A fashionable woman's corset exerted, on the average, 21lb (9kg) of pressure on her internal organs, and extremes of up to 88lb (39kg) were measured. Add to this the fact that a well dressed woman wore an average of 37lb (16kg) of street clothing in winter, of which 19lb (8kg) were suspended from her tortured waist. Some of the short term results of tight lacing were shortness of breath, constipation, weakness and a tendency to violent indigestion. Among the long term effects were bent or fractured ribs, displacement of the liver and uterine prolapse. In some cases the uterus would be gradually forced, by the pressure of the corset, out of the vagina.[1]

Nowadays women often give the following reasons for wearing tight constricting clothes:

- it's sexy;
- it's fashionable;
- I look better when I look thin;
- blokes like thinner girls;
- it will encourage me to diet; and
- all the others do it as well.

- Have things changed at all since Victorian times?

- Do any of the statements above ring true for you?

- If any of the statements above *were* relevant to you and you feel you have changed in your attitudes, why do you think you changed?

- Can you think of other examples from other cultures or periods of time when women suffered to be 'beautiful'?

[1] From Ehrenreich, B, and English, D, *For Her Own Good* (1979), Pluto Press.

WORKSHEET *5.11*

Fat and thin

In Western society, there are many pressures on women to be slim. It may help us to remember that it was once fashionable for women to be big, rounded and buxom, and that large women are still considered the most attractive in some societies.

The late 1960s was the era of fashion models like Twiggy, who at 6½ stone (40kg) was the first in a line of skinny, leggy models. Girls' and women's magazines are full of these images, although the popular press also present images of sexy, buxom women – we are, it seems, expected to be both skinny and buxom!

The slimming industry continues to grow and make profits – slimming is now another commodity we are encouraged to spend money on, and there always seems to be another miracle slimming diet to try. Yet research shows that the majority of those who diet will eventually put weight back on.

Other studies have shown that about half the UK's female population takes a size 16 and over – does this surprise you?

And now health and fitness has become another profit-making industry – we are encouraged to buy jogging outfits, aerobics sessions and sign up for the new local health club. On a positive note, this now emphasises *health*, not simply losing weight to look more attractive. Yet it may also provide another pressure for women.

Who are women doing this for? For ourselves – or for others?

What words come to mind when you think of thin women and fat women? Put down as many as you can.

THIN WOMEN   FAT WOMEN

RESOURCES

For contact details of distributors and organisations listed here, see Chapter 11 *General resources*.

Publications

Bovey, Shelley, *Being Fat is Not a Sin* (1989), Pandora, £5.99.
Easy-to-read book about the diet industry, surgery, the tyranny of fashion. Looks at 'the fat personality'.

Browne, Susan, Conners, Debra and Stern, Nanci, *With the Power of Each Breath: a Disabled Women's Anthology* (1985), Cleis, £8.95.
Women with disabilities talk about their lives, self-image, struggles, relationships and other topics. American.

Buckroyd, Julia, *Eating Your Heart Out: the Emotional Meaning of Eating Disorders* (1989), Optima, £5.99.
Looks at the issues from both traditional and feminist perspectives.

Centre Prise Trust, *Breaking the Silence* (1984), £2.45.
Experience of women with a range of backgrounds giving insight into the lives of Asian women in Britain.

Chapkis, W, *Beauty Secrets: Women and the Politics of Appearance* (1988), Women's Press, £5.95
Interviews with different women about how they see themselves. This is then analysed in terms of the way such visual statements are statements about power within a divided society. Wonderful photographs.

Chernin, Kim, *Womansize: the Tyranny of Slenderness* (1983), Women's Press, £5.95.
A theoretical study of woman's image and society.

Dally, Peter and Gomez, Joan, *Anorexia and Obesity: a Sense of Proportion* (1990), Faber, £4.99.
Advice and information on dealing with the difference between these issues.

Dyson, Sue, *A Weight Off Your Mind: How to Stop Worrying About Your Body Size* (1991), Sheldon, £4.99.
A look at the success of various diet plans, attitudes of fitness, self and media image and how to build up a positive image.

Greaves, M, *Big and Beautiful* (1990), Grafton Books, £6.99.
Challenges the view that only slim women are attractive, successful and healthy. Practical advice to ward off others' prejudices and to enable large women to develop positive self-image.

Hutchinson, Marcia Germaine, *Transforming Body Image: Learning to Love the Body You Have* (1985), Crossing Press, £6.95.
A guide to developing an improved sense of self.

Lyons, Pat and Burgard, Debby, *Great Shape: the First Fitness Guide for Large Women* (1990), Bull, £10.95.
Puts emphasis on fun. Includes a range of fitness and esteem boosting activities and a guide to looking your best. Includes resources in Britain. American.

Monro, Maroushka, *Talking About Anorexia* (1992), Sheldon, £3.99.
Introduction to the subject with personal stories and how to cope with stress without starving. Deals with sexual abuse, relationships, breaking up, and more.

Morris, Jenny, *Pride Against Prejudice: Transforming Attitudes to Disability* (1991), Women's Press, £6.95.
Confronts the nature of prejudice against disabled people.

Orbach, Susie, *Fat is a Feminist Issue I* (1988), Arrow, £3.50.
Second revised edition of a book that looks at women's relationships to food, particularly as related to body image, compulsive eating and slimming.

Orbach, Susie, *Fat is a Feminist Issue II* (1984), Arrow, £3.50.
Self-help for compulsive eaters.

Roth, Geneen, *Feeding the Hungry Heart: the Experience of Compulsive Eating* (1983), Signet, £4.99.
Writings by women and how they dealt with compulsive eating.

Singh, Jasbindar and Rosier, Pat, *Nobody's Perfect: Dealing with Food Problems* (1989), Attic, £4.99.
Guide with activities for individuals and groups.

Wolf, Naomi, *The Beauty Myth* (1990), Vintage, £6.99.
An analysis of work, culture, religion, sex, hunger and violence in light of the author's analysis of beauty, women and society.

Videos

Brief lives: Catherine and the Story behind Catherine (1987), Academy Television, 91 minutes.
The story of Catherine Dunbar and her fight against anorexia nervosa.

Looking in the Fridge for Feelings, Concord. 30 minutes.
Discusses dieting, compulsive eating therapy, and the emotional reasons for overeating.

The Waistland (1985), Concord. Two programmes of 23 minutes. Titles: *Eating Disorders; Why Diets Don't Work*.

Organisations

Eating Disorders Association

Support and information for sufferers of anorexia and bulimia and their families. National network of self-help groups with membership scheme.

Women's Therapy Centre

Workshops and therapy on a range of topics, including eating disorders.

6 Female cycles

INTRODUCTION

This chapter consists of three sections: *Knowing our bodies, The menstrual cycle,* and *The menopause.*

These three sections have been put together because they focus on the part of a woman's body which is about reproduction. Very often, women's health is taken to be only about reproductive health, covering such topics as pregnancy, periods and menopause. In fact women's health is much wider and concerns the whole woman, including physical and social environments and relationships.

The working of the female body involves complex biological and hormonal interactions, and so discussion of reproductive health may be very medicalised. Health professionals often use Latin names to describe parts of the body. This can make women feel unknowledgeable, and they may be reluctant to admit not understanding what has been said. This chapter attempts to present information in an accessible way.

There are many different taboos surrounding women's reproductive cycles and these vary from culture to culture. Women can learn from each other across different ages and cultures to expand knowledge of how our bodies work. Having such knowledge enables us to have more control in decisions that affect our health.

Knowing our bodies

BACKGROUND INFORMATION

- This section is about the parts of a woman's body which include sexual organs and reproductive organs (the pelvic area). It aims to help women understand how this part of their body works and to discover what is normal for themselves.

- Many women do not normally examine their own genitals. There are taboos within different cultures that restrict exploration of this part of women's bodies. Women may feel uncomfortable and embarrassed about it.

- The pelvic area is associated with birth, periods, discharges, and internal examinations which can be embarrassing. It is commonly associated with infections such as cystitis and thrush which may be painful, yet is also associated with intense pleasurable sexual feeling.

- It is empowering for women to know about their genital and reproductive organs. Finding out just what is normal for themselves may enable them to use self-help measures, and improve their decision making.

PRACTICAL POINTS

- As a tutor consider what your own concerns are about your own pelvic area, and be aware of what you are prepared to discuss and what you would want to avoid in discussion and disclosure.

- Be aware that this is a sensitive intimate topic for many women, which they may never have discussed with others.

- Be prepared for women to learn/participate in their own way. Some groups of women may prefer to watch a video and have a discussion rather than exchange personal information.

- Use both Latin and common names for parts of the body and for medical procedures where possible, to demystify terminology.

- Focus upon gaps in understanding.

- Use resources such as books, leaflets and videos with the group in order for them to find out information themselves, and provide leaflets to take home.

- This topic may bring up negative experiences which women have had with the medical profession.

- End on a positive note, focusing on what women can do for themselves to promote their own health, such as pelvic floor exercises (see Information Sheet 6.3).

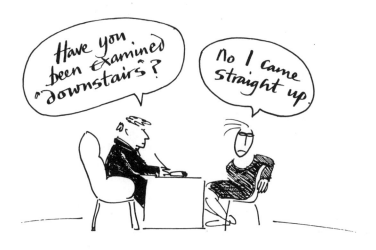

INFORMATION SHEET *6.1*

Understanding reproductive anatomy

Ovaries

Thousands of egg cells are spread in the ovaries. In response to a chemical message from the brain (from the pituitary gland at the base of the skull) ovaries produce the female hormones, oestrogen and progesterone, responsible for the menstrual cycle. Females are born with their supply of eggs. Males produce sperm as they go along.

The ovaries are greyish white, almond shaped, about two inches (5 cm) long and less than an inch (2 cm) thick. The surface is covered by a white membrane – an egg breaks through and is caught by the fimbria which draws the egg into the fallopian tube.

A woman needs only a portion of the ovary to be there for her still to be fertile and produce hormones.

Fallopian tubes

The fallopian tubes are about five inches (12 cm) long and very narrow. They are the place where egg and sperm meet, and move in waves to ensure the fertilised egg moves down to the uterus.

Tubes can become blocked or scarred from pelvic infections. If tubes are 'tied' (i.e. if a woman is sterilised) or damaged then the sperm cannot swim up and the egg cannot move down, but hormonal production remains normal, and periods will still happen.

Uterus or womb

The womb is pear-shaped, about the size of a clenched fist, made of three strong layers of muscle woven together, supported by strong supple ligaments. In the non-pregnant state, the uterine cavity would hold a teaspoon of water but in nine months it can accommodate a fully grown foetus.

Normally the uterus rests on top of the bladder, at a right-angle to the vagina. When the bladder is full the uterus is pushed back and when it is empty the uterus drops forward. One in five women have a retroverted uterus which tilts backwards but can still function normally. If the uterus is removed (hysterectomy), other organs, such as the bowel, move in to take its place.

▷

▷ 6.1 cont.

The uterus is the most muscular organ in the body apart from the heart. During labour the whole uterus contracts to push the baby out. The inner lining is called the endometrium. It is full of blood vessels and thickens to receive a fertilised egg and is shed during menstruation if conception doesn't occur.

Cervix

The cervix has a firm, smooth and rubbery surface like the tip of the nose. The small dimple at the centre is the os. This is the opening of the cervical canal which leads to the womb. The opening may be as small as the head of a match; however, it dilates (opens) to let the baby out. (That is what, for example, 4 inches (10cm) dilation refers to during labour.)

Sperm swim up through the os. It is impossible for a finger, tampon or penis to go through. A cervical smear is taken from the inside of the cervix.

The opening (os) varies according to the time of the month and the number of children a woman has had. The os is more open at menstruation; and in women who have had several children it can be a small slit rather than a pinhole opening.

Vagina

The vagina is a soft, elastic, wet, muscular tube, about four inches long and one inch in diameter, but it expands during sexual arousal and for birth. Secretions are produced which provide lubrication and help to keep the vagina clean and acid. The opening of the vagina is sensitive with nerve endings.

Hymen

The hymen is a thin strip of membrane which lies across the lower part of the vaginal opening in a virgin (although some women have a stretched hymen even when they are no longer virgins). The hymen can also be stretched by fingers or tampons. The absence of a hymen is also possible without having experienced intercourse.

Vulva

The vulva is the area on the outside of the vagina. There are two flaps of skin, the outer one covered with pubic hair. The vulva varies in size and colour from woman to woman.

▷

▷ 6.1 cont.

Perineum

This is the area of skin which links the vulva and anus, often cut at childbirth to avoid tearing during the delivery of the baby. Afterwards, it is stitched back together.

Clitoris

The inner lips of the vulva join to form the hood of the clitoris. The hood covers a highly sensitive little bulb, which fills with blood and becomes erect when aroused. It is the primary source of the female orgasm.

Urethra

The tubal passage which carries urine from the bladder.

Bladder and rectum

The floor of the bladder lies against the roof of the vagina and the floor of the vagina lies against the roof of the rectum. The tissues separating the bladder and vagina are only a fraction of an inch thick, so pressure on the floor of the vagina puts pressure on the bladder – sometimes experienced during intercourse or when inserting tampons.

Pelvic floor

See Information Sheet 6.3, *Pelvic floor exercises*.

INFORMATION SHEET *6.2*

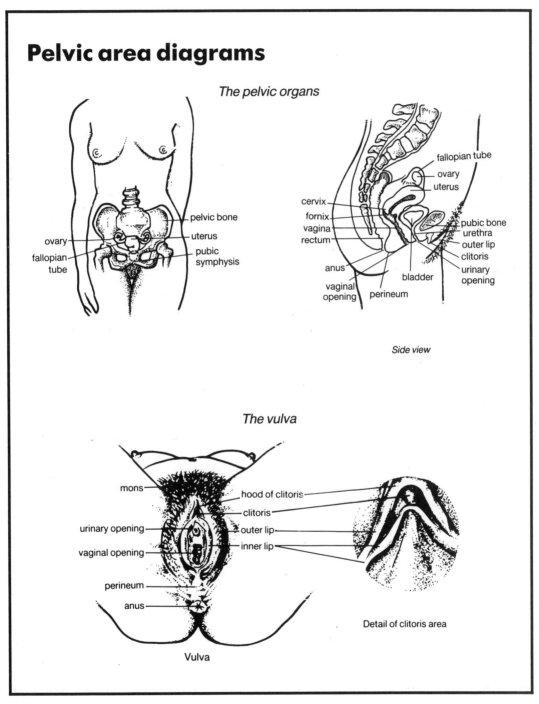

Pelvic area diagrams

The pelvic organs

ovary

fallopian tube

pelvic bone

uterus

pubic symphysis

fallopian tube

ovary

uterus

cervix

fornix

vagina

rectum

pubic bone

urethra

outer lip

clitoris

urinary opening

anus

vaginal opening

perineum

bladder

Side view

The vulva

mons

urinary opening

vaginal opening

perineum

anus

hood of clitoris

clitoris

outer lip

inner lip

Vulva

Detail of clitoris area

INFORMATION SHEET *6.3*

Pelvic floor exercises

What is the pelvic floor?

The pelvic floor consists of layers of muscle stretching like a hammock from the pubic bone (in the front) to the end of the backbone (see below). These muscles hold the bladder, uterus and bowel in place.

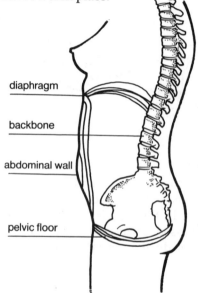

diaphragm

backbone

abdominal wall

pelvic floor

Boundaries of the pelvic cavity

The muscle sheet has three openings for the urethra, the vagina, and the anus. Muscle fibres circle around these openings forming sphincters which act like valves, e.g. the urinary sphincter stops and starts the flow of urine. The muscles form a figure of eight around these three openings.

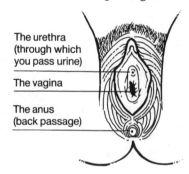

The urethra
(through which
you pass urine)

The vagina

The anus
(back passage)

▷

▷ 6.3 cont.

How does the pelvic floor work?

Ideally the muscle floor is a firm supportive hammock forming a straight line from the pubic bone to the end of the backbone (see below). The contraction of the pelvic floor is a combination of several movements of different muscles. The muscles at the side of the pelvic floor move up and in, causing a squeezing and lifting effect.

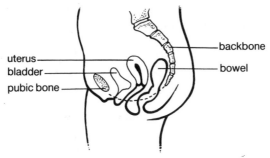

uterus
bladder
pubic bone

backbone
bowel

Good pelvic floor support with organs in place

The muscles are always slightly tense and the sphincters are normally closed. When you pass urine or faeces (bowel movement), the muscle floor relaxes and the sphincter opens. Afterwards, the muscles contract again and the sphincter closes. These muscles can be tensed or relaxed at will, for example when gripping a partner's fingers or penis during sexual excitement, or to relax muscles for a vaginal examination.

Why do pelvic floor exercises?

A healthy active pelvic floor has a normal firmness which responds to stretch and movement. Weakness or injury, due to lack of exercise, childbirth or the ageing process causes the pelvic floor to sag.

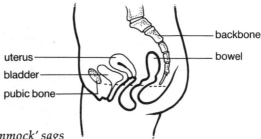

uterus
bladder
pubic bone

backbone
bowel

Inadequate support, and the 'hammock' sags

▷

▷ 6.3 cont.

This may result in one or more of the following conditions: loose vaginal walls, prolapse of the uterus, constipation, incomplete emptying of the bladder, leaking of urine under pressure (e.g. when coughing, sneezing or laughing) and other problems.

Three benefits of pelvic floor exercises

1 Your sex life may improve:

- increased awareness of these muscles may increase the pleasure you feel; and

- the vagina becomes more snug as muscles improve in strength and thickness.

2 It helps your body to cope with the physical demand of a pregnancy:

- firmer support for the uterus and other organs during pregnancy;

- greater relaxation in childbirth, because of increased suppleness and muscle control;

- healthy exercised muscles lead to quicker healing after birth;

- if these exercises are not done the muscles remain stretched and become further weakened as you resume activities involving lifting and straining.

3 It may improve urinary control in women suffering from stress incontinence. Stress incontinence is the leaking of urine when the pressure on the pelvic floor is suddenly increased (e.g. by coughing or sneezing):

- if you have trouble reaching the toilet first thing in the morning, it will help to do a few pelvic contractions before you stand up;

- if after practising the following exercises for a month or so, your symptoms do not improve, seek medical advice. In severe cases, surgical correction may be the only answer.

How to do pelvic floor exercises

All the following activities involve the action of lifting up the pelvic floor and tightening the sphincters. These exercises will centre on the front loop of muscle which controls the vaginal and urinary openings. First you need to identify the muscles you are trying to strengthen. The pelvic floor muscles can be tensed when you try to interrupt the flow of urine. Imagine yourself stopping the urine flow, and concentrate on the muscles you are using. This is one way to gain awareness and control of these muscles.

▷

▷ 6.3 cont.

A good test of muscle strength is stopping and starting the urine flow. If your pelvic floor is weak, you may have difficulty even slowing down the flow of urine. If this is so do not continue with this test, especially with a full bladder, as it may further weaken the muscles. A pelvic floor that is undergoing re-education must be treated with care.

You can feel the pelvic floor muscles working, by placing one or two fingers in your vagina and tensing. You may like to try this during sex, and get more feedback and encouragement from your partner. You will notice after a small number of contractions that they decrease in strength. This is quite normal.

Position

Start by lying down as there will be less pressure on the pelvic floor, from the weight of the pelvic organs. If you cannot feel the muscle working in this position, raise your buttocks on a pillow, and use gravity to assist. The pelvic floor will sink into your body closer to the position you are trying to achieve (see Figure 6.5 p. 207). As you progress, and the pelvic floor strengthens, you will be able to do your exercises, standing or sitting, at any time of the day.

Exercise 1

Contract or draw up the pelvic floor, hold for three seconds, relax and repeat five times. Continue this during the day building up to ten groups of five contractions. Overworking this muscle may result in soreness. If this happens, reduce the number you do or stop the exercises for a day or two, until temporary soreness disappears, and then increase gradually.

Exercise 2

Imagine you are riding in a lift and as you go up, try to draw in the muscles gradually. When you reach your limit, don't just let go, you must go down, floor by floor again, gradually relaxing the muscles in stages. When you reach basement, let go of all the tension and think release. Then come back up to the first floor again, so the pelvic floor is slightly tense, and able to hold the pelvic organs firmly in place.

Exercise 3

Raise the entire pelvic area as though sucking water into the vagina. Relax and repeat five times. To feel this action you can insert a finger and feel the vagina drawing in. This series of five contractions may be repeated four to six times a day building up to twenty to thirty contractions a day.

▷

▷ 6.3 cont.

Each of these exercises has a similar effect of strengthening the pelvic floor. You may choose to focus on one particular exercise or use a combination. It is important not to strain or overwork your pelvic floor, so try to keep to no more than fifty contractions a day.

Remember

Pelvic floor contractions are entirely private and can be performed at any time and in any place or position that you fancy. Do about five in a series, holding each contraction for about three to five seconds, then rest a while. Always end with an uplifting contraction, to ensure support for your pelvic organs.

Reprinted with permission from: Adelaide Women's Community Health Centre, 64 Pennington Terrace, North Adelaide, Australia.

INFORMATION SHEET *6.4*

Hysterectomy

What is a hysterectomy?

A hysterectomy is the surgical removal of the womb, or uterus. There are different types of hysterectomies (see Information Sheet 6.5; *Hysterectomy diagram*):

- removal of the womb only – **subtotal or partial hysterectomy**;

- removal of both womb and cervix – **total hysterectomy**;

- removal of womb, cervix, fallopian tubes and ovaries – **unilateral or bilateral salpingo-oophorectomy**; and

- removal of womb, cervix, fallopian tubes, ovaries and top of vagina – **radical or Werthiems hysterectomy** (used for invasive cancer of the cervix).

How is it done?

Hysterectomies are most commonly performed by cutting into the lower abdomen. Sometimes they are done vaginally.

The vaginal method is thought to lead to more post-operative bleeding and a greater risk of infections, yet the healing time is much reduced and there is no visible scar. Ideally the decision would be made by the woman and the surgeon based upon which method is best for that individual woman.

How necessary are hysterectomies?

They can be life-saving operations as well as removing much pain, discomfort and infection. However, up to one third of hysterectomies done in the USA have been seen to be unnecessary. In the UK figures are much smaller yet some women undergo unnecessary hysterectomies.

Situations which may justify or require a hysterectomy are:

- cancer of cervix, fallopian tubes, or ovaries;

- severe pelvic inflammatory disease (PID) – a general name for infections which affect the fallopian tubes, ovaries, and womb;

- severe bleeding;

- severe prolapse of the womb (womb dropping due to damaged muscles);

▷

© Health Education Authority, 1993

▷ 6.4 cont.
- fibroid tumours;

- severe endometritis (where tissue which lines the womb is found growing in other parts of the body, usually in the pelvic area); and

- some pre-cancerous changes.

Sometimes hysterectomies are performed unnecessarily. This can happen for the following reasons:

- to prevent future pregnancies where birth control is not sanctioned;

- to prevent future uterine cancer;

- to end menstruation for women who no longer want children; and

- prevention of ovarian cancer may be given as the reason for hysterectomy, but we need to consider the risks of surgery together with associated risks of hormone replacement therapy (HRT).

Risks and complications

- Infections following surgery.

- Urinary-tract complications.

- Bleeding.

- Slight chance of premature menopause where there is no removal of ovaries.

- Depression – mainly with women who had unnecessary hysterectomies or who have not had proper counselling before the operation.

Sexual after-effects

- Loss of sensation of uterine contraction at orgasm.

- Vaginal dryness after removal of ovaries.

- Local effects of surgery such as a shortened vagina and scar tissue at the top of the vagina.

What you can do

Before the operation

- Seek a second opinion if you are not happy that this is the right choice for you, especially if removal of the ovaries is suggested.

▷

▷ 6.4 cont.

- Take someone with you when discussing options with a doctor.

- Contact other women who have had hysterectomies.

- Search out up-to-date information.

- Be aware of your rights even when in hospital.

- Reduce your own stress as much as possible – organise others to take over some of the things you currently do.

- Talk to others about what your options are.

After the operation

- Find out exactly what has been done and why.

- Menstruation will stop and fertility will end, so there will be no more need for contraception. Condoms can still contribute to safer sex.

- If the ovaries have been removed, there will be severe menopausal symptoms which should be discussed before the operation.

- Ask your GP about counselling or contact a local hysterectomy support group.

- Do gentle exercise such as walking, cycling, swimming and yoga, building up gradually.

- Take time over resuming sexual activity. Doctors advise waiting six to eight weeks before intercourse. You may find that you need more arousal using such things as books, massage, candlelight and fantasies. Use KY jelly if you have vaginal dryness.

- Investigate your need for hormone replacement therapy.

- Do not lift heavy items for at least four weeks after the operation.

- Ask others to do things for you.

INFORMATION SHEET *6.5*

Hysterectomy diagram

Total hysterectomy – uterus and cervix removed. Ovaries and tubes are then attached to the top of the vagina.

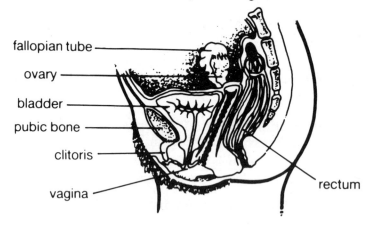

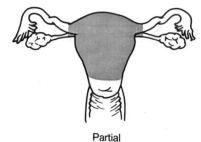

Partial

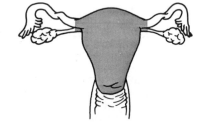

Total

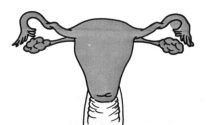

Total with removal of ovaries and fallopian tubes

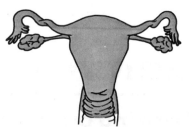

Radical with removal of top of vagina

Source: Phillips & Rakusan, *Our Bodies, Ourselves* (1989).

ACTIVITY *6.1*

Getting to know our bodies

Aims

- To familiarise women with the anatomy of their reproductive, genital and urinary system.

- To demystify the size, location and function of the various organs.

- To provide a basic understanding which can enable women to ask more questions, understand what has happened or will happen with certain surgical procedures, and feel more in touch with their bodies.

Materials

A copy of Information Sheets 6.1 *Understanding reproductive anatomy* and 6.2 *Pelvic area diagrams* for each woman; a pelvic model (if available).

Method

Use the information sheets and, if possible, a pelvic model, to talk about the pelvic area, with questions and discussions.

Discussion points

- Women are not encouraged to get to know their pelvic area and they may feel uncomfortable and separate from this part of their body. Why is this so?

- The vaginal opening, urethra and anus are very close together. This is why women are so much more susceptible than men to cross-infections.

- What are the names given to various parts of our bodies? How has this affected the way we think of our genital area?

*ACTIVITY *6.2*

Drawing our reproductive anatomy

Aims

- To find out the gaps in knowledge.

- To share information and understanding.

Materials

Large sheets of paper and pens, copies of Information Sheet 6.2 *Pelvic area diagrams* for each woman; flipchart.

Method

1 Brainstorm all the anatomical words used to describe women's sexual and reproductive areas, and write them on the flipchart.

2 In pairs, women draw the pelvic area, to include:

– uterus;
– ovaries and fallopian tubes;
– cervix and os;
– vagina.

3 Pairs join to make groups of four and draw a plan of the area around the vagina to include:

– anus and urinary opening;
– labia (inner and outer lips);
– clitoris and hood;
– mons;
– vaginal opening.

4 Put all the papers on wall or floor, and take time to look at them.

5 Discuss, possibly using the information sheet to check accuracy.

Discussion points

- Was the activity difficult to do?

- Did any differences arise between the drawings?

- Was anything learnt or clarified within the group – what was it?

- How often do women examine their pelvic area?

- Have any women ever examined themselves with a mirror?

ACTIVITY *6.3*

What were we told?

Aim

- To share experiences of finding out about how the sexual and reproductive system works.

Materials

Flipchart and pens; a copy of Worksheet 6.1 *What were we told?* for each woman.

Method

1 In small groups ask women to go through the worksheet and then share what feels comfortable.

2 In the large group, discuss the issues raised.

Discussion points

- Was the general experience of the group positive or negative?

- Have attitudes about talking of female sexual anatomy changed over the years or not?

- What is the best way to pass on this information to young women?

- It may be useful to have books and information about sexual and reproductive anatomy and physiology available for women to look through.

WORKSHEET *6.1*

What were we told?

- At what age did you really start to understand your sexual and reproductive anatomy?

- How did you find out? Was it a positive experience?

- Has anyone ever explained what a female orgasm is and what happens to your body during one?

RESOURCES

For contact details of distributors and organisations listed here, see Chapter 11 *General resources*.

Publications

Dennerstein, Lorraine, Wood, Carol and Burroughs, Graham, *Hysterectomy: How to Deal with the Physical and Emotional Aspects* (1986), Oxford University, £7.95.
A comprehensive, in depth look at hysterectomy. Australian.

Goldfarb, H, *The No-Hysterectomy Option* (1990), John Wiley & Sons, £11.45.
Written by a gynaecologist surgeon, this book alerts women – and their doctors – to the options and alternatives to hysterectomy.

Haslett, Sally and Jenkins, Molly, *Hysterectomy and Vaginal Repair* (1992), Beaconsfield, £1.95.
Third revised edition of the guide to preparation for the operation and recovery.

Hayman, Suzie, *Hysterectomy: What is it and How to Cope with it Successfully* (1989), Sheldon, £3.50.
An easy-to-read guide to the problems associated with hysterectomy, including your partner's fears, what to do after the operation, and effects of the various procedures.

Hufnagel, Vicki, *No more Hysterectomies* (1990), Thorsons, £6.99.
A woman surgeon explains how unnecessary hysterectomies can – and should – be avoided, and gives straightforward advice on the latest alternatives – both preventive and reconstructive. Describes many treatments as yet unavailable in Britain.

Martin, Emily, *The Woman in the Body: a Cultural Analysis of Reproduction* (1989), Open University Press.
Looks at menstruation, childbirth and the menopause. Contrasts the views of ordinary women and medical science.

Webb, Ann *Experiences of Hysterectomy* (1989), Optima, £4.99.
Women describe their experiences. Published in association with the Hysterectomy Support Group.

Video

Hysterectomy (1992), (available in Bengali, English, Gujarati, Hindi, Punjabi and Urdu), 20 minutes, £37.25 inclusive. Available from N. Films.

The menstrual cycle

BACKGROUND INFORMATION

- For some women their periods are trouble-free and for others there are problems of pain, heavy bleeding, irregular periods, cessation of periods and emotional mood swings.

- Many things influence how women regard their periods. These include the culture within which women live, their own experiences, how they found out about menstruation and how well prepared they were when it started.

- Women are presented with many conflicting messages from the media and from doctors about the role which hormones play in both their physical and emotional health. If women have an understanding of their own cycles, they are better placed to judge whether symptoms are hormonally or emotionally based.

- The ways in which women have coped with their periods have changed over the years with the development of a variety of products. Although many of these are convenient they may also carry risks (see Information Sheet 6.9 *Health and sanitary protection*).

- Menstruation is viewed differently in different cultures. In some cultures it is seen as the onset of fertility and may sometimes be associated with preparations for marriage. In others it is not given much social significance and is viewed as a private matter. Activity 6.5 *Menstruation – myths and taboos* looks at how culture and wider society views menstruation. With multi-cultural groups there will be a richness of information from doing this activity.

- Information about premenstrual syndrome (PMS) is in Chapter 10 *Staying healthy*.

PRACTICAL POINTS

- This can be a unifying topic of common interest for a group to look at. It is particulary relevant for the start of a women and health course, and can lead on quite naturally to other topics such as contraception, reproductive rights, menopause and premenstrual syndrome.

- It is important that women understand why and how their bodies change and respond to the menstrual cycle. It is not relevant to include complex biological and biochemical processes.

- Tutors who feel they need more information about the physical/biological aspects of this topic will find appropriate resources at the end of the section.

- Depending upon the language and literacy skills of the group it is useful for women to research the menstrual cycle for themselves either using books brought to the group, or local libraries and other sources of information outside the group.

- It is important to balance positive and negative experiences of, and attitudes to, menstruation. It is not a good idea to dwell too long upon the bad experiences or health problems of individual women. If women have particular concerns, suggest they seek advice from their GP or local well-women centre.

- The focus needs to be centred upon learning from sharing experiences and reducing taboos about talking of such topics.

INFORMATION SHEET *6.6*

The menstrual cycle – hormonal changes

Where are hormones originally produced?

At the base of the skull is the pituitary gland, which is responsible for the production of hormones.

What are hormones?

Hormones are chemical messengers carried through the bloodstream and targeted towards specific parts of the body.

What are the main hormones involved in the menstrual cycle?

The pituitary gland sends a message to the ovaries to produce two main types of hormones which are primarily responsible for the changes during the menstrual cycle. These are called *oestrogen* and *progesterone*.

What happens during the cycle?

At the beginning of the cycle (day 1 being the first day of menstruation) there is a low level production of oestrogen and progesterone. Gradually the oestrogen level increases. By about mid-cycle oestrogen levels are high enough so that the ovary releases the egg. This is known as *ovulation*. Once this has happened, the level of oestrogen is reduced and the production of progesterone increases.

What happens if the egg is fertilised (if conception takes place)?

If the egg is fertilised, progesterone continues to be produced until three months of pregnancy, after which the placenta, the life support system of the baby, takes over hormone production.

What happens if conception does not take place?

If conception does not take place the progesterone level drops, and the lining of the womb (the *endometrium*) is shed and lost through the vagina as menstrual bleeding. ▷

▷ 6.6 cont.

What are some functions of oestrogen?

- To prepare the ovaries to release the egg.

- To build up the lining of the womb to receive the fertilised egg.

- To change the texture of the cervical mucus to assist the transportation of the sperm.

What are some functions of progesterone?

- To make the womb lining a nutritious environment for conception to take place.

- To cause the tubes to contract to assist transporting the sperm and egg.

- To raise the body's temperature in preparation for pregnancy.

- To change the texture of cervical mucus to make it more difficult for sperm to enter the uterus.

What is the average length of the cycle?

The length of the cycle varies from woman to woman: 28 days is only an average and it is normal to have a shorter or longer cycle. Day 1 is counted as the first day of menstruation, so the length of your cycle is measured from the first day of your period to the start of your next period.

Does ovulation always occur on day 14?

Ovulation (when the egg is released and we are fertile) is often said to occur on day 14. In fact, it only occurs on about day 14 if the cycle is 28 days. Otherwise it occurs approximately 14 days before your next period. So for instance if you have a cycle of 32 days, ovulation occurs on approximately day 18 of your cycle.

How can we tell when we are fertile?

Fertilisation can take place only if an egg is produced (during ovulation). The egg can survive and be fertilised for up to 48 hours.

One way is to use a calendar to estimate when ovulation occurs based on the average cycle length. Another method is to record our temperature each day. A half a degree drop in temperature followed by a minute rise indicates that ovulation has occurred. It is a complicated and often inaccurate method.

Perhaps the simplest and most accurate way of predicting when ovulation will occur is to observe changes in vaginal secretions. During ovulation, mucus is clear,

▷

▷ 6.6 cont.

slippery and stretchy. Once ovulation has occurred the mucus becomes thick and sticky (see Information Sheets 6.7 and 6.8 *Diagram of the menstrual cycle 1* and *2*).

The techniques of using fertility awareness as a means of natural birth control need to be learned carefully (for more information contact the Family Planning Association or the Catholic Marriage Advisory Council).

Do hormones affect only the uterus, ovaries and mucus?

Hormone production affects various parts of our bodies. Other changes may occur in addition to the changes in our ovaries, uterus and cervical mucus. For example, changes in our appetite, mood, sleep patterns, weight, breasts, nipples and skin. Some of these are more marked before our periods and during the menopause.

When do girls begin their periods?

Periods can begin anywhere between 8 and 18 years. It is interesting to note that girls are starting to menstruate at a younger age. One factor triggering the start of periods is relative body weight. Improvements and changes in diet mean that girls today reach that triggering weight earlier than in previous generations.

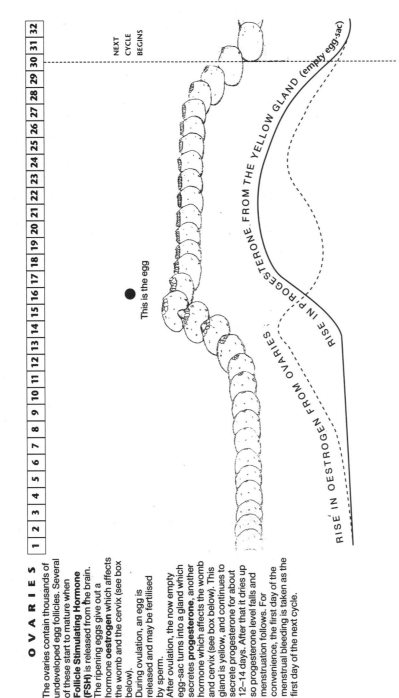

INFORMATION SHEET *6.7*

Diagram of the menstrual cycle 1

© Health Education Authority, 1993

OVARIES 1 2 3 4 5 6 7 8 9 10 11 12 13 14 15 16 17 18 19 20 21 22 23 24 25 26 27 28 29 30 31 32

The ovaries contain thousands of undeveloped egg follicles. Several of these start to mature when **Follicle Stimulating Hormone (FSH)** is released from the brain. The ripening eggs give out a hormone **oestrogen** which affects the womb and the cervix (see box below).

During ovulation, an egg is released and may be fertilised by sperm.

After ovulation, the now empty egg-sac turns into a gland which secretes **progesterone**, another hormone which affects the womb and cervix (see box below). This gland is yellow, and continues to secrete progesterone for about 12–14 days. After that it dries up so progesterone level falls and menstruation follows. For convenience, the first day of the menstrual bleeding is taken as the first day of the next cycle.

This is the egg

NEXT CYCLE BEGINS

RISE IN OESTROGEN FROM OVARIES

RISE IN PROGESTERONE FROM THE YELLOW GLAND (empty egg-sac)

Diagram of the menstrual cycle 1 *cont.*

1	2	3	4	5	6	7	8	9	10	11	12	13	14	15	16	17	18	19	20	21	22	23	24	25	26	27	28	29	30	31	32

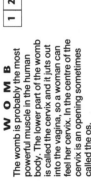

This is the womb at different stages of the menstrual cycle

This shows mucus glands

W O M B

The womb is probably the most powerful muscle in the human body. The lower part of the womb is called the cervix and it juts out into the vagina, so a woman can feel her cervix. In the centre of the cervix is an opening sometimes called the os.

The effects of **oestrogen** on the womb and cervix are quite noticeable:
- the womb may change position generally moving upwards
- the cervix becomes soft
- the os opens
- the numerous mucus glands in the opening become very active and secrete a lot of mucus.

This mucus can protect, guide, nourish and prepare sperm for fertilisation. The mucus can help keep sperm alive for up to three to five days.

Once ovulation has occurred, progesterone is secreted.

The affects of **progesterone** on the womb are also noticeable:
- the womb generally moves downward or changes position
- the cervix becomes firmer
- the os closes up often very abruptly within a matter of hours
- the mucus glands stop producing fertile mucus and a thick plug forms in the opening
- the lining inside the womb is built up and completed.

Progesterone levels fall when the yellow gland dries up. The lining of the womb then becomes thinner and bleeds during menstruation.

The length of a menstrual cycle is strongly influenced by this early phase of the cycle. Women who have short menstrual cycles may start to become fertile towards the end of bleeding, perhaps as early as day 3 or 4.

A very slow or interrupted build-up to ovulation may be normal for some women but it can also be the result of stress, poor diet, drugs or breast feeding.

The time from ovulation to menstruation usually runs in a consistent pattern for long spells of time in a particular individual. A common pattern is 12–16 days from ovulation to menstruation.

Puberty, breast feeding and the changes coming up to the menopause can affect this phase of this cycle. Women who have recently come off the pill or who are in poor health may also find this phase of their cycle is shorter.

Diagram of the menstrual cycle 1 *cont.*

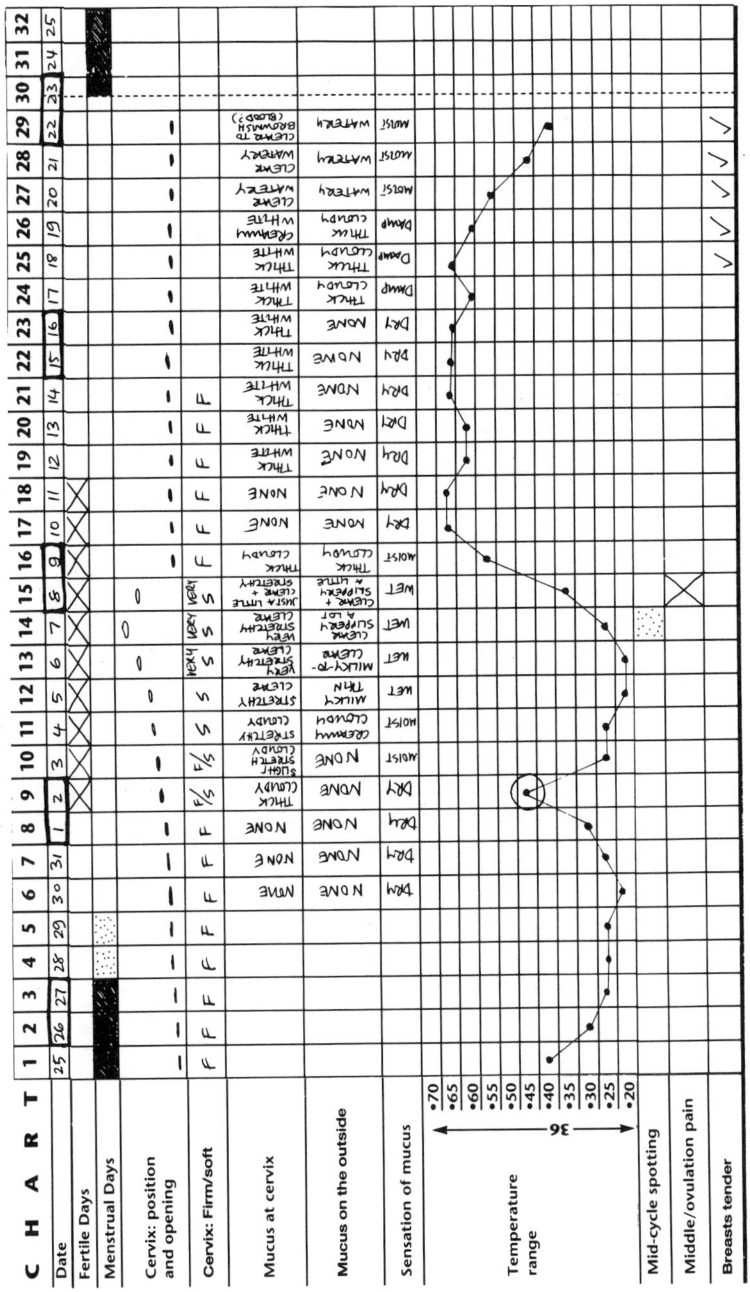

Row labels (chart):

- C H A R T
- Date
- Fertile Days
- Menstrual Days
- Cervix: position and opening
- Cervix: Firm/soft
- Mucus at cervix
- Mucus on the outside
- Sensation of mucus
- Temperature range
- Mid-cycle spotting
- Middle/ovulation pain
- Breasts tender

INFORMATION SHEET *6.8*

Diagram of the menstrual cycle 2

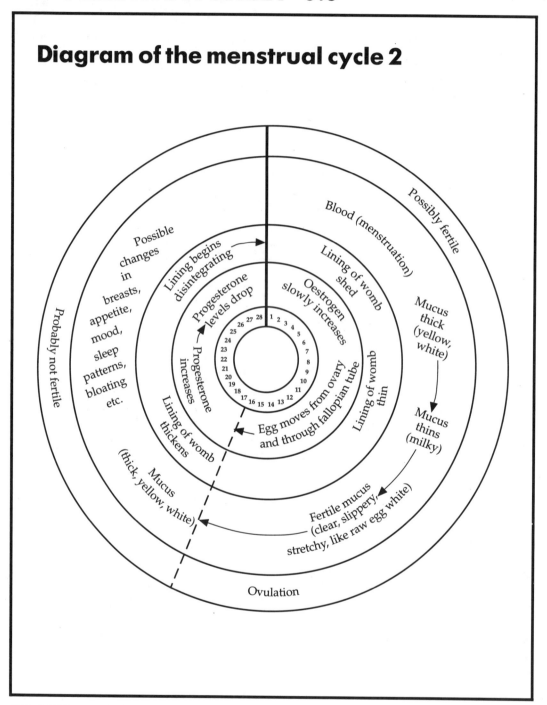

INFORMATION SHEET *6.9*

Health and sanitary protection

In the UK there are about 14 million menstruating women who spend £150 million a year on disposable sanitary protection: 44% on tampons; 40% on towels (looped or press-on); and 16% on mini-pads.

Manufacturing and disposal risks

Sanitary towels

Until the late 1980s these were made from chlorine bleached wood pulp which produced dioxins. This had health risks and environmental effects. Recently safer methods have been devised which include: chemo-thermo mechanical pulp (CTMP) – a safer process to bleach wood pulp; oxygen bleaching – which leaves some chlorine gas in the atmosphere; and using recycled pulp.

Sanitary towels generally have an inner plastic lining which gets flushed down the toilet and pollutes beaches and oceans indefinitely. Half a billion sanitary towels are washed into the sea each year as part of untreated sewage.

Tampons

Tampons are made from cotton and rayon mix. The cotton is usually grown in the Third World using pesticides not used in this country. This affects land and workers in these countries as well as being a health risk for the user. Tampons are not sterile and are not regulated by government safety standard controls.

Tampons are also flushed away down toilets and, together with sanitary towels, cause an estimated 75% of blocked drains in this country. The UK is the only EC country that permits disposal of sanitary products by flushing down the toilet.

Health risks from tampon use

- Epithelial layering – where the outer cells of the vagina flake off.
- Ulceration of the vaginal passage causing bleeding and admission of toxins to the bloodstream. Tampons absorb 65% blood and 35% vaginal secretion, leading to vaginal dryness.
- Toxic shock syndrome (TSS).

▷

▷ 6.9 cont.

Toxic shock syndrome

This is related to tampon absorbency. For every one gram increase in absorbency the risk of illness increases by 37%. It was first made public in the USA in 1980 and it is estimated that up to 15 per 100,000 women experience this illness, which can be fatal. Since 1980, twelve young women in the UK have died from TSS.

It is caused by tampons creating a local environment suitable for the growth of a certain strain of bacteria called *Staphylococcus*, which produces a toxin (TssT-1).

Symptoms of TSS are flu-like and include:

- high temperature;
- vomiting and diarrhoea;
- sore throat and aching muscles;
- headache, stiff or tender neck;
- dizziness and fainting; and
- sunburn-like peeling rash on feet, hands or trunk of body.

This can rapidly develop into loss of blood-pressure, septicaemia, shedding skin and respiratory and kidney failure.

What you can do to protect yourself and the environment

- Don't flush towels or tampons down the toilet.
- Buy towels without plastic liners.
- Avoid towels with deodorants.
- Use unbleached towels.
- Write to manufacturers requesting unbleached recycled products.
- Write to your MP asking for VAT to be removed from sanitary protection.
- Use no tampons or low absorbency tampons during heaviest flow.
- Use tampons less frequently and use towels at night.
- Use re-usable sanitary protection (see Personal Hygiene Supplies p 630).
- If you feel you have symptoms of TSS, remove tampon and seek medical advice.

Source: All factual information contained in this sheet is from: Costello, Alison, Vallely, Bernadette and Young, Josa, *The Sanitary Protection Scandal* (1989), Women's Environmental Network.

ACTIVITY *6.4*

Experiences of periods

Aims

- To explore society's attitude towards menstruation.

- To share common experiences about early womanhood and starting periods.

- To increase awareness of how society's attitudes and our early experiences influence our own feelings about our periods.

Materials

Flipchart paper, pens, copies of Worksheet 6.2 *Experiences of periods* for each woman.

Method

1 Share and write up on the flipchart all the words women have heard of to describe menstruation.

2 Ask women to work through the worksheet individually and then discuss in groups of two or three.

3 Feed back in the large group, and discuss.

Discussion points

- How do the words used to describe periods influence the way women might feel about their periods?

- In some societies the onset of menstruation is cause for celebration. How does this compare with western society's attitudes?

- Many girls first hear about periods from friends or sisters, not from parents or teachers. This kind of sharing of experience is often devalued as 'women's talk', although it can be an important source of learning between women. What other examples of this informal learning between women can you think of?

ACTIVITY *6.5*

Menstruation – myths and taboos

Aims

- To explore attitudes, myths and taboos surrounding periods.

- To identify some positive beliefs and feelings about menstruation

Materials

Flipchart paper, pens.

Method

1 On the flipchart, list all the myths, taboos, prohibitions and religious laws the group have heard of for menstruating women.

2 Go through each one and see which the women believe are true and which can be dispelled. Discuss how certain taboos, prohibitions or laws may have evolved.

3 Now list all the positive beliefs and feelings surrounding periods.

Discussion points

- In some societies men have associated menstruation with power and danger, because of women's special ability to have periods and bear children. How far does this go to explain some of the taboos listed?

- There are many taboos and prohibitions which on closer examination have no sound basis, e.g. there is no health reason why women should not wash their hair, swim or bathe while menstruating. Having intercourse during menstruation is a matter of personal preference rather than danger to one's health. However, some studies have shown recently that intercourse during menstruation facilitates transmission of sexually transmitted diseases, especially HIV. How have these taboos and prohibitions developed over time?

- Multi-cultural groups may find this a very rewarding activity. Different religions and cultures promote different beliefs about menstruation.

ACTIVITY *6.6*

Do's and don'ts about periods

Aims

- To look at the different 'do's' and 'don'ts' women have been told about periods.

- To see which have got factual basis.

Materials

Flipchart paper and pens.

Method

1 In small groups, use flipchart paper and brainstorm all the different things women have been told or know of about menstruation, under the headings 'do's' and 'don'ts'.

2 In the large group, share ideas and combine them on one flipchart.

3 Discuss.

Discussion points

- Are there more do's than don'ts?

- Can women remember how they found out or who told them about them?

- Do some of the do's and don'ts originate from cultural taboos? (See Activity 6.5 *Menstruation – myths and taboos*.)

Source: Adapted from Ealing Health Authority, *Female Cycles* (1991).

ACTIVITY *6.7*

Using a menstrual calendar

Aims

- To enable women to become more familiar with their bodily changes.

- To help women determine which changes are clustered around the time before their periods and which occur randomly throughout the month.

Materials

A copy of Worksheet 6.3 *Using a menstrual calendar* for each woman; pens.

Method

1 Give a copy of menstrual calendar to each woman, and explain to the group how to use it.

2 Women fill in menstrual calendar over a few months, for their own personal information.

Discussion points

- Do cycles differ from month to month?

- Do events in one's life have an effect on the cycle, e.g. stress, late nights, illness etc?

- How can getting to know one's own cycle make it easier to sort out what is due to PMS and what is due to outside factors in women's lives?

- In what ways can greater familiarity with one's cycle have other gains? For example, encouraging women to feel more in touch with their body, increasing understanding of their own fertility.

ACTIVITY *6.8*

Changing lives

Aims

- To examine how the changing lives of women over time and cultures has meant a change in menstruation patterns.

- To look at the implications this has for women's lives.

Materials

A copy of Worksheet 6.4 *Changing lives* for each woman; flipchart paper, markers, blutack.

Method

1 Go through the worksheet either individually, or with younger and older women interviewing each other.

2 In the large group, feed back and write up on the flipchart.

3 Display the flipchart, and discuss.

Variation: Women may use the worksheet as an interview tool with younger/older women outside the group, or as part of a group project.

Discussion points
- Childbearing alters menstrual cycles: more children mean different cycles and associated problems.

- How have maternity services and benefits changed since your grandmother's day, and what effect has this had on women's lives?

- Did our grandmothers experience PMS?

- What kind of differences are there between women of your grandmother's age and yourself?

- If your grandmother lived in a different country or within another culture to yourself, are there even more differences between your experiences?

- What differences are there among group members?

- What role does either race, class or status play in this discussion?

ACTIVITY *6.9*

Images of menstruation

Aim
- To explore images of menstruation.

Materials
Women's magazines (ask the group to collect some), scissors, glue, large sheets of paper, blutack.

Method
1 In small groups, cut out advertisements about sanitary protection and make collages.
2 Display them on a wall, and discuss in the large group.

Discussion points
- How positive or negative were the adverts in general?

- What ideas were used to get you to buy the products – effectiveness, deodorisation, fear of being seen wearing sanitary protection?

- Do any of the adverts give information about environmental or health risks associated with their products?

- Do you agree with the sale of sanitary products, or should they be free?

- What type of woman is used in adverts? Is she big, Black, thin, small, skinny, in a wheelchair? Why?

- See also Information Sheet 6.9 *Health and sanitary protection.*

Source: Adapted from Ealing Health Authority, *Female Cycles* (1991).

WORKSHEET *6.2*

Experiences of periods

1 How did you first learn about periods?

2 How old were you when you started menstruating?

3 Were you prepared?

4 Were you aware of your mother having periods?

5 Has sanitary equipment changed since you were young?

6 If you have daughters will you talk, or have you talked, to them about periods? If so, at what age and how?

WORKSHEET *6.3*

Using a menstrual calendar

Place a p for the first day of your period. If you want to see how long your period lasts, continue placing p's until your period is finished. The length of your cycle is counted from the first day of one period to the first day of your next period. Enter a symbol for the symptoms that you experience (e.g. H for headache) on the days that you experience them.

Length of Cycle	1	2	3	4	5	6	7	8	9	10	11	12	13	14	15	16	17	18	19	20	21	22	23	24	25	26	27	28	29	30	31
January																															
February																															
March																															
April																															
May																															
June																															
July																															
August																															
September																															
October																															
November																															
December																															

WORKSHEET *6.4*

Changing lives

Use your imagination to fill in the questions below, or interview someone who is younger or older than you.

	Yourself	*Women your grandmother's or granddaughter's age*
Age when periods began		
Age at first pregnancy		
Number of children		
Time between pregnancies		
Children – breast/bottle fed		
How long breast fed		
Approximate number of periods in life		
Sort of sanitary protection used		

RESOURCES

For contact details of distributors and organisations listed here, see Chapter 11 *General resources*.

Publications

Birke, Lynda and Gardner, Katy, *Why Suffer: Periods and Their Problems* (1982), Virago, £4.50.
Covers both physical and emotional changes through the menstrual cycle. Includes a self-help approach. Second revised edition.

Costello, A, Vallely, B and Young, J, *The Sanitary Protection Scandal* (1989), Women's Environmental Network, £5.95.
Manufacturers have no legal obligation to reveal how their products are made. This book explores the manufacturing processes and spells out the implications for women and children, as users of sanitary products, and for the environment. Re-usable sanitary protection available from Personal Hygiene supplies.

Delaney, Janice, Lupton, Mary Jane and Toth, Emily, *The Curse: a Cultural History of Menstruation* (1988), Illini, £10.85.

Kingston, Beryl, *Lifting the Curse: How to Relieve Painful Periods* (1984), Sheldon, £2.50.
Clear, thorough, easy-to-read guide to the subject. Out of print but available at Healthwise.

Laws, S, *Issues of Blood: the Politics of Menstruation* (1990), MacMillan, £9.99.
A unique approach to menstruation – investigation of what men really think and feel about it, and how as lovers, fathers, husbands, doctors or experts, they impose their views on women.

Sanders, Diana, *Coping with Periods* (1985), Chambers, £3.95.
Readable book, based on research and women's experiences. Deals with a broad range of problems from a medical and self-help perspective. Resources somewhat out of date.

Shuttle, Penelope and Redgrove, Peter, *The Wise Wound: Menstruation and Every-woman* (1989), Paladin, £4.99.
An historical and cultural view of menstruation. Encourages women to get in touch with inner energies.

Stead, Martine, *Female Cycles: a Resource Pack for Working with Girls and Women* (1991), Ealing Health Promotion Unit, Ealing Health Authority. £20.00. Available from West London Health Promotion Agency. Ring binder resource pack.

Women's Health. Send s.a.e. for individual orders, for the following leaflets available from Women's Health: *Painful Periods* (30p), *Heavy Bleeding* (40p), *Knowing Your Cycle* (40p).

The menopause

BACKGROUND INFORMATION

- All women will have the menopause if they live long enough, yet it is not always talked about openly. Some women may experience some or all of the symptoms associated with the menopause, while others experience none.

- Younger women sense a mystery, a taboo subject, and often older women don't feel able to discuss it with them. Yet times are changing and many more women now share experiences of the menopause.

- Sometimes when women in their 40s and 50s go to their GP with problems, they are told 'it's just your age'. This is seen as a catch-all phrase to cover physical, emotional and social problems experienced by women of this age.

- A common name for the menopause is the 'change of life'. This is because many changes seem to take place in women's lives around the general time of the menopause. These may include children growing up and leaving home, changing relationships with partners, a questioning of their role at home and possible paid work outside the home.

- This period in a woman's life can also be extremely interesting and stimulating and there is often time available now to experience new things. However, it can also be a time when women are caring and supporting others with little recognition – especially in the case of looking after elderly relatives or young grandchildren.

- For some women the menopause can mean freedom from using contraception, for others it can be a distressing time as it signals the end of fertile years. This can be especially significant for women whose culture favours male children but who have not had sons themselves.

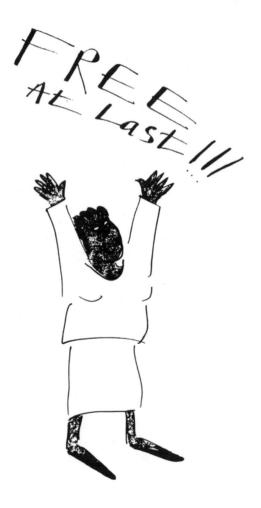

- Menopause is invariably linked to growing older and this can raise many different and contradictory feelings. Although a woman may feel comfortable with herself growing older the images that we are given of older women in this culture are generally negative.

PRACTICAL POINTS

- Sessions about the menopause often generate much discussion and sharing of experiences, especially if women are experiencing or have already gone through the menopause.

- Information can be given in the form of handouts at the end of the session, so that the sharing of experiences and discussion is not hindered.

- Tutors who have not themselves experienced the menopause may feel that they are not able to do a session about it. However your role would be to provide information and to generate and facilitate discussion around this topic. You may not have had direct experience but you can usefully comment upon some women's experiences based upon your own knowledge. This can be useful if women who have had awful experiences scare others into believing it is always like that, or when women who have had no problems give the impression to others that too much fuss is being made about it.

- When working with groups with a wide age span, there may be women who have not even begun to think about the menopause while for others it is an everyday reality. In order to keep the session interesting for all women it may be useful to focus upon feelings about the menopause and becoming older in general. This would encourage everyone to contribute. Women may also be able to reflect upon the time when their mothers would have gone through the menopause and whether it was apparent or not.

- It is useful to bear in mind that women may be wary about discussing the menopause with a doctor who she feels uncomfortable with. While this could be any doctor, some women may experience more embarrassment with either male doctors or white doctors depending upon their past experiences and expectations.

INFORMATION SHEET *6.10*

What is the menopause?

What is the menopause?

It is the process of the ending of menstruation. The menopause is a natural event in the life of every woman who lives long enough. It occurs when our level of hormone production, which has been slowly declining, drops too low to maintain the menstrual cycle and the ovaries stop releasing eggs. Hormone levels fluctuate during the menopause often producing very unpredictable periods and other symptoms. After the menopause we continue to produce female hormones such as oestrogen, but at much lower levels.

At what age does the menopause start and how long does it last?

For most women the menopause takes place between 45 and 55 but it could be earlier or later. There does not seem to be any connection between the age of starting periods and the onset of the menopause. The length of the menopause also varies. For some women periods are regular until they suddenly cease, but for most there is a phase of irregularity and perhaps other symptoms, lasting from a few months to several years.

Women who have had their ovaries removed will have an early and accelerated menopause unless they are given hormone replacement treatment.

What are the symptoms of the menopause?

Many people, including doctors, blame any physical or emotional problems of middle-aged women on the menopause – the 'it's just your age' syndrome. In fact there are few real symptoms of the menopause, and not every woman will be affected by them all.

- Irregular and unpredictable periods, sometimes accompanied by increased premenstrual syndrome (PMS).

- Hot flushes.

- Vaginal dryness.

- Osteoporosis. (This is more a part of the general process of ageing than a

▷

▷ 6.10 cont.

distinctive symptom of the menopause. It is included here because for some women the process is accelerated during the menopause.)

Any other symptoms – such as very heavy periods, bleeding between periods or any other irregularities should always be investigated by a doctor.

Why has my PMS worsened during the menopause?

If you are generally affected by PMS it could become prolonged when periods are delayed or missed during menopause. Hormone levels which are too low to start a period can still produce premenstrual symptoms. See the section on premenstrual syndrome in Chapter 10 *Staying healthy* p 479.

What are hot flushes and do all women get them?

A hot flush is a wave of heat passing over the body, sometimes accompanied by redness, sweating or tingling. Hot flushes at night may be called night sweats. Chills often follow hot flushes. The frequency and intensity of flushes and sweats varies enormously – some women never experience them, others have flushes occasionally, while a minority of women feel their lives are disrupted by flushes. Flushes are caused in some way by the fluctuating levels of hormones, but there are conflicting theories as to exactly how.

Will everyone notice when I have a hot flush?

Hot flushes are not as obvious to everyone else as to the woman having one, and for many women the anxiety about having a flush in a public place is worse than experiencing the flush itself. Nevertheless, hot flushes are the only outward sign of the menopause so they raise emotional and social issues for us. How do we feel about work colleagues or friends knowing we are in the menopause? How will they react if we ask for special consideration, such as a few minutes break, when we have a hot flush?

Is there any treatment for hot flushes?

The treatment usually offered by doctors for hot flushes and other menopausal symptoms is hormone replacement therapy (HRT). There are some side effects involved in this and it is important to have enough information to make an informed decision. See Information Sheet 6.12 *HRT – for and against* and Resources for further reading.

There are ways we can help ourselves to have a more comfortable menopause – see Information Sheet 6.13 *Self-help ideas for menopause and osteoporosis.*

▷

▷ 6.10 cont.

Is vaginal dryness inevitable during the menopause?

Most but not all women experience some degree of vaginal dryness during the menopause and for some this can cause problems. The vagina needs lubrication to cleanse, and fight infection – vaginal dryness can make us prone to vaginal and urinary infections. See the section on vaginal health in Chapter 10 *Staying healthy* for information on preventing and treating these infections.

Doctors may offer oestrogen cream for vaginal dryness; see Information Sheets 6.12 *HRT – for and against* and 6.13 *Self-help ideas for menopause and osteoporosis.*

Will vaginal dryness affect my sex life?

Vaginal secretion is decreased in most women after the menopause. Vaginal dryness can make penetration painful and difficult, but other forms of sexual or sensual activity could ease the dryness by increasing vaginal lubrication.

Am I likely to become depressed during the menopause?

Depression may be a symptom of the menopause, but women can become depressed at any point in life. For some of us the menopause symbolises the beginning of getting older. If we have fears about ageing we may become depressed during the menopause, particularly if it coincides with other changes in our lives such as our parents dying or becoming infirm, loss of a job, or children leaving home.

Our mental and physical health are closely related, so a woman who has severe physical symptoms in the menopause may become depressed. And a woman who is feeling very positive about her menopause and busy enjoying life may cope more easily with physical symptoms than one who dreaded the menopause.

INFORMATION SHEET *6.11*

Osteoporosis

Osteoporosis is a disease of the bones, in which they become too porous so that they break easily. It affects more than one woman in four, and one man in twenty. The condition develops silently over many years, gradually and without discomfort. It will usually show up after the age of fifty, but maybe as early as the late thirties. You may become aware of it suddenly, with a painful fracture after only a slight fall or awkward movement. Or your clothes may appear not to fit any more because your spine is starting to curve.

Women are at far greater risk of osteoporosis than men because as the woman approaches the menopause, the level of the hormone oestrogen declines, slowing down calcium absorption and speeding up the loss of bone mass.

Other factors which may increase the risk of osteoporosis include:
early menopause (naturally or after hysterectomy) before 45 years;
prolonged loss of periods (e.g. from anorexia or bulimia nervosa);
family history of osteoporosis;
low calcium intake or absorption;
lack of exercise;
tobacco abuse.

Prevention of osteoporosis is important for everyone:

Keeping active – Bones need steady regular exercise to help build strong bones and reduce bone loss. Walking, using the stairs, dancing, cycling, tennis or running are all good examples. It's best to do a little steady exercise every day.

Diet – Eat plenty of foods rich in calcium, particularly cheese, milk and yoghurt. Low fat versions have more calcium. Other good sources include nuts, canned fish and dark green leafy vegetables such as broccoli.

Avoid smoking – Smoking accelerates the onset of the menopause by two to five years, and may suppress new bone growth. Passive smoking can also have a bad effect on bones.

Hormone replacement therapy – This may be an appropriate treatment to prevent osteoporosis in women who have a high risk of developing the disease. It may also be used to reduce further bone loss in women suffering from osteoporosis. If you want to consider using HRT it is essential to ask your doctor. For more information see Information Sheet 6.12 *HRT – for and against*.

Source: based on information from the National Osteoporosis Society.

INFORMATION SHEET *6.12*

HRT – for and against

Hormone·replacement therapy (HRT) is used to treat the symptoms of the menopause with oestrogen and progestogen, or oestrogen alone when a woman has had a hysterectomy. Treatment can be in the form of pills, skin patches, creams or implants under the skin.

It has been talked about as a 'cure' for the menopause and sometimes as a way of holding back the ageing process. It is a controversial treatment and, as such, women need to be able to make decisions about whether or not to use it. However, the reality for many women is that their GP will prescribe HRT with or without discussion of possible side effects. Alternatively, they may not be offered HRT because their GP does not believe in it, or feels the risks outweigh the benefits.

What HRT can do

- Relieve such short-term menopausal symptoms as hot flushes, sweats and vaginal dryness.

- Reduce the long-term risks of osteoporosis, heart attacks and stroke.

- Relieve the after-effects of hysterectomy and removal of ovaries.

HRT can also help with depression, insomnia, loss of self-confidence and migraine. Reducing the disturbing effects of night sweats and hot flushes promotes better sleep.

HRT can also increase fluid retention and so 'puff' out the skin and reduce wrinkle lines. Because of this it has sometimes been described, particularly in the USA , as a 'youth' drug. In reality, it can improve the health of women who need it, particularly those at high risk of osteoporosis and heart disease. Women who have not had a hysterectomy must take progestogen as well as oestrogen and will therefore in most cases have a monthly bleed. Regular medical checks are given to women prescribed HRT.

Side effects of using HRT

- Possible increased risk of breast cancer when taken for ten years or more.

- Resumption of menstruation for women who have not had a hysterectomy.

- Minor effects such as breast tenderness, weight gain, and other premenstrual

▷

▷ 6.12 cont.

syndrome type symptoms. These should disappear after the first two months, and if not the dose or type of HRT should be changed.

What HRT cannot do

- It cannot totally reverse the process of bone loss, and cannot replace bone if the osteoporosis is advanced. It is mainly a preventive treatment.

- It cannot make a woman a different person than she was before her oestrogen was lost, but it can restore her self-confidence, and her libido and interest in sex by helping with vaginal lubrication.

When is the use of HRT appropriate

HRT may be appropriate for:

- women who have had ovaries and womb removed before the menopause (especially before age 45 years). Women who have had their ovaries removed are particularly at risk from osteoporosis;

- women suffering from osteoporosis, to reduce further bone loss;

- women with a family history of osteoporosis;

- women who have a high risk of osteoporosis detected by bone scan; and

- women with a history of loss of periods (anorexia or bulimia nervosa sufferers particularly).

HRT may not be appropriate for women with the following:

- history of oestrogen-dependent tumours of genital tract or breast;

- family history of breast cancer;

- undiagnosed irregular bleeding;

- pregnancy;

- uncontrolled hypertension;

- fibroids;

- endometriosis;

- recent thrombo-embolic disease.

▷

▷ 6.12 cont.

Asking your doctor

If you feel you want to consider using HRT, it is essential to ask your doctor:

- what medical checks you will need;
- how often these need to be done;
- what checks to do for yourself;
- what type of preparation you will need;
- whether you will have bleeding;
- side effects that need reporting back; and
- length of treatment.

Women starting to take HRT should have their blood pressure checked, a pelvic and breast examination and a urine test. Some doctors may also recommend a screening test for thyroid problems.

INFORMATION SHEET *6.13*

Self-help ideas for menopause and osteoporosis

The views expressed here are those of the authors and do not necessarily reflect the views or policies of the Health Education Authority

What alternatives are there either to taking hormones or to putting up with uncomfortable symptoms of the menopause? There are ways we can help ourselves to have a happier and more comfortable menopause – including making changes in our lives, exercise, diet, and natural remedies. This list of ideas is not a 'prescription' for a healthy menopause, merely some suggestions you may like to follow up yourself. You can find more information about these ideas and remedies in *Menopause: A Positive Approach*, and other books in the Resources section.

Look after yourself

- Put your own needs first for a change.

- Try to identify and reduce stress in your life (see the sections on *Stress* and *Relaxation and massage* in Chapter 4 *Mental health*).

- Make some time for yourself, to relax or follow your own interests.

- Take some regular exercise, for example swimming, yoga, dancing, keep-fit classes or walking.

- Eat a balanced diet with as much fresh fruit and vegetables as you can afford. Make sure you are getting enough calcium (see the section on osteoporosis, below).

- Start something new just for yourself – learn a skill you've always wanted to, join a class or group, begin a new hobby or interest or take up one you dropped because of other commitments.

- Strengthen the relationships and friendships that are important to you.

- Be open to making new friends.

Hot flushes and night sweats

- Try to cut out or down on cigarettes and sugar (these can cause sweating and

▷

▷ 6.13 cont.

flushes in people not having the menopause), alcohol, tea and coffee. See the activities for reducing stress in Chapter 4, *Mental health*.

- Check with your doctor if any drugs you are taking could be making your flushes worse. You can also look up side-effects of drugs in the paperback, *Medicine: A Guide for Everyone* by Peter Paris (Penguin).

- Tell your family or those you live with (if you feel you can) what hot flushes are and how you feel when you have them. Explain that at times you may need to switch heating off or on and that you expect their co-operation and understanding.

- Ensure that you will be able to adjust your temperature if you need to by dressing in easily removed layers, and sleeping with the bedding loose.

- Avoid artificial fibres (for example, nylon) for your clothes and bedding as they increase sweating. Wear natural fibres as much as possible (cotton or wool, or mixtures with some natural fibres in them) and use cotton sheets.

- When you feel a hot flush coming on, don't fight it, just let it wash over you. Try to relax with some deep breathing.

- Place the insides of your wrists and arms on a cold surface or under running water during a flush or sweat.

- Keep a change of night clothes and bedding and some talcum powder or cologne handy in case of a severe night sweat. You will get back to sleep more quickly if you feel comfortable.

Vaginal dryness

Doing pelvic floor (or Kegel) exercises can increase the suppleness and elasticity of the vagina and other internal organs. (See Information Sheet 6.3 *Pelvic floor exercises*.) More imaginative and tender love-making, or masturbation, will increase vaginal secretions and reduce the likelihood of infections.

There is much you can do to prevent vaginal and urinary infections – see the section on vaginal health in Chapter 10, *Staying healthy*. A cream or jelly could help. There are several available: for example, Aci-jel is a jelly which is slightly acid to restore the vagina to its natural acidic balance and so prevent infection. It is available over the counter from your chemist, and may be suggested for thrush. KY jelly is a simple lubricant which is often used to help penetrative sex be more comfortable.

▷

▷ 6.13 cont.

Osteoporosis

A balanced diet which is rich in calcium is important for all women, but particularly those around or beyond the menopause. Calcium-rich foods include milk, cheese, yoghurt and green vegetables. Calcium supplements, such as Dolomite, are available from chemists or health food shops and can also reduce symptoms such as night cramps which disturb sleep.

Vigorous activity such as a brisk walk, keep-fit classes, running, dancing or cycling will help to strengthen bones and reduce calcium loss. Swimming is good for internal organs and muscle and skin tone, but does not exercise bones or prevent bone loss because the weight of your body is supported by the water.

ACTIVITY *6.10*

Feelings about the menopause

Aims

- To identify and discuss our feelings about the menopause.

- To encourage a sharing of feelings and experiences between women who have not yet reached the menopause and those who have.

- To explore the source of our feelings about the menopause.

Materials

A copy of Worksheet 6.5 *Feelings about the menopause* for each woman; flipchart, markers, pens.

Method

1 In small groups fill in and discuss the sentences on the worksheet.
   Option: Pair women who have been through the menopause with those who have not. Ask the women to interview each other using the worksheet.

2 In large group make two lists on a flipchart of positive and negative thoughts about the menopause and discuss where some of our ideas and feelings come from.

Discussion points

- Are there more positive than negative thoughts?

- Where do our negative feelings about the menopause come from? What are they based on?

- What would increase our positive feelings about the menopause?

ACTIVITY *6.11*

Talking about the menopause

Aim

- To look at the difficulties and benefits of talking about the menopause.

Materials

A copy of Worksheet 6.6 *Talking about the menopause* for each woman; pens.

Method

1 Ask each woman to read through the worksheet.

2 Discuss the issues raised, and the questions identified on the worksheet.

Discussion point

Do you think the menopause should be more widely discussed? What effect do you think this would have?

WORKSHEET *6.5*

Feelings about the menopause

Complete these sentences and discuss them in your group.

For women who have not yet reached the menopause

When I think about the menopause:

I most look forward to

I fear

I am bothered about

I want to know more about

For me the menopause means

For women who are in or have been through the menopause

What the menopause meant for me was

The best thing about the menopause was

The worst thing about the menopause was

Before the menopause, I expected it to be

WORKSHEET *6.6*

Talking about the menopause

A considerate woman usually makes a valiant effort to disguise the fact that she is 'going through the Change of Life'. Sheer pride: pride in keeping young, pride in not talking about bodily ailments, pride in adjusting well to Nature's demands – these keep her lips glued and help her hold her head high through the months when she experiences new, unusual feelings . . . Talk makes mountains out of molehills.[1]

Talking about the menopause is the best thing a woman can do. By talking to a sympathetic listener, you can begin to look at how you feel about it. When I became convinced that talking about the menopause would make the experience more positive for me, I found that my life began to change . . . I was able to learn what feelings other women were experiencing about menopause, as well as about ageing, love, sex, health, and even work and children, for those areas were also involved.[2]

- Do you agree with either of these views?

- Have you ever discussed the menopause with your:
  - partner?
  - mother?
  - daughter?
  - friends?
  - work colleagues?

- Has it been useful for you to talk about the menopause? In what ways?

[1] From Lincoln, Miriam, *You'll Live Through It* (1950).
[2] From Reitz, Rosetta, *Menopause – A Positive Approach* (1983), Unwin.

RESOURCES

For contact details of distributors and organisations listed here, see Chapter 11 *General resources*.

Publications

Arnold, June, *Sister Gin* (1979), Women's Press, £3.95.
A novel about a woman experiencing the menopause.

Coope, Jean, *The Menopause: Coping with the Change* (1989), Optima, £6.99.
Useful general guide to the menopause and HRT. Includes tips on fitness, sex, avoiding osteoporosis and much more.

Cooper, Wendy, *No Change: a Biological Revolution for Women* (1990), Arrow, £3.99.
Promotes the use of HRT. Fourth revised edition.

Dickson, Anne and Henriques, Nikki, *Menopause: the Women's View* (1987), Grapevine, £2.99.
Brief, overall guide to the topic.

Fairlie, Judi, Nelson, Jayne and Popplestone, Ruth, *Menopause: a Time for Positive Change* (1988), Javelin, £2.00. Available from Women's Health.
Useful information on the menopause. Attempts to combat negative attitudes. Provides health advice.

Greenwood, Sadja, *Menopause the Natural Way* (1990), Optima, £7.99.
A holistic look at the menopause, including an evaluation of whether to use HRT.

Greer, G, *The Change: Women, Ageing and the Menopause* (1991), Hamish Hamilton, £16.99 (hardback).
This is a dense, challenging book which includes a comprehensive study of the fundamental change which women experience during the menopause and which needs mental preparation for acceptance.

Kahn, Ada and Holt, Linda, *Menopause: the Best Years of Your Life?* (1987), Bloomsbury, £4.99.
Detailed guide to the emotional and health issues for women in and after the menopause. American.

Mackenzie, Raewyn, *Menopause: a Practical Self-help Guide for Women* (1990), Sheldon, £3.99.
A chatty book on the physical and emotional changes associated with the menopause. New Zealand.

Ojeda, Linda, *Menopause without Medicine: Feel Healthy, Look Younger, Live Longer* (1990), Thorsons, £6.99.
Holistic information and advice on staying healthy through the menopause.

Reitz, R, *Menopause: a Positive Approach* (1979), Unwin, £2.95.
Remains an early, classic positive approach to dealing with the menopause, packed with information and discussion of wider issues such as self-esteem, sexuality, nutrition.

Shreeve, C, *Overcoming the Menopause Naturally* (1986), Century Arrow, £2.95.
Positive approach to menopause as an important milestone that marks a stage of physical and emotional maturity and the beginning of the prime of a woman's life. Advice on the use of complementary therapies and relaxation techniques, without resorting to artificial hormones.

Taylor, Dena and Sumrall, Amber Coverdale (eds), *Women of the 14th Moon: Writings on Menopause* (1991), Crossing Press, £9.95.
Spirituality and the menopause. Writings by a number of American women.

Wellwomen Information, *Multi-lingual Menopause Leaflets*, 60p each plus postage. Available from Wellwomen Information, Bristol, in Urdu, Punjabi, Hindi, Bengali, Gujarati, Vietnamese and Chinese.

Women's Health. Send SAE for individual orders of the following leaflets available from Women's Health: *Hormone Replacement Therapy* (30p), *Menopause broadsheet* (general discussion) (40p), *Menopause leaflet* (practical suggestions) (40p).

Videos

Is it Hot in Here? (A film about menopause) (1989), 37 minutes, National Film Board of Canada, £75 plus VAT and p&p. Available from Educational Media International.

That Funny Age: Women and the Menopause (1989), 27 minutes, £25 plus VAT. Available from Video in Pilton.
Made with women in Lothian health projects this video looks at local women's experience of the menopause and of entering their middle years. Women talk about their physical changes against the background of their lives as a whole.

The Menopause (1992) (available in Urdu, Bengali, Gujarati, Hindi, Punjabi and English), 20 minutes, £37.25 inclusive. Available from N Films.

Organisations

Menopause Clinics
Specialist clinics exist in many parts of the UK. For information and addresses, contact Women's Health, the Family Planning Association, or your local Community Health Council.

Menopause Support Groups
There are many local menopause support self-help groups throughout the UK. For addresses, contact Women's Health.

Menopause Society
A medically oriented organisation which looks at the menopause and ageing.

Older Feminists Network
Has information about local groups.

Women's Health Concern
Information and advice on women's health with an emphasis on menopausal and post-menopausal problems. Provides leaflets. Send stamped SAE for publications list.

Women's Nutritional Advisory Service
An advisory service which is diet-based for women suffering from the menopause. Fee paying.

7 Motherhood

BACKGROUND INFORMATION

- Motherhood stirs our deepest emotions. It can raise feelings about our own childhood. The concept of motherhood, its roles and responsibilities, is a social and political issue.

- Becoming a mother involves profound changes in status, identity, self-esteem and lifestyle. Both the rewards from, and costs of, motherhood can be enormous.

- Mothering is grossly undervalued in British Society. Society is not 'children-friendly' in the sense that children may be seen as a nuisance in public places, there is a lack of good childcare provision, and little support for mothers.

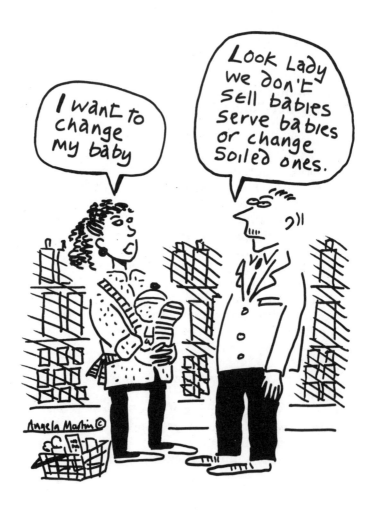

- New mothers are often given lots of prescriptive and 'expert' advice on the 'right' way to bring up children which can be confusing. Mothers have to make choices on behalf of their children, for example over breastfeeding, child immunisation and child safety.

- Mothering takes place within different family structures, each with advantages and disadvantages, and their own values and norms.

- If, when and how to have children is a huge political issue. Some women decide they do not wish to parent. Others wanting children may find they are unable to. Medical technology means that assisted conception techniques are available to some women – but such techniques themselves raise intense ethical, social, legal and political concerns.

PRACTICAL POINTS

- As with most women's health issues, motherhood is a very emotive area. Establish ground rules within the group.

- Acknowledge your own position as to whether or not you are a mother. Emphasise a non-expert approach. Acknowledge feelings and experiences – you don't have to be a mother yourself to feel strongly about it.

- Encourage women to focus on themselves as mothers, not just on their children.

- You will need to be aware of different family structures. Not all activities will be appropriate for all groups. There may be different cultural and class issues within the group which will affect women's views of motherhood.

- Be aware of lack of choice for some women to have children. Also, in any group there may be women who have had miscarriages, babies who died, whose children are fostered or adopted, who gave up children for fostering and adoption, who are infertile, and so on.

- It may be helpful to provide a list of useful local or national contacts.

INFORMATION SHEET *7.1*

Family structures

We all have beliefs about families and the way we think they should be, including:

- size of family;
- emotional relationships within it;
- responsibilities of each member of the family;
- support from other family members;
- who makes decisions in the family; and
- independence of individual family members.

The organisation of the typical Western family is just one of a variety of possible approaches. Families in Britain with different structures and cultural norms from the majority may find that health care services are not geared to their particular needs. Western culture emphasises the right of the individual over the family. This is not necessarily so in other cultural groups, where the family unit itself may contain three or four generations and more than one married couple; where children may be raised by all the adults, or by elder women.

Different minority ethnic communities may believe in some of the following:

- the pivot of the family may be the mother, grandmother, grandparents, parents, or the wider extended family;
- the priorities and values of individual members may be closely tied up with those of the family, and decisions may be made by the whole family rather than the individual;
- it may be the duty of older family members to make all important decisions (even if they themselves do not live in Britain);
- individuals may feel they are part of the wider family for most of their lives;
- roles and aspirations of men and women within the family may be different;
- the family may have honour and reputation to maintain;
- marriage may be seen as a bond between two families rather than just between two individuals;
- marriage may not be considered particularly important.

▷

▷ 7.1 cont.

Some issues relevant to different family structures in Britain

- In some cultures it is not the traditional role of women to make major decisions.

- In many societies men and women lead separate lives. Pregnancy and child-birth may be seen as 'women's' matters only, and women may wish to have other female relatives with them.

- Different cultures raise children in different ways. For example, in some Asian families girls may be regarded as vulnerable, and male members of the family may be very protective. For historical reasons, girls in African-Caribbean families may be raised to be independent and self-sufficient.

- Mothers may feel a conflict in raising children in Britain 'between two cultures'. They may wish to retain traditional family values and be concerned at the effect of Western culture on their children.

- If women are used to an extended family where childcare is shared between several adults, they can miss the family support if it is no longer available in Britain.

INFORMATION SHEET 7.2

Reproductive technology

Below are the most common 'assisted conception' techniques used in Britain. The issue of reproductive technology is a hotly contested one with moral, ethical and political aspects.

Procedures such as IVF (in vitro fertilisation) and GIFT (gamete intrafallopian transfer) are expensive (and not often available on the NHS) and do not have a high success rate. Such techniques are usually available only to heterosexual couples living in a 'stable relationship'. They are controlled through licensing bodies and the law.

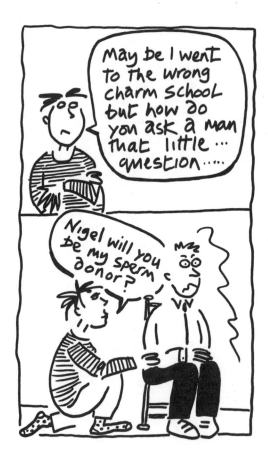

▷ 7.2 cont.

Artificial insemination with donor (AID)

This is a very simple technique where semen from a donor is put into a woman's vagina.

It is used by women when:

- their male partner is infertile;

- there is chance of a genetic condition being passed on;

- they are single; or

- they choose not to have sex with men.

Frozen semen is usually used as a precaution against HIV. This allows a three month period following donation of semen when a follow-up HIV test may be taken to ensure that the donor is HIV negative. This procedure is so simple that it can be done by a woman herself without medical intervention. However, with the advent of HIV, many women are now reluctant to use the semen of 'informal' donors. Single women are often unable to obtain AID through official services.

In vitro fertilisation (IVF)

IVF is a technique used when a woman has fallopian tubes which are either damaged or missing, but who still ovulates. An egg is fertilised with semen outside of the body, in a special culture medium, and left to develop into an embryo. The embryo is then transferred to the mother's womb (more than one embryo may be transferred).

Usually the ovaries are stimulated (with drugs) to produce more than one egg at a time – 'superovulation' – in order to maximise chances of producing embryos.

- *IVF with woman's egg, partner's sperm*: when a woman has damaged or missing fallopian tubes and the partner's sperm is OK. This is the most usual situation in Britain.

- *IVF with donor sperm*: allows a woman's egg to be fertilised with donor sperm (in cases of abnormal sperm in her partner).

- *IVF with donor egg*: fertilisation of an egg which has been donated by another woman, with sperm from the partner in the couple (when a woman cannot give her own egg, because of no ovaries/malfunctioning ovaries/or if she is the carrier of a genetic disease).

- *IVF with donor embryo*: fertilisation of a donor egg with donor sperm (when there is serious infertility on the part of both partners in the couple).

▷

▷ 7.2 cont.

Gamete intrafallopian transfer (GIFT)

In this method, both egg and sperm are put into the woman's fallopian tube (which is where fertilisation normally occurs). After superovulation, usually two eggs are removed from the woman's ovary and mixed with the partner's sperm. Sperm and eggs are drawn into a thin tube and put directly into the fallopian tubes; fertilisation takes place inside the woman's body.

This method is useful when:

- there are immune factors which prevent conception in the usual way;

- the male partner has low sperm count;

- the woman suffers from endometriosis; or

- there is unexplained infertility.

Surrogacy

Surrogacy is an agreement where a woman gets pregnant with the intention of giving up the baby to a couple who want a child but are unable (for a variety of reasons) to have one themselves. The pregnancy can be achieved through sexual intercourse, but is more usually arranged through artificial insemination with the semen of the male of the couple. In this case the baby is genetically the result of the male and the surrogate mother.

The pregnancy can also be arranged via IVF using an egg from the 'commissioning' mother and the semen from her male partner. The surrogate mother will bear the baby but will not be its genetic mother. There are laws controlling surrogacy (see Information Sheet *7.3 Timetable of reproductive technology*).

Freezing of embryos

Embryos that have reached the eight-cell stage of development can be frozen (in liquid nitrogen) and thawed when needed. Embryo freezing makes possible:

- the donation of eggs from another woman; and

- storage for future use (in case the first attempt is unsuccessful, or for a second pregnancy).

Sex determination

Using a genetic DNA probe, the male Y chromosome can be identified in embryos 4-8 days old. This method can be used to screen embryos and prevent sex-linked disorders such as haemophilia by not transferring male embryos.

INFORMATION SHEET *7.3*

Timetable of reproductive technology

1978 **Louise Brown**, the first 'test-tube' baby born in Britain.

1984 **Warnock Report** published:

Terms of reference: 'To consider recent and potential developments in medicine and science related to human fertilisation and embryology; to consider what policies and safeguards should be applied, including consideration of the social, ethical and legal implications of these developments, and to make recommendations'.

Particular interests: artificial insemination by donor (AID), in vitro fertilisation (IVF), and embryo donation.

Possible options for controlling the above: control by the Secretary of State, reliance on voluntary self-regulation, or a statutory licensing authority.

1985 **Kim Cotton**, Britain's first known commercially arranged surrogate mother. Social services put a place of safety order on the baby, who stayed in hospital for 10 days while the legal wrangle was sorted out.

1985 **Surrogacy Arrangements Act**, prompted by the Kim Cotton case:

- illegal for a third party (e.g. an agency) to receive payment;

- illegal to advertise to be a surrogate mother, or find a surrogate (even without payment);

- payment to a surrogate mother is not illegal, but under adoption laws any payment of expenses would make it difficult for a 'commissioning' mother to adopt the child legally.

1985 **Private Members' Bills to prohibit human embryo research** introduced into the House of Commons. The one causing most controversy was Enoch Powell's *Unborn Children (Protection) Bill*. All Bills failed to become Acts of Parliament due to lack of time.

1985 **Voluntary licensing authority** set up (jointly sponsored by the Medical Research Council and the Royal College of Obstetricians & Gynaecologists) to control embryo research and IVF.

1987 **Baby M case – surrogacy**: the widely publicised case in America of surrogate mother – Mary Beth Whitehead – who changed her mind about giving up the baby to the 'commissioning' parents, declining the payment agreed. The

▷

▷ 7.3 cont.

court awarded custody to the father. This case raised the issue of a middle-class 'commissioning' couple in comfortable circumstances versus a working-class woman on limited means, in terms of what each could give the child.

1987 **Legislation on human infertility services and embryo research**, a consultative document issued by Government. The main issues covered were:

- licensing body;
- membership of licensing authority;
- anonymity of donors;
- embryo research; and
- surrogacy.

1990 **Human Fertilisation and Embryology Act** passed.

1990 **Statutory Licensing Authority** set up.

ACTIVITY 7.1

My children/me as a child

Aims

- To introduce women to the issue of motherhood by sharing information on their own children and/or what they themselves were like as children.

- To find out the age range of children of women in the group (to help the tutor choose subsequent activities to offer the group).

Materials

A flipchart and pens.

Method

1 Go round the group, asking women to share the names and ages of their children. Write these on the flipchart.

2 Go round the group again, asking women to share any nickname they had as a child, and think back to what they remember about themselves when they were 5 or 6 years old.

Discussion points

- Did some women remember how they looked physically, or what their particular interests were at the time?

- If there is a wide age range of women in the group, did older women remember different things from younger women?

Note for tutor

Remembering back to childhood may be painful for some women, particularly if they did not have a happy childhood. You will need to be sensitive to how women are responding to this activity.

Source: adapted from *Women Learning Together*, Salford Women's Education Forum.

ACTIVITY 7.2

Liking/not liking being a mother

Aim

- To enable women to begin thinking about the advantages and disadvantages of being a mother.

Materials

Flipchart paper (one sheet headed 'like', one sheet headed 'don't like'), post-it notes.

Method

1 Give two post-it notes to each woman.

2 Ask them to write down something they like about being a mother on one, and something they don't like about being a mother on the other.

3 Ask women to place their 'likes' and 'don't likes' on the appropriate flipchart sheet.

4 Sort similar responses together, and discuss the findings.

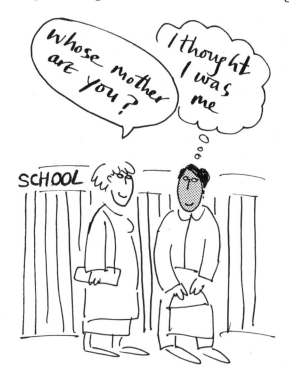

Discussion points

- Did some women find it easier to decide what they didn't like about being a mother? Why was this?

- Were there similar responses to 'like'?

- Were there similar responses to 'don't like'?

- Did the advantages outweigh the disadvantages? What might this depend on (e.g. having chosen to have children/ children being healthy/ help from others/having enough money/ages of children/adequate housing/support etc.)?

- Did anyone change their mind about the advantages and disadvantages of being a mother while doing this activity?

Source: adapted from *Women Learning Together*. Salford Women's Education Forum.

ACTIVITY 7.3

My mother

Aim

- To help women reflect on their own upbringing in order to consider whether they are parenting differently from their own mother.

Materials

Flipchart, markers, pens and paper for each woman.

Method

1 Write the following two statements on a flipchart: *As a child, what I liked about my mother was . . .* , and *As a child, what I didn't like about my mother was . . .*

2 Each woman writes down her responses on paper. Stress that what she writes will not be shared with the group (some women may choose to work in pairs to prompt each other).

3 In the large group

- Ask women what life was like for their own mothers. Is it any different now? Flipchart the responses.

- Ask women what they want to do differently from their own mothers. Why? Flipchart the responses.

Discussion points

- Was life different for our mothers, for example, now that:
  - we have labour saving devices for housework;
  - men help more in the house and with childcare;
  - women are more likely to have paid work outside the home (rather than, say, taking in washing);
  - we live in a generally more affluent society; and
  - we have better contraceptive methods?

- Is it easier to be a mother these days? Why? Why not?

- What are the kinds of things we want to do differently from our own mothers? Are we succeeding? If not, why not?

Notes for tutor

- If you have group members who are related to each other (e.g. mother and daughter), this can affect the group dynamics!

- Be sensitive – some women may not have been brought up primarily by their mother because she died, they were adopted, or for other reasons.

ACTIVITY 7.4

Motherhood then and now

Aims

- To compare motherhood now with what it was like for our grand-mothers.

- To look at the changing standards and expectations of motherhood.

- To share experiences and feelings about being a mother.

Materials

A copy of Worksheet 7.1 *Motherhood then and now* for each woman; flipchart paper and pens.

Method

1 Give out the worksheet. Divide the group into two, half discussing motherhood in the past, the others motherhood now, and listing the main points on flipchart paper.

2 After about twenty minutes get the group back together to pool their ideas.

Discussion points
- What main issues make motherhood difficult today? How can we cope with them?

  - What support can we get in being parents? Where can we go for advice about problems with our children:
    - local helping agencies;
    - voluntary or self-help groups?

ACTIVITY *7.5*

More than just a mother

Aims
- To explore constraints on women.
- To consider the changing structure of family life in Britain and abroad.
- To examine feelings about being a wife, partner, daughter, housewife – as well as being a mother.
- To consider the value given to unpaid housework.

Materials
None.

Method
1 Divide the women into two groups.

2 Ask one group to consider the advantages of the extended family, and the second group the disadvantages.

3 In the large group, share findings and discuss.

Discussion points
- Do the advantages of the extended family outweigh the disadvantages?
- How do women feel about being:

  - a mother?
  - a daughter?
  - a wife?
  - a mother-in-law?
  - a daughter-in law?

- How much power do women have as mothers?

- What can women do if they are subjected to violence within the home?

- What are the pressures on women to behave according to family and traditional values? Does this conflict with the values regarding women in the wider society?

- How do we relate to our daughters?

- How do we get recognition for all the unpaid housework we do? Should there be wages for housework?

- How can we make changes which would improve our position as women, e.g.

  – adequate childcare provision;
  – laws to protect us against violence in the home?

ACTIVITY 7.6

The job of mothering

Aims

- To enable women to realise the skills they have to be a mother.

- To show the complexities of being a mother.

Materials

Post-it notes, a large circle of flipchart paper for each small group, flipchart, pens.

Method

1 Divide women into small groups.

2 Give each small group some post-it notes and a circle of flipchart paper.

3 Ask women to think about all the tasks involved in being a mother and write one down on each post-it.

4 Place the post-its on the circle of paper, with the most important one in the centre, the others in outer circles.

5 Feed back to the large group. Together construct a job advert for a mother, including:

- tasks (already identified on post-its);

- skills needed;

- hours of employment;

- length of contract;

- conditions of service; and

- pay!

Flipchart responses.

Discussion points

- Was there agreement between groups on:

  - kinds of tasks? What sort of categories emerged (e.g. 'caring', 'practical', 'educational', 'domestic')?
  - which tasks were central?

- Was the group surprised at the responses?

- Given the wide range of tasks a mother needs to do, the skills required, and conditions of service, why do we do it?

- How could women use the skills they have developed through being a mother as the basis of acknowledging existing skills if planning to return to paid employment, or listing them in job applications?

ACTIVITY 7.7

Choosing to be a mother

Aim

To clarify what 'choice' means in becoming a mother.

Materials

Flipchart, pens.

Method

1 In pairs, ask women to discuss:

- whether they have positively chosen to have children;

- whether they got pregnant intentionally;

- whether they have decided to have children but have been unable to (either because of infertility or lack of opportunity); or

- whether they have made a positive choice not to have children.

2 Feed back to the large group and discuss.

Discussion points

- For women who have positively chosen to be a mother, what did they base that choice on (e.g. expected of women/makes a relationship with partner better/wanted to give partner a child/wanted something to love/thought they'd enjoy it/pressure from family)?

- For women who have become pregnant unintentionally, how did they feel about becoming mothers?

- For women who have decided to have children, but for some reason have not been able to, how do they feel about not being mothers? How do they feel others view them?

- For women who have positively chosen not to be a mother, what did they base that choice on (e.g. lack of money/didn't want to do it alone/don't like children/career takes precedence/not right at this time/partner doesn't want children)? How do they feel others view them?

Note for tutor

It may be painful for some women to do this activity, and you need to be sensitive to women's needs. Stress that women should only share what they feel comfortable with.

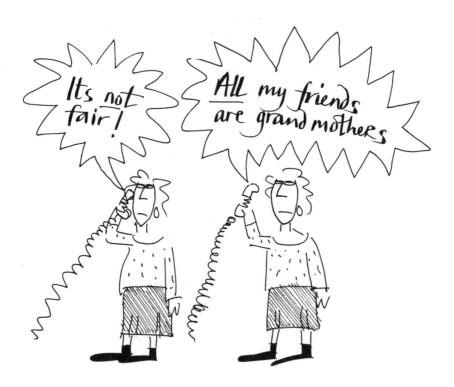

ACTIVITY 7.8

Ways of becoming a mother

Aim

- To consider whether motherhood is a biological or social concept.

Materials

Flipchart, pens; a copy of Information Sheet 7.2 *Reproductive technology* for each woman.

Method:

1 In the large group, brainstorm all the possible ways of becoming a mother, for example:

- sexual intercourse with a fertile male;

- self-insemination;

- reproductive technology (AID, IVF/GIFT);

- surrogacy;

- fostering; and

- adoption.

2 In the large group, discuss the different methods, and their acceptability to individuals in the group.

3 Give out the information sheet.

Discussion points

- Why do some of us feel comfortable about some methods of becoming a mother, and not about other methods?

  Some women may feel they would only consider having children through sexual intercourse within a heterosexual couple. Others may feel prepared, if necessary, to achieve pregnancy using sperm other than their partner's. Others still would be prepared to use medical intervention to have a child not necessarily genetically 'theirs'. Some single women may take a pragmatic view and be happy about using AID, others may feel that however much they wanted children, motherhood would have to take place within a heterosexual couple.

  What influences our views on what is acceptable to us?

- Is motherhood a biological or social concept? That is, are we a mother as a result of physically going through pregnancy and giving birth, or because we rear babies through childhood to adulthood?

- What anxieties do women have about reproductive technology, and why?

- Do all women have the opportunity to have children if they want:
  - married women?
  - single women?
  - young women (under 16)?
  - older women (over 40)?
  - lesbian women?
  - women with a physical disability?
  - women with learning difficulties?

Why? Why not?

ACTIVITY *7.9*

Fit to be a mother

Aims

- To enable women to consider who in our society is encouraged to be a mother.

- To promote discussion on whether or not all women should be able to have children if they wish.

Materials

A copy of Worksheet 7.2 *Fit to be a mother* for the tutor, two (A4) sheets of paper for each woman, markers, sellotape. Enough room for women to stand in one line.

Method

1 From the list of categories below, write one category on each of two A4 sheets.

Married women, single women, young women (under 16), older women (over 40), lesbians, Black women, women with physical disabilities, women with learning difficulties. If there are more than eight women in the group, devise more categories e.g. married with learning difficulties, older lesbians.

2 Give each woman her two sheets, and ask her to attach them to her front and back with sellotape.

3 Ask the women to stand in a long line, all facing you.

4 Read out questions from the worksheet, and for each question, ask women to step forward if the category they are wearing is appropriate.

5 After women have stepped forward, ask others if they agree.

6 Move on to the next question, until all have been dealt with.

7 In the large group, discuss issues raised.

Discussion points

- It may have been difficult for women to decide in some instances whether or not to take a step forward. Some questions provoke a clearcut response, others are not so straightforward.

- Women often fit into more than one category, which makes answers more complex.

- Are there certain categories of women who are encouraged to be mothers? Are some actively discouraged? Why should this be so?

- Should all women be able to be mothers if they wish?

ACTIVITY *7.10*

Coping with feeling angry

Aim

- To help women focus on an aspect of their child's behaviour which makes them angry, and share how best to deal with it.

Materials

A copy of Worksheet 7.3 *Coping with feeling angry* for each woman. A sheet of flipchart paper with the diagram from the worksheet drawn on, markers.

Method

1 Give the worksheet to each woman. Ask her to think of a current behaviour exhibited by one of her children which makes her angry. Fill in the worksheet clockwise. Women may want to pair up to prompt each other.

2 Each woman reads out her worksheet. The tutor fills in each woman's responses in turn on the flipchart.

3 As each woman gives her responses, the rest of the group offer suggestions of what they might do in these circumstances.

Discussion points

- If women do not have children themselves, they may want to think about ways in which other people's children make them feel angry.

- Are there common behaviours which make women angry?

- Do women deal with these differently?

- Do the ages of our children make any difference? Do we get angry over different things depending upon whether our children are younger, or teenagers?

- How could we deal with the anger in future?

Source: adapted from *Women learning together*, Salford Women's Education Forum.

ACTIVITY *7.11*

Coping with children

Aims

- To stimulate discussion about some important issues for parents.

- To explore a range of possible ways of coping with children.

Materials

A copy of Worksheet 7.4 *Coping with children – case studies* for each woman; flipchart, markers.

Method

1 Introduce the activity making it clear you are not expecting 'the answer' to each problem to emerge.

2 Use the case studies and talking points on the worksheet for discussion in the large group or smaller groups.

Option: you could ask women to select the particular case studies they wish to discuss.

3 Begin to make a list of advice and helping agencies or support groups as suggestions arise from discussion.

Discussion points

- Often it is assumed that women are 'natural' mothers rather than having to learn. How do we learn to be a mother?

- How does having children affect our relationships – with our partner, parents and friends?

- Why is it hard to ask for help over problems with our children?

- What help is available in our area?

ACTIVITY *7.12*

My relationship with my children

Aims

- To explore the generation gaps between parents and children.

- To consider the development of children within the family.

- To consider the possible clash of cultures between family and wider society.

Materials

The following prompt questions written up on a flipchart.

- How much time do you spend with your children out of school?

- How much affection, cuddling, touching do you share with your children?

- How much time do you spend talking with your children?

- How do you relate to your child if s/he faces racism and a clash of cultures in school?

Method

1 In pairs, ask women to discuss the questions on the flipchart.

2 In the large group, discuss and share experiences.

Discussion points

- How difficult is it to achieve 'quality' time with our children? What might prevent us?

- Are our children faced with a clash between family values and those within wider society? How are our own values challenged by our children growing up in the West?

- How can we help our children if they are confronted with racism outside the home?

- If we live in an extended family, how do we cope with pressures from the rest of the family, or relations in our home country, about ways of raising our children?

ACTIVITY *7.13*

Occupying children

Aims

- To consider the positive development of children within the family.

- To explore outside influences that can create barriers within family structures.

Materials

A copy of Worksheet 7.5 *Occupying children* for each woman; pens.

Method

1 Give each woman a worksheet.

2 In small groups, ask women to think about how they keep their children occupied at home.

3 List the activities on a worksheet according to whether they see them as positive or negative for their child's development.

4 In the large group, discuss issues raised.

Discussion points

- Do we sometimes arrange activities for our children that are to suit *us* rather than to benefit our children? If so, why might we do this?

- Do we sometimes arrange activities for our children because they wish to do them, in spite of our belief that they are not particularly good for the child? Might this involve a clash with traditional family values?

- Do we change our attitude to enable us to relate to our children growing up in the West?

ACTIVITY *7.14*

Older children and change

Aim

- To explore how the role of mother might change as children get older.

Materials

Paper, pens, a flipchart with the following headings written on:

Think about the role of a mother, and what changes and stays the same between the ages of 3 and 16?

Stays the same	**Changes**

Method

1 In small groups, discuss the question on the flipchart, and make lists of things that change, and things that stay the same.

2 Feed back to the large group.

Discussion points

Some things that do not change are the need for love, emotional support, food and clothes, but the form of some things change, for example:

- children are always expensive (initially for equipment like prams and cots, later on for fashionable clothes);
- you protect them always, but in a different way as they get older;
- you still need to be there for them emotionally as they get older, but the need is a different one;
- friendship is always there, but it changes;
- children always take up time, but for different reasons as they get older.

Other things may change more:

- swapping of roles (they can take care of you);
- they go out more (but they give you no free time/space);
- they question you;
- they might contribute to the household tasks; and
- the way you discipline them changes.

ACTIVITY *7.15*

Coping with young teenagers

Aims

- To raise some of the issues in living with and parenting young teenagers.

- To discuss options for dealing with some of the difficulties and dilemmas.

Materials

A copy of Worksheet 7.6 *Coping with young teenagers – case studies* for each woman; pens.

Method

1 Divide into small groups, and share out the case studies between groups. Discuss them in the small groups.

2 In the large group, feed back the main points about each case study.

ACTIVITY *7.16*

Motherhood – visions of the future

Aims

- To encourage reflection about the long term changes that might make motherhood more attractive and fulfilling.

- To produce a visual representation of the future to share with other women.

Materials

Flipchart, markers, flipchart paper, women's magazines, glue, scissors, coloured pens, crayons, blutack.

Method

1 Write the following on a flipchart:
Imagine a time in the future – and it's a really good time for women. No

money problems, good health services, good public services. What would life be like for mothers and children? Would more women choose to have children? Where would you be? What choices would you have?

2 Divide women into small groups. Each small group is given sheet(s) of flipchart paper. Ask each group to use the materials available to produce a picture or collage of their future vision. Stress that the activity is to promote discussion, and that you are not looking for works of art!

3 Put the flipcharts on the wall, and encourage women to look at the other groups' collages.

4 In the large group, discuss similarities and differences between the artwork.

Discussion points

- What similarities and differences did the visions have?

- Was it difficult to 'let go' and fantasise like that? If so, why might this be so?

- How can we move towards making our visions/fantasies a reality?

WORKSHEET *7.1*

Motherhood then and now

Group 1

Read the following extracts. Discuss what motherhood was like in our grand-mothers' days and list the difficulties and hardships.

Utterly overdone

When he was six years old, I had my fifth baby, and had also a miscarriage, and then I went on strike. My life was not worth living at this rate, as my husband was only a working man, out of work when wet or bad weather, and also in times of depression. I had all my own household work to do, washing, mending, making clothes, baking, cooking and everything else.

In those six years I never knew what it was to have a proper night's sleep, for if I had not a baby on the breast I was pregnant, and how could you expect children to be healthy, as I always seemed to be tired. If I sat down, I very often fell asleep through the day.

I knew very little about feeding children; when they cried, I gave them the breast. If I had known then what I know now, perhaps my children would have been living. I was ignorant and had to suffer severely for it, for it nearly cost me my life, and also those of my children.[1]

A miserable experience

I am really not a delicate woman, but having a large family, and so fast, pulled me down very much. I used to suffer very much with bad legs; and my husband was laid out of work most winters, so I had a great deal of poverty to deal with.

Nearly all my children were delicate, and being badly off, very often I could not get or do what I would like to for them. I lost four out of ten, and had a very great difficulty in rearing some of the others. They were nearly all two years before they ran; my eldest girl was three years before she ran; I never thought she could live, but, thank God, she has lived, and is nearly twenty-two. If something could be done for poor women with large families, I think it would be a good thing; for a

▷

[1] Source: Reprinted with permission from Llewellyn Davies, Margaret (ed.), *Maternity: Letters from Working Women*, Virago publishers.

▷ 7.1 cont.

woman's life is not much when she is in poverty and got sickly children, and never knows what an hour's liberty is. It is keep on work with no rest days, and not much nights very often.[1]

Group 2

You young mothers have it easy nowadays, what with your smaller families, more money, washing machines and playgroups.

But is it really easier being a mother today?

Discuss what it is like being a mother today and list some of the problems and difficulties.

[1] Source: As previous page.

WORKSHEET 7.2

Fit to be a mother

Read out each question in turn and allow women to respond.

- Who is encouraged to use contraception?
- Who is encouraged to have children?
- Who is encouraged to terminate a pregnancy?
- Who has access to infertility treatment:
  - AID?
  - IVF/GIFT?
- Who is encouraged to foster children?
- Who is encouraged to adopt children?

WORKSHEET *7.3*

Coping with feeling angry

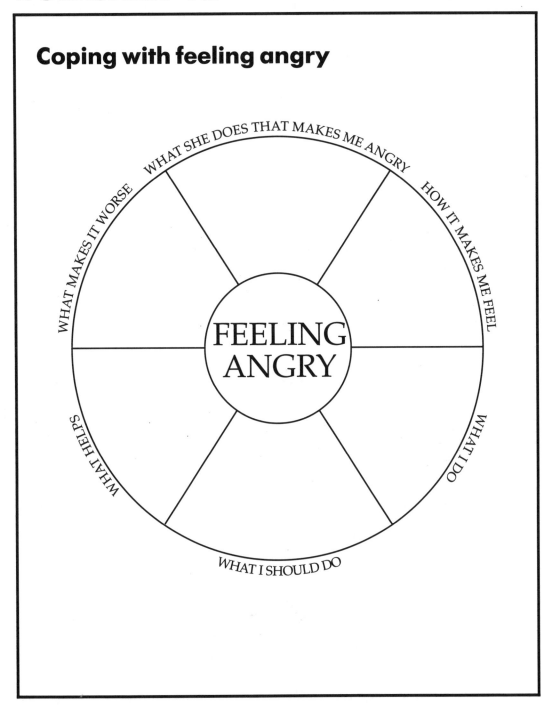

WORKSHEET 7.4

Coping with children – case studies

1 Linda is a young mother with her first baby, Andrew. She does not feel very confident about looking after him as she has had very little experience of babies before he was born. Andrew is two months old and cries a lot. Linda is getting depressed and anxious. The doctor says it's just colic and Andrew will grow out of it in a month or two. How can Linda cope now?

   - How can Linda become more confident as a mother?
   - Is there anywhere she could meet other mothers, or get practical help?

2 Katy is four and a lively and wilful child. She seems to do the opposite to what her parents, Jill and Paul ask her to do. Jill thinks Katy is highly strung, perhaps upset by their recent move of house, and needs extra love and attention. Paul says Katy is naughty and they should be stricter with her. How can they improve the situation?

   - What is 'naughty' behaviour in a small child?
   - How are disagreements between parents (or relatives) about behaviour sorted out?

3 Firdos has what she assumes are the usual tantrum problems with her two-year-old, Fatima. She can cope at home, but if they are out other people start making comments and telling her what she should do, e.g. 'That child needs a good smacking' or 'Poor little thing'. Firdos is very confused by this and is losing confidence in her own judgement.

   - How can we cope with tantrums?
   - What kind of behaviour do we expect of our children in public places?
   - What is the best way to respond to interference from passers-by or relatives?

4 Since Amrit started at secondary school her family have been very worried about her. They think her friends have a bad influence on her. She has begun to swear a lot, refuses to do her homework, and is often in minor scrapes at school. She has also begun to be very negative about family values.

   - How can the family deal with this situation?

5 There is a family in your street who you feel neglect their children. The children are left on their own sometimes in the evening and you and other neighbours often give them snacks as they always seem hungry.

   - What responsibility do we have for other people's children?

▷

▷ 7.4 cont.

- How can we watch out for and care for the children in our community?
- At what point does caring become interfering?

6 Nicola is 11 and grown-up for her age. She is an independent girl and there are constant arguments about when and where she can go, on her own or with her friends. Her friends' parents all seem to have different rules. Nicola's parents want to allow her some freedom and responsibility for herself, but know there are dangers for children out without adults. Where do they draw the line?

- How can we best protect our children from today's dangers?
- How do we decide how much freedom to give them as they grow older?

7 John is becoming a difficult teenager. His mother is a single parent, and is finding his behaviour difficult to cope with on her own. One of John's group of friends has been in trouble with the police for shop-lifting, and John's mother suspects they are all glue-sniffing.

- What can John's mother do?
- How can we help keep teenage children out of trouble?
- What could we do if we suspected our child was glue-sniffing/drinking/ taking drugs?

8 Jan and David have two daughters aged 15 and 13. Both are grown-up for their age and the elder one has a steady boyfriend. They worry about the possibility of her getting pregnant, but wonder if discussing contraceptives with her may encourage her to start having sex too young.

- How can we talk about emotions and morality with our children?
- When and what do we tell our children about sex, relationships, contraception and sexually transmitted diseases?

WORKSHEET 7.5

Occupying children

List the different activities you use to occupy your children at home, under the headings positive and negative.

Positive   Negative

WORKSHEET *7.6*

Coping with young teenagers – case studies

1 Your teenage daughter often comes home with lots of new things. Given the amount of pocket money she gets, you are puzzled as to how she can afford them. You are worried she may be shop-lifting. How might you tackle this?

2 Over the past few months your relationship with your partner has been rocky, but you think you have managed to hide this from the kids. It now seems that a separation will happen. What do you say to the kids?

3 You have lots of financial worries, debts are piling up. Should you tell your teenage children?

   • Is it appropriate to tell young teenagers about your own feelings and worries?
   • At what age are they capable of dealing with them?
   • How could it be done?
   • Do we deal with this situation differently with sons and with daughters?

4 Your 16-year-old chooses to stay up late watching TV in the sitting room, and gets up early in the morning to do homework. You are feeling you have no space or time to yourself. What can you do?

5 A group of teenagers wants to go away for the weekend camping. Your daughter says she is going too.

   • How does this make you feel?
   • How much control do you have in this situation?
   • How could you approach it?
   • Are there any differences between sons and daughters in this situation?

6 Although doing well at school, your son/daughter says s/he can't be bothered to take the exams, and wants to leave school as soon as possible. What do you do?

7 You have found an empty condom packet in your teenager's bedroom. You have not discussed any sexual relationship before.

   • What is your first reaction?
   • What do you do?
   • Does your reaction depend on whether your teenager is a boy or a girl?

8 You do not like the group of friends your teenager is going around with. You think your child is easily led, and you are worried that s/he will get up to no good. What can you do?

RESOURCES

For contact details of distributors and organisations listed here, see Chapter 11 *General resources*.

Publications

Apter, Terri, *Altered Loves: Mothers and Daughters During Adolescence* (1990), Harvester/Wheatsheaf.
Research into the sensitive relationship between women and their daughters.

Arcana, Judith, *Every Mother's Son – the Role of Mothers in the Making of Men* (1983), Anchor Press/Doubleday, New York, £5.95.
How can women challenge male stereotypes within their own families with their own sons? Is it possible to care for a son without reinforcing the image of women serving men? This book explores these issues and others which can arise from rearing a son within a deeply patriarchal society.

Arcana, Judith, *Our Mothers' Daughters* (1981), Women's Press, £5.95.
Explores the relationship between mothers and daughters through interviews with 120 women.

Arditti, Rita, Klein, Renate Duelli, and Minden, Shelley, *Test Tube Woman: What Future for Women* (1989), Pandora, £4.99.
A look at the negative aspects of reproductive technology.

Bedford Square Press/Gingerbread/Community Education Development Centre, *Just Me and the Kids: A Manual for Lone Parents* (1990), £4.95, ISBN 0 7199 1266 0.
Available from booksellers or from Plymbridge Distributors Ltd.
Written by and for lone parents, this handbook offers practical suggestions to help explore ideas and feelings about lone parenting. It questions the myth of the "typical" lone parent and is relevant to lone fathers and mothers, as well as teenagers, Black people, gay men, lesbians and disabled people.

Bethune, Helen, *Positive Parent Power: a Seven Part Programme* (1991), Thorsons, £6.99.
A guide to parenting: rights and responsibilities.

Bettelheim, Bruno, *A Good Enough Parent*, Pan Books.
A book about parenting which promotes the view that all parents do the best they can, and that parental self-awareness and understanding of a child's perspective are important qualities for parents.

Billingham, Kate, *Learning Together: a Health Resource Pack for Working with Groups* (1990), Nottingham Community Unit, price on application. Available from Nottingham Community Unit.
Designed for those in voluntary or statutory sectors wanting to work with parents

on issues of parenting and child health, and aimed at those new to the field as well as those with some experience. Includes materials on pregnancy and childbirth, young women, pregnant women, and childcare. Well written and clearly presented.

Birke, Lynda, Himmelweit, Susan and Vines, Gail, *Tomorrow's Child: Reproductive Technologies in the 90s* (1990), Virago, £9.99.
An analysis of the hazards and benefits of reproductive technology. Shows how women can take positive control of the processes.

Comport, M, *Surviving Motherhood* (1990), Ashgrove, £5.99.
A guide to parenting and dealing with post-natal depression.

Corea, G, *The Mother Machine* (1988), Women's Press, £6.95.
An early book considering reproductive technologies from artificial insemination to artificial wombs, written from a point of view that women have no control over the techniques (which can exploit them) and therefore there should be more safeguards for women.

Dworick, Stephanie and Grundberg, Sibyl (eds), *Why Children?* (1980), Women's Press, £2.75.
Women write about their choices of whether to have children.

Edwards, Harriet, *How Could You? Mothers Without Custody of Their Children* (1989), Crossing Press, £9.95.
Guide for mothers who have given up or lost custody of their children.

Fletcher, Gillian, *Get into Shape after Childbirth*, (1991), National Childbirth Trust, Ebury Press, £7.99, ISBN 0 85223 988 2. Available from booksellers or from National Childbirth Trust.
Provides an illustrated exercise plan to help women tone up after childbirth. It also offers advice on dealing with stress, healthy eating, weight control, and returning to work. Additional information is given for mothers with a variety of disabilities.

Gieve, Katherine (ed), *Balancing Acts: on Being a Mother* (1989), Virago, £5.99.
A personal experience of motherhood.

Hanscombe, Gillian and Forster, Jackie, *Rocking the Cradle: Lesbian Mothers – a Challenge in Family Living* (c1982), Peter Owen, £12.95.
A look at lesbian mothering, the joys and difficulties.

Health Education Authority, *Birth to Five – A Guide to the First Five Years of Being a Parent* (1989), ISBN 1 85448 070 7. Free to first time parents and distributed by Health Visitors. Can also be purchased from booksellers at £5.99.
Excellent book for parents about the first five years of life with babies and small children. Reassuring, practical advice and information. Easy to read, lots of cartoons and photographs, takes a multicultural approach.

Hey, V, Itzin, C, Saunders, L, and Speakman, M (eds), *Hidden Loss: Miscarriage and Ectopic Pregnancy* (1989), Women's Press, £5.95.
Includes what happens and why; medical viewpoints; women's own experiences;

process of grieving; future pregnancies; self-help possibilities; addresses/ resources/contacts.

Hodder, Elizabeth, *Stepfamilies Talking* (1989), Optima, £4.99.
Case studies and information about new families.

Jones, Maggie, *Infertility: Modern Treatments and the Issues they Raise* (1991), Piatkus, £6.99.
Information on causes, test and options. Looks at stresses and discusses emotional and ethical problems.

Klein, Renate (ed), *Infertility: Women Speak Out about their Experience of Reproductive Medicine* (1989), Pandora, £4.95.
International perspective on infertility.

Laskeer, Judith N, and Borg, S, *In Search of Parenthood: Coping with Infertility and High Tech Conception* (1989), Pandora, £5.99.
An in depth view of new technology, its effects, availability and what women go through emotionally, financially and otherwise when embarking on a high tech pregnancy.

Levene, Sarah, *Play it Safe – the Complete Guide to Child Accident Prevention* (1992), BBC, £3.99, ISBN 0 563 36300 2.
Written to accompany the BBC series. A comprehensive overview of accidents inside and outside the home. Written for parents but of interest to health workers too. Contains many practical suggestions for accident prevention.

Llewllyn Davies, Margaret, *Maternity: Letters from Working Women* (1978), Virago, £5.50.
First published in 1915. Letters from members of the Women's Co-operative Guild about their experiences of motherhood.

Macdonald, Fiona, *The Parents' Directory* (1989), Bedford Square Press, £6.95. ISBN 0 7199 1235 0. Available from bookshops or from Plymbridge Distributors Ltd.
Details of help, advice and information that voluntary organisations can give to parents. Divided into sections: family welfare, health, handicap, education and leisure, with contact lists.

Mencap, *Ordinary Everyday Families – Action for Families and Their Young Children with Special Needs, Disabilities and Learning Difficulties* (1990), Mencap London Division, £5. Available from: Under Fives Project, Mencap London Division.
Aimed at parents, professionals and policy-makers the report builds upon good practice and makes suggestions whereby everyone involved can be better supported and enabled to work in partnership.

McKeith, P, Phillipson R, and Rowe, A, *45 Cope Street. Young Mothers learning through Groupwork. An Evaluation Report* (1991), Nottingham Community Health.

Oakley, A, McPherson, A and Roberts, H, *Miscarriage* (1990), Penguin, £4.99.
Deals with not only physical realities – giving up-to-date information and medical detail – but also considers the emotional and psychological effects of one of the

commonest yet most hidden areas of women's reproductive experience. Based on case histories.

Open University (see Chapter 11 *General resources*) has a number of packs relating to parenting, including: *Living with Babies and Toddlers, Family Lifestyles, Childhood, The Pre-school Child, Women and Young Children, and Parents Talking.*

Pfeffer, N and Woollett, A, *The Experience of Infertility* (1983), Virago, £3.50.
Written by two women who have been through infertility investigations; provides a guide to sterility, subfertility and miscarriage, with the emphasis on women's emotional, sexual and physical response. Confronts the notion that infertility is assumed to be only a woman's problem.

Peck, Frances, *Handbook for Young Mothers* (1990), The Rainer Foundation, £4.95.
ISBN 09516498 09. Available from bookshops or the Rainer Foundation.
An attractive book, designed to meet the needs of teenage and young mothers. Lots of information, easy to read format, multicultural approach.

Phillips, Angela, *Until they are Five* (1989), Pandora.
A book for parents that recognises that there is no one 'right' way of caring for children. Full of humour and good sense.

Price, Jane, *Motherhood: What it Does to Your Mind* (1990), Pandora, £4.99.
A guide to the effects of motherhood, looking at sexuality, jealousy, guilt, post-natal depression and more.

Saffron, L, *Getting Pregnant Our Own Way: a Guide to Alternative Insemination* (1986), Women's Health, £5. Available from Women's Health.

Whitehead, M B, *A Mother's Story* (1990), Arrow Books, £3.99.
The story of the Baby M case – from the mother's point of view. Mary Beth Whitehead elected to become a surrogate mother for a price. When her daughter was born, she changed her mind. The consequences of her decision are described.

Videos

Help for Parents of Children with Special Needs (Bengali, Gujarati, Hindi, Punjabi, Urdu and English). There is also an accompanying booklet available in the same languages. English video £12; other languages £10; booklet 50p each. Available from AWAAZ.

Isobel's Baby: a Disabled Woman's Experience of Pregnancy and Early Motherhood. 42 minutes, £21 + VAT. Available from Arrowhead Productions.
Follows the experience of Isobel Ward who has multiple sclerosis. It features discussions with health professionals and with Isobel and her husband about their concerns, preparations and experiences.

My Mum Thinks She's Funny: An Introduction to Services for Parents with Young Children, 20 minutes. Hire £20 per week. Sale £40 to VOLCOF members or £50 to non-members. All prices include ten copies of the booklet, extra booklets £1 each. Available from VOLCOF.

ITV (Academy Television), *Surrogate Mothers* (undated), 25 minutes.
Women who have been surrogate mothers talk about their feelings.

ITV (Academy Television), *Who's your Mother?* (undated), 25 minutes.
A look at how reproductive technology is changing the way people look at making babies.

Organisations

Birthright
Produces information on gynaecological problems, healthy eating, infertility and more.

Child Abuse Studies Unit, The University of North London
Courses and conferences, research training and consultancy from a feminist perspective.

Child Poverty Action Group
Helps families on low income to get their full entitlement to welfare benefits. Produces publications.

Exploring Parenthood
National charity which brings together professionals and parents to discuss problems and pleasures of parenting. Adviceline, publications.

Gingerbread
Self-help organisation for lone parents. Has lists of local support groups.

Maternity Alliance
Multi-lingual information leaflets, newsletter, books and reports.

Meet-A-Mum Association (MAMA)
Aims to provide a network of care to help all mums and mums-to-be. Facilitates the setting up of local self-help groups to alleviate feelings of isolation, loneliness, and depression. Newsletter, starter pack, meetings and conferences.

Miscarriage Association
Information and support during and after miscarriage.

National Childbirth Trust
Publications, training and information on choice in pregnancy, childbirth and early parenthood.

National Childcare Campaign
Mass national childcare campaign around demand for flexible, free childcare facilities. Newsletter, leaflets, support and advice to campaigns.

National Council of One Parent Families
Information and training services for one-parent families.

Parent Network
National network of parent education and support groups to improve relationships between children and adults.

Parentline: Organisation for Parents Under Stress
Network of self-help groups in England, Scotland and Ireland for parents under stress. Has numbers of local groups.

Rights of Women
Information and advice to women on legal matters, particularly relating to parenting issues.

Single Parent Network
A multi-racial, anti-racist group of single parents working to improve the lives of one-parent families in Britain. Quarterly bulletin.

8 Older women's health

BACKGROUND INFORMATION

- How old is an older woman? There are many different definitions, for example the National Health Service defines two age groups of 60–74 years, and over 75 years; social services define older as over 65 years; the University of Third Age defines older as over 50 years. For the purposes of this book we are referring to women of 45 years and over.

- For most women, there is a huge age span between 45 years and the end of their life, and at different stages women may have different needs and interests over and above the differences between individuals. People, especially women, are living longer. Women are a disproportionately large percentage of the elderly population.

- Getting older is often seen as a 'problem' by authorities and professionals, and by society in general.

- Older women are subjected to ageism as well as sexism. Black women can be further disadvantaged through racism.

- Included in this chapter are activities of particular relevance to older women on the following themes:

  – definitions of older women;
  – advantages and disadvantages of growing older;
  – images of older women;
  – making the most of your time;
  – sexuality;
  – retirement;
  – coping with loss;
  – carers; and
  – celebration of older women.

- In addition to this chapter, all other chapters in the book may be of relevance and interest to older women.

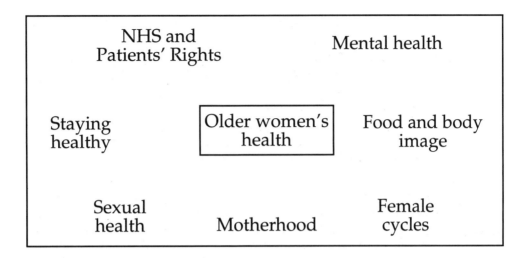

PRACTICAL POINTS

- Think about whether you are planning a single session or a course of several sessions on older women's health; and what age-group of women you are targeting.

- Older women's health courses may be difficult to recruit. When targeting older women, you will need to think about issues such as:

  - how and where you publicise the course;
  - what you call your course – because of some negative connotations to the word 'older', be creative with your title;
  - accessibility of venue;
  - needs of women with mobility impairments;
  - position of the toilets;
  - comfortable chairs;
  - acoustics of the room – some women may have hearing problems;
  - good lighting and reliable heating;
  - access to refreshments;
  - timing of the course;
  - carers allowance?
  - creche for grandchildren?

- Older women can bring many positive qualities to enhance a course:

  - lively minds;
  - acceptance of others;
  - support for each other;
  - a wealth of experience and skills; and
  - a willingness to develop in new directions.

- Some older women may not have had the benefit of much formal learning, so you may need to be sensitive to literacy issues.

- Some older women may have experienced learning methods such as group work, but others may be unused to the approach, and may be seeking an 'expert' who can provide solutions to problems. Older women may want lots of medical information. You will need to be clear about the aims of the group, and your role as a tutor. Also, be sensitive about the style you adopt: for example, some older women prefer to be referred to as 'ladies' rather than women.

- Carefully consider the methods you will use in your sessions and don't be too ambitious. Older women may appreciate the chance to get together and just talk (which can be fine), and may be reluctant to get on with the activity in hand. If there is resistance to splitting into small groups, start with pairs first, then gradually use small groups as appropriate. Methods using games may not be appreciated, and guided fantasies may be resisted. Methods involving a lot of reading or writing may be off-putting – questionnaires to tick may be better. Women may prefer to take a worksheet home to fill in and return completed the following session. Videos can be useful for stimulating discussion. Outside speakers on specific topics can be warmly received. Back-up information in the form of articles or leaflets to take home and read at leisure are often appreciated.

- Within a group of older women, there may be a large span of ages. Some activities may seem more appropriate for older age groups; but those at the 'younger' end of the scale may feel it useful to be thinking ahead.

- If the group seems to be coming up with lots of negative aspects of ageing, have positive prompts ready to redress the balance.

- Some topics and issues may be particularly sensitive, and need careful facilitation. Some older women may be less used to talking about sexuality, for example. Discussions around loss or bereavement may be threatening. While there are no 'neutral' topics in women's health, it may be better to start a course with topics such as 'food and healthy eating' or 'making the most of your time' until the group members know each other better and feel safer.

- If you are a younger tutor, you may need to think about how you could be received by older women in the group and how you feel about this. Older women will have more experience than you, and do you feel comfortable about challenging their responses?

INFORMATION SHEET *8.1*

Using outside speakers

At your first meeting with a group, it may be useful to find out what topics group members would like to cover. You could brainstorm this, or provide a list of topics for the group to choose from and add to. Having identified specialist topics, you may want to consider bringing in outside speakers, especially for those areas in which you feel you lack expertise. Many organisations and firms are willing to provide speakers. Some will do it as part of their job, others may need a small fee and/or expenses. Below are some suggestions of where to find speakers.

Before the session, you will need to discuss with the speaker details of your course generally, and what group members want from her session. Check any materials or equipment she might need. Some speakers may appreciate beforehand a list of questions which the group would like answering. It is useful to confirm arrangements with a speaker in writing. If a booking is being made for some time ahead, a reminder phone call just before the date is reassuring. Don't forget to send explicit details of how to find the venue. Have a member of the group available to welcome the speaker.

Popular topics

The following topics, popular in older women's health groups, may benefit from an outside speaker.

Medical Information	*Alternative Medicine*	*Social Issues*
osteoporosis	reflexology	carers
arthritis	osteopathy	welfare benefits
cancer	yoga and relaxation	retirement
hysterectomy	massage	education in later life
coronary heart disease	homeopathy	leisure/recreational
Alzheimer's disease		activities
incontinence		

▷

▷ 8.3 cont.

Finding your speakers

Many national organisations will have a local group in your area. Your local reference library, local volunteer bureau, or local Council for Voluntary Service may be able to provide you with a list (failing this, ask to look at the *Voluntary Agencies Directory* or the *Charities Digest*, which will give you national contact numbers (see Information Sheets 8.2 and 8.3 *Useful national organisations*).

- Your local *Health Promotion Department* may be able to provide speakers, information on where you might find speakers, and resources, e.g. videos and leaflets. Contact your Health Authority (from the phone book) and ask for the Health Promotion Department.

- *Health visitors or community nurses* may be willing to give talks on relevant topics – especially if they have a remit for older people. They may be found through the Community Unit of the local Health Authority, or attached to GP surgeries or health centres.

- *Well-women clinics* exist in many parts of the country. Their volunteers may be willing to come and talk to your group. Check in the phone book.

- The *social services department* of your local authority might be able to give you details of carers' groups, groups for older people, etc. The local authority *leisure and recreational department* may be a useful contact too. Check in the phone book.

- Your local *Community Health Council* should be able to advise you of contacts. Check in the phone book, or through your local Health Authority.

- Your local *Family Health Services Authority* may be able to advise you. Check in the phone book.

- *Voluntary organisations*
  - CRUSE may be able to supply a speaker on bereavement.
  - Age Concern may be able to provide a speaker, and help with leaflets.
  - Your Citizens' Advice Bureau will probably be able to provide a speaker on welfare rights relevant to older people (e.g. pensions, disablement allowance, and making a will).
  - MIND has local branches, which may be able to help with talks on depression, anxiety, tranquillisers, or issues such as 'care in the community' schemes.

- *Firms*
  - Body Shop will give a free demonstration and talk on aromatherapy (with specimens to test) and on make-up. Contact the manager of your local shop.
  - Scholl foot and leg care centres will provide a demonstration of chiropody and advice on shoe-fitting. This is free to groups who can visit their centres. Contact the manager of your local shop.

INFORMATION SHEET 8.2
Useful national organisations – general services

Organisation	Subjects	Local groups	Infor-mation	Helpline	Advice	Other
Age Concern (England) Astral House 1268 London Road London SW16 4ER 081 679 8000	Welfare rights Health Housing Money matters	✓	✓		✓	Produce free factsheets on a wide range of topics
Age Concern (Scotland) 54a Fountainbridge, Edinburgh EH3 9TT 031 228 5656						
Age Exchange 11 Blackheath Village, London SE3 9LA 081 318 9105	Theatrical group					Museum of 1920s/1930s free to the public Tours, mainly to sheltered accommodation and hospitals
Asian Women's Resource Centre 134 Minet Avenue London NW10 081 961 6549	Welfare rights Housing Domestic violence Developmental work Activities at the centre		✓		✓	Health worker available

△

△ 8.2 cont.

Organisation	Subjects	Local groups	Information	Helpline	Advice	Other
Bangladeshi Women's Association 91 Highbury Hill London N5 1SX 071 359 5836	Adult education classes Library		✓			Female doctor available
Black Women's Action 76 Elsted Street Walworth London SE17 1QT 071 708 1643	Welfare rights		About other organisations			
British Geriatrics Society 1 St Andrews Place Regents Park London NW1 4LB 071 935 4004	Professional association for the elderly		Factsheets			
Carers National Association 29 Chilworth Mews London W2 3RG 071 724 7776	Support for carers	✓	✓			Speakers Membership: £3.00 p.a. journal
Counsel and Care Twyman House 16 Bonny Street London NW1 9LR 071 485 1566	Advice and information on residential care			10.30 am– 3.00pm Mon–Thurs		

△

▷ 8.2 cont.

Organisation	Subjects	Local groups	Information	Helpline	Advice	Other
Cruse Cruse House 126 Sheen Road Richmond Surrey TW9 1UR 081 940 4818	Bereavement care	✓			Free counselling through local branches	
Elderly Accommodation Council 46a Chiswick High Road London W4 1SZ 081 995 8320 081 742 1182	Information on nursing homes, residential homes, sheltered accommodation		✓			
Help the Aged 16–18 St James Walk London EC1R 0BE 071 253 0253	Fundraising charity provides: daycentres, minibuses, hospices, education, information	Local fundraisers	✓	Senior Line 0800 289404		
Keep Fit Association Francis House Francis Street London SW1P 1DE 071 233 8898	Keep fit classes (all ages)	✓				

© Health Education Authority, 1993

△ 8.2 cont.

Organisation	Subjects	Local groups	Information	Helpline	Advice	Other
Law Centres Federation Duchess House 18–19 Warren Street London W1P 5DB 071 387 8570	Legal advice		✓			Keeps a list of local law centres
Midlifestyle Birmingham Settlement 318 Summer Lane Birmingham B19 3RL 021 359 2113	Run courses of 8–12 weeks on assertiveness etc.		✓			Newsletter
National Association of Widows (NAW) 54–57 Allison Street Digbeth Birmingham B5 5TH 021 643 8348	Social support	✓	✓		✓	Membership £5.00 p.a. Newsletter
National Council for the Divorced and Separated (address for correspondence:) 13 High Street Little Shelford Cambs CB2 5ES 0533 700 595	Social support	✓			✓	A voluntary body, so the correspondence address may change annually.

△ 8.2 cont.

Organisation	Subjects	Local groups	Infor-mation	Helpline	Advice	Other
National Federation of Retirement Pensions Association Melling House 14 St Peter Street Blackburn BB2 2HD 0254 52606	Welfare rights Social support	✓	✓		✓	Membership £6 p.a. Newspaper *Pensioners Voice*
Occupational Pensions Advisory Service 11 Belgrave Road London SW1V 1RB 071 233 8080	Pension advice	Local advisors (contact central office)			✓	
Older Feminists Network c/o 54 Gordon Road London N3 1EP 081 346 1900	Discussion group (London based)					Newsletter £5 p.a.
Pre-Retirement Association (PRA) Nodus Centre University Campus Guildford Surrey GU2 5RX 0483 39390	Preparation for retirement	Local associations	✓			Run training courses throughout the country

△

△ 8.2 cont.

Organisation	Subjects	Local groups	Information	Helpline	Advice	Other
Relate Herbert Gray College Little Church Street Rugby Warwickshire CV21 3AP 0788 573241	Relationship counselling	Relate centres (in local telephone directory)				
Research into Ageing 49 Queen Victoria Street London EC4N 4SA 071 236 4365	Medical research on age-related ailments	Some	✓		✓	Speakers
Shelter 88 Old Street London EC1V 8HU 071 253 0202	Housing	Regional housing aid centres	✓	in London 6pm–9am 0800 446 441	At local centres	
Society of Pension Consultants Ludgate House Ludgate Circus London EC4 071 353 1688	Pension advice	Contact central office for local consultant				
Wireless for the Bedridden 159a High Street Hornchurch Essex RM11 3YB 0708 621101	Radios and TVs for the housebound					Write for application form – only available for those in financial need (proof of this is necessary)

© Health Education Authority, 1993

△

△ 8.2 cont.

Organisation	Subjects	Local groups	Information	Helpline	Advice	Other
Women's Health (formerly Women's Health and Reproductive Rights Information Centre WHRRIC) 52–54 Featherstone Street London EC1Y 8RT 071 251 6580	Health		✓	Phones open Mon, Wed, Thurs, Fri 11am–5pm		
Women's Nutritional Advisory Service (WNAS) PO Box 268 Hove East Sussex BN3 1RW 0273 771366	Menopause advisory service				By phone	Clinics in London and Hove. Sponsor programme if on low income – send s.a.e.
Women's Therapy Centre 6–9 Manor Gardens London N7 6LA 071 263 6200	Mental and emotional health			2–4.30pm		

INFORMATION SHEET 8.3
Useful national organisations – specific services

Organisation	Subjects	Local groups	Infor-mation	Helpline	Advice	Other
Alzheimer's Disease Society 158/160 Balham High Road London SW12 9BN 081 675 6557/8/9	Alzheimer's Disease	✓	✓		✓	
Arthritis and Rheumatism Council Copeman House St Mary's Court St Mary's Gate Chesterfield Derbyshire S41 7TD 0246 558033	Arthritis and rheumatism		✓			
Arthritis Care 6 Grosvenor Crescent London SW1X 7ER 071 235 0902	Arthritis	✓	✓		✓	Holiday section Counsellors Welfare advice Membership £3 p.a. Newsletter
Asthma Research Council National Asthma Campaign 300 Upper Street London N1 2XX 071 226 2260	Asthma	✓	✓	Mon–Fri 1–9pm 0345 010203	✓	Newsletter £5 p.a.

△ 8.3 cont.

Organisation	Subjects	Local groups	Information	Helpline	Advice	Other
Back Pain Association 31–33 Park Road Teddington Middlesex TW11 0AB 081 977 5474	Back pain	✓	✓			
Breast Care and Mastectomy Association of Great Britain 15–19 Britten Street London SW3 3TZ 071 867 1103	Breast care and mastectomy	Cancer Link has local groups (see below)	✓	✓	✓	Speakers, videos, prostheses
Bristol Cancer Help Centre Grove House Cornwallis Grove Clifton Bristol BS8 4PG 0272 743216	Cancer	✓	✓		✓	
British Association of Cancer United Patients (BACUP) 121/123 Charterhouse Street London EC1M 6AA 071 608 1785	Cancer	✓	Resource directory 071 608 1661 (within London) 0800 181199 (outside London)	Counselling service in London only 071 608 1038		Local speakers

△ 8.3 cont.

Organisation	Subjects	Local groups	Infor-mation	Helpline	Advice	Other
British Colostomy Association 15 Station Road Reading Berkshire RG1 1LG 0734 391537	Colostomy	Area organisers work under head office and with health care teams	✓			
British Diabetic Association 10 Queen Anne Street London W1M 0BD 071 323 1531	Diabetes	✓	✓		✓	Local speakers
British Heart Foundation 14 Fitzhardinge Street London W1H 4DH 071 935 0185	Heart disease	✓	✓			Videos for hire Speakers
British Migraine Association 178a High Road Weybridge Surrey KT14 7ED 09323 52468	Migraine	Very few	✓		By phone	£3 p.a. for newsletter
Cancer Link 17 Britannia Street London WC1X 9JN 071 833 2451	Cancer	✓	✓			Offer training, speakers

△

△ 8.3 cont.

Organisation	Subjects	Local groups	Information	Helpline	Advice	Other
Cancer Link (Scotland) 9 Castle Terrace Edinburgh EH1 2DP 031 228 5557	Cancer	✓	✓			Offer training, speakers
Council for Complementary and Alternative Medicine 179 Gloucester Place London NW1 6DX 071 724 9103	Alternative medicine					Provides list of practitioners Send s.a.e. and 50p
Council for Involuntary Tranquilliser Addiction Cavendish House Brighton Road Liverpool L22 5NQ 051 949 0102	Tranquilliser addiction	✓	✓	✓	✓	Speakers
Food and Chemical Allergy Association 27 Ferringham Lane Ferring by Sea West Sussex BN12 5NB 0903 694205	Allergies		Books			Send s.a.e. and £2.00 for booklet *Understanding Allergies*

© Health Education Authority, 1993

△

△ 8.3 cont.

Organisation	Subjects	Local groups	Information	Helpline	Advice	Other
Ileostomy Association Amblehurst House Black Scotch Lane Mansfield Notts NG18 4DF 0623 28099	Ileostomy	√	Publish a journal		√	Membership £8 p.a. – journal quarterly
Migraine Trust 45 Great Ormond Street London WC1N 3DH 071 278 2676	Migraine	Very few	√	√	At specialist clinics	£10 p.a. for newsletter
MIND, National Association for Mental Health 22 Harley Street London W1N 2ED 071 637 0741	Mental health	√	√			
Multiple Sclerosis Society 25 Effie Road Fulham London SW6 1EE 071 736 6267	Multiple sclerosis	√	√	Welfare Advice 10am–5pm Mon–Fri 071 371 8000	√	Volunteer speakers

△

△

△ 8.3 cont.

Organisation	Subjects	Local groups	Information	Helpline	Advice	Other
Myalgic Encephalomyelitis (ME) Association Stanhope House High Street Stanford le Hope Essex SS17 0HA 0375 642466	ME	Will put people in touch when they join the association	✓	Ring central office 2–4pm advice line 7–10pm listening ear	✓	Speakers Membership £12 p.a. Quarterly newsletter
National Institute of Medical Herbalists 0392 426 022	Herbalism		✓			List of practitioners
National Osteoporosis Society PO Box 10 1 Riverside Radstock Bath, Avon BA3 3YB 0761 432472	Osteoporosis	✓	✓		✓	Send A4 s.a.e. for information
Pain Research Institute Rice Lane Walton Liverpool Merseyside L9 1AE 051 523 1486	Pain	Pain clinics – ask GP	✓	Self-help in pain, Walton Hospital Liverpool 051 525 3611	At the pain clinics	Speakers. Send A4 s.a.e. for information
Parkinson's Disease Society 22 Upper Woburn Place London WC1H 0RA 071 383 3513	Parkinson's disease	✓	✓	10am–12 noon, 2–4pm Tues & Thurs	Welfare Department	

△ 8.3 cont.

Organisation	Subjects	Local groups	Information	Helpline	Advice	Other
Stroke Association CHSA House Whitecross Street London EC1Y 8JJ 071 490 7999	Stroke illness – research and rehabilitation	✓	✓		Advisory service in London office and regional centres	Family support scheme
Tinnitus Association Royal National Institute for the Deaf 105 Gower Street London WC1E 6AH 071 387 8033	Tinnitus Ménières disease	✓	✓	0345 090210 (Voice/ Minicom) 10am–3pm, then answer-phone	✓	
Women's Alcohol Centre 66a Drayton Park London N5 1ND 071 226 4581	Alcohol problems		✓	✓	✓	Counselling at the centre in Islington. Self-referrals accepted Creche available Support for children
Women's Nationwide Cancer Control Campaign Suna House 128–130 Curtain Road London EC2 3AR 071 729 4688	Cancer		Information on breast-screening 071 729 4915 cervical screening 071 729 5061	071 729 2229		Information leaflets in 9 languages 5 mobile screening units

INFORMATION SHEET 8.4
Factors which may affect sexuality

Factors	*Possible effects*	*Possible action*
Social		
• Social beliefs about sexuality and ageing	• Live the myths of old age	• Information/support
• Women's own beliefs	• Feel asexual, unattractive	• Challenge negative attitudes and stereotypes
• Family, friends' attitudes	• Rejection, disinterest	• Explore issues with friends and partner
• Lack of available partners	• Self-esteem, confidence decreases	• Define and enjoy own sexuality
• Partner is uncooperative, ill, has a disability	• Anger, fear, loneliness	• Improve communication, explore possibilities
Health problems		
• Surgery	• Emotional anxiety, fear of rejection, feel less attractive	• Information about effects on sexuality and changes needed to accommodate them
• Drugs/alcohol	• Sexual desire decreases	• Information about effects on sexuality and changes needed to accommodate them
• Chronic fatigue	• Sexual desire decreases	• Information about effects on sexuality and changes needed to accommodate them
• Arthritis	• Joint pain, physical limitations	• Co-operation from partner
• Heart disease	• Fear of another attack	• Information/co-operation from partner
• Urinary incontinence	• Anxiety, fear of rejection	• Pelvic floor exercises

△ 8.4 cont.

Factors

Factors	Possible effects	Possible action
Health problems		
• Body changes	• Loss of fatty tissue in breasts, hips and genital area	• Self-acceptance, talk to partner, friends
	• Thinning of pubic hair	• Redefining meaning of beauty
	• Weight increase	• Diet and exercise
		• Positively take care of yourself
Physical changes		
• Vaginal lubrication decrease	• Possibility of painful penetrative sex	• Use extra lubrication
		• Talk to partner if relevant
• Thinning of vaginal walls	• Risk of vaginitis and infection increases	• Acknowledge change has occurred
		• Pelvic floor exercises
• Vagina becomes shorter and narrower		• Take more time with sexual activity
• Size of clitoral hood decreases		• Consider complementary therapies
• Response to sexual stimulation decreases	• Worry about sexuality and performance	• Acknowledge change
• Shorter duration of orgasm		• Talk about it
• Intensity of desire and frequency of sexual activity decreases		• Take more time with non-genital sexual expression

ACTIVITY *8.1*

Who is an older woman? 1

Aims

- To encourage discussion about relative ages.

- To illustrate that the term 'older woman' has different definitions depending upon context.

Materials

Pens, post-its, bag, flipchart paper.

Method

1 Ask each woman to write down her own definition of the term 'older woman' on a post-it. Stress that what she writes will be shared with the group anonymously.

2 Fold post-its and put into a bag. Women each pick one exchanging it for another if they pick their own.

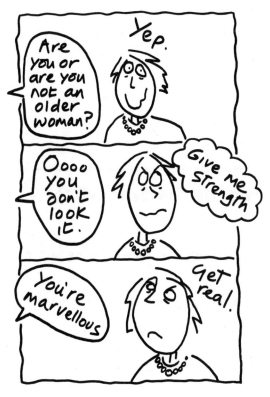

3 Each woman reads from her post-it.

4 Group uses post-its to make an age continuum on flipchart paper. Note span of ages and other specific details such as having experienced the menopause or children left home.

5 Discuss issues raised.

Discussion points

- How different are these definitions? Is this due to ages of women in the group?

- Are there common threads?

- Are groupings related to life events such as menopause or children leaving home or are they age related?

- Overall are the definitions positive or negative? If a lot of them are negative it may be useful to follow this activity with Activity 8.6 *Issues for older women*.

Notes for tutor

- Responses will vary depending upon ages of women in the group. For example, women in their mid-40s may use retirement as the definition for being older; women 60+ may focus upon being 'old and frail'.

- It may be useful to provide some background information on the changes in life expectancy for women, in order to put discussions about what is and isn't 'older' into perspective.

ACTIVITY *8.2*

Who is an older woman? 2

Aim

- To explore what defines a woman as being 'older'.

Materials

Copies of Worksheet 8.1 *Who is an older woman?* for each woman; pens, flipchart paper, markers.

Method

1 Ask women to go through the worksheet in pairs or small groups noting responses.

2 Report back to the large group, flipcharting responses, and discuss.

Discussion points

- How alike are the group's ideas?

- How important is age compared to other aspects such as experience or attitudes? Is there a close fit?

Note for tutors

- Some older women may not be interested in this activity (use it with a group you know and who you feel will be receptive to it).

- It may be useful to use this activity to show there is no need for a definition since this may merely reinforce stereotypes and ageist attitudes.

ACTIVITY *8.3*

What is a 'senior citizen'?

Aims

- To focus older women on their ability to adapt to change in the past.

- To consider changes which they may face in the future.

Materials

A copy of Worksheet 8.2 *What is a 'senior citizen'?* for each woman; flipchart, markers.

Method

1 Give each woman a copy of the worksheet, and read them individually, or as a group.

2 Discuss issues raised.

3 Ask women to talk about the kind of changes they themselves have experienced (e.g. technological, social, economic, political) and flipchart responses.

4 Flipchart possible changes which they feel might face them in the future, and discuss how they might adapt to these (in the light of their earlier experiences of change).

Discussion points
- Highlight how women have adapted positively to changes in the past, and how they can draw on these earlier experiences of dealing with change?

- The statutory definition of 'senior citizen' for women is age 60 or over (although they may see themselves merely as 'recycled teenagers'!). What are the implications in terms of pensions; national insurance; divorce/death of spouse; changes in married women's contributions and husbands' contributions?

ACTIVITY 8.4

Lifeline

Aim
- To stimulate thought and discussion about ageing and life changes.

Materials

A copy of Worksheet 8.3 *Lifeline* for each woman; different coloured pens.

Method

1 Individually or in pairs, fill in the worksheet.

2 Discuss in the large group.

Discussion points
- Are there similarities in women's life changes?

- Which life changes do women feel have been most significant for them personally?

- How do women feel about the changes in the future which they have indicated on their lifeline?

- Which future changes do women see as positive? Why is this?

- Which future changes do women envisage will be negative? Why should this be?

ACTIVITY *8.5*

Benefits and challenges of becoming older

Aim
- To provide the opportunity to evaluate the types of changes which happen to women as a result of becoming older.

Materials
Prompt questions (see below) written up on a flipchart, or on paper for each small group; paper and pens, flipchart paper, markers.

Method
1 In small groups, women work through the prompt questions, noting responses.

2 In the large group, feed back and flipchart, grouping responses under the headings of 'personal factors' and 'social factors'. Discuss.

Prompt questions
- What are the benefits of being an older woman?

- What do you think are the particular challenges associated with being an older woman?

Discussion points
- It is useful to group responses into personal factors such as health, changing relationships, and social factors such as economics, status.

- How much control can women have in their lives?

- What is the balance between the challenges and the opportunities? How can women turn challenges into opportunities?

ACTIVITY *8.6*

Issues for older women

Aim
- To enable women to consider physical, intellectual, emotional, spiritual and social aspects of ageing.

Materials

A copy of Worksheet 8.4 *Issues for older women ('SLOT')* for each woman; pens.

Method

1 Working in small groups; give each woman a worksheet, and ask them to consider what *strengths* they have as older women, what *opportunities* do they foresee, what might be the *limitations* and *threats* as they get older?

2 Feed back to the large group and flipchart, identifying common themes.

3 Discuss ways of dealing with limitations and threats.

Discussion points

Strengths might include:

- coping and survival skills;
- breadth of skills and experience;
- previous experience of change;
- adaptability;
- time management skills;
- friendships and supportive networks;
- good health;
- physical endurance; and
- experience of relationships.

Opportunities might include:

- time;
- concessions (travel/social activities/educational opportunities);
- social activities, e.g. pensioners' clubs;
- being yourself, not having to conform;
- new relationships;
- grandchildren;
- adult education;
- hobbies;
- voluntary work;
- being able to please yourself about what to spend time on; and

- divorce from an estranged partner (including feeling able to divorce once children have left home).

Limitations might include:

- lack of money;
- ill-health;
- less mobility;
- loneliness; and
- not being accepted as a person in your own right.

Threats might include:

- poverty;
- illness;
- loss of a loved one;
- ageism;
- sexism;
- racism;
- becoming dependent on others;
- loss of a home base; and
- being perceived as incapable of making decisions for yourself and others.

ACTIVITY *8.7*

Images of older women

Aims

- To discuss the feelings and attitudes we have about ageing.
- To promote a positive image of older women.

Materials

Copies of Worksheets 8.5 and 8.6 *Images of older women 1* and *2* for each woman; pens.

Method

1 In small groups, read through the case study on Worksheet 8.5, discuss the questions and note responses.

2 In the large group, share findings.

3 Read out the poem *Warning* by Jenny Joseph on Worksheet 8.6, and discuss the questions together.

Discussion point

For a group with a big span of ages, what are the similarities and differences about how women want to look, and the images presented.

Variation: It might be useful to follow this up by making a collage of positive images of older women by collecting pictures from magazines, health leaflets and other sources.

ACTIVITY *8.8*

Making the most of your time 1

Aim

- To explore possible ways of reducing isolation, boredom and gaining confidence and self-esteem.

Materials

Post-its, flipchart paper, pens, blutack.

Method

1 Give each woman several post-its and ask them to write ideas about what you can do, either for yourself or for others. These can be from experience or from what others have told you.

2 Women stick their post-its onto two separate flipchart sheets on the wall, one headed 'for self' and one 'for others'.

3 Take time to look at everybody's ideas.

4 Discuss.

Discussion points

- Have you come across any new ideas or any that appeal to you?

- Has this sparked off any other ideas you might want to add to the lists?

- Are some things more suited to you than others?

Notes for tutors
- Some women may express a lack of confidence in starting new things.

- Some women may be in the position of constantly caring for others and may need to consider the availability of respite care; others may not be able to take advantage of respite care.

- For some women choice may be limited, for example due to mobility or disability.

ACTIVITY *8.9*

Making the most of your time 2

Aim
- To explore possible ways of reducing isolation, boredom and gaining confidence and self-esteem.

Materials

A selection of different magazines, scissors, glue, large sheets of paper, pens, flipchart, markers.

Method
1 Individually or in pairs women use images in magazines to make a collage on the theme of: 'What things have you always wanted to do with your time?'

2 Spend time looking at the collages.

3 In the large group, discuss, and flipchart the main issues and activities portrayed.

Discussion points
- Women may prefer to use images in magazines as a trigger, and spend time reflecting rather than making a collage.

- Are women surprised by the range of activities?

- What prevented you from doing them up to now, and how might you still do them?

- What do you see as constraints now and how could these be overcome?

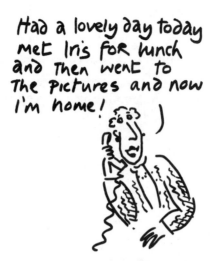

Had a lovely day today
met Iris for lunch
and then went to
the pictures and now
I'm home!

ACTIVITY *8.10*

Making the most of your time 3

Aim

- To find out about local opportunities for 'doing' things.

Materials

Flipchart paper, markers.

Method

1 The week before, ask women to work individually or in pairs to find out what they can about their area in terms of:

- leisure and sports courses for older women;

- education classes;

- voluntary work;

- free concerts/talks/lectures; and

- other activities.

2 The following week, women share their findings. Record information on a flipchart.

Variation: Women may feel they want to make a booklet about local provision for other women to use.

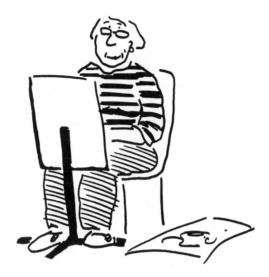

Discussion points

- Does the provision of leisure and sports courses for women seem to be increasing or decreasing?

- Do opportunities for older women exist in both statutory and voluntary sectors?

- What were the best sources of information on what is available: libraries, leisure centres, the local council, or others?

- How could provision be improved?

- What can women do to improve what is available: by individuals writing letters, working together as a group campaigning, or enlisting the help of others with influence, for example, local councillors?

*ACTIVITY 8.11

Older women and attitudes to sexuality

Aim

- To acknowledge and explore social attitudes towards older women and sexuality.

Materials

A copy of Worksheet 8.7 *Older women and attitudes to sexuality* for each woman; pens, flipchart paper, markers.

Method

1 Ask women to go through the worksheet in small groups, noting their responses.

2 In the large group, share ideas, taking responses to each question from each group in turn, and writing main points on the flipchart.

3 Discuss issues raised.

Discussion points

● Have these types of attitudes influenced how older women view their sexual needs?

● What can be done to counteract such attitudes?

● For some women, the idea that sexuality decreases with age reduces the pressures to be sexually active and is a relief.

● For some women there is little choice about being sexually active with a partner, either because of widowhood, divorce, separation or ill health. However, feelings of attraction and sexuality are just as valid.

● Older women are just as likely to see themselves as lesbian, bisexual or celibate as younger women.

Note for tutor

Sessions dealing with sexuality may need sensitive facilitation.

*ACTIVITY 8.12

Change and sexuality 1

Aims

● To begin discussion about change, age and sexuality.

● To explore what changes come as a surprise and what are expected.

Materials

Post-its, pens, flipchart paper, markers, copies of prompt questions, blutack.

Method

1 Head one sheet of flipchart paper 'SURPRISE' and one sheet 'PREPARED FOR' and divide each sheet into three columns: physical changes, emotional changes and social changes. Stick the two sheets up on the wall.

2 In pairs or small groups, go through the prompt questions (below) noting responses on individual post-its.

3 Ask groups to put their post-its on the appropriate flipchart papers on the wall.

4 Take time to read through the two sheets, and discuss.

Discussion points

- Is this a difficult activity to do? Why?

- Are you surprised by some of the post-its?

- Are women generally well prepared for changes associated with ageing?

- Are these changes social or personal in nature?

Prompt questions

In terms of sexuality and growing older, what physical, emotional and social changes:

- took you by surprise?

- were you prepared for in some way or had some idea about?

Notes for tutor

- Make it clear that women only need talk about what they feel comfortable with.

- Be aware of group pressure on individuals.

ACTIVITY 8.13

Change and sexuality 2

Aims

- To provide some background information on physical changes associated with growing older.

- To explore some effects upon women's own ideas of sexuality.

- To consider what action women can take for themselves.

Materials

Copies of Information Sheet 8.4 *Factors which may affect sexuality*, and Worksheet 8.8 *Change and sexuality – true or false?*; paper and pens.

Method

1 In pairs, go through the worksheet.

2 Join pairs to make foursomes, and give out the information sheet. Compare responses to the information sheet.

3 Discuss in the large group.

Discussion points

- Were you surprised about any of the changes described in the information sheet?

- What else besides physical factors might affect older women's sexuality:

    – the 'double standard' between men and women and what is seen as acceptable behaviour?
    – family attitudes to a grandmother/mother who might be thought of as 'past it' by the rest of her family?

- What might be the benefits of being sexually active when you are older:

    – the fear of pregnancy removed?
    – time for exploring your sexuality?
    – using a wealth of experience?

ACTIVITY *8.14*

Space invader

Aim

- To enable women whose male partners will be retiring from a lifetime of paid work:

    – to reflect on what effect his retirement might have on her life; and
    – to consider advantages and disadvantages of having a partner more often at home.

Materials

A copy of Worksheet 8.9 *Space invader* for each woman; flipchart, markers.

Method

 1 Give each woman a copy of the worksheet to read, or read it aloud in the group.

 2 In small groups, discuss issues which this article raises.

 3 Report back to the large group, and flipchart the main points.

Discussion points

 • Can women identify with the author's feelings?

 • Has any woman in the group experienced something similar? How did they feel? How did they deal with it?

 • What does the author appear to be most fearful of?

 • Why does she talk about being 'selfish', 'feeling guilty'?

 • How could she deal with her situation?

 • Is such a 'spouse-in-the-house' syndrome common?

 • What is the situation when *women* retire from paid employment?

ACTIVITY *8.15*

After retirement

Aims

 • To enable women to reflect on how they and their partner spend their time.

 • To allow women to identify any changes they would like, and to share strategies for change.

Materials

A copy of Worksheet 8.10 *After retirement* for each woman; flipchart, markers.

Method

 1 Explain the activity to the group the week before you intend to do it. Give each woman a copy of the worksheet, and ask her to record how she and her partner have spent the week, and bring the completed worksheet to the following session.

2 At the session, ask women to compare their worksheets in small groups and identify any changes they would like.

3 In the large group, discuss women's experiences.

Discussion points

● Were women surprised by how they and their partner tend to spend the week? What were the main differences?

● Were women content with existing arrangements?

● Were there similarities between women in how they spent their week and how their partners spent the week? Did this depend on whether the partner was a man or a woman? If so, why might this be so?

● If women would like other arrangements, how might they approach their partner with regard to making changes?

*ACTIVITY *8.16*

Relationships

Aim

● To enable women to consider their existing relationships, to project future relationships, and think through what kinds of relationships they might want.

Materials

A copy of Worksheet 8.11 *Relationships* for each woman; pens, flipchart, markers.

Method

1 Give each woman a copy of the worksheet, and ask them to work in pairs and complete it.

2 Feed back to the large group.

3 Discuss the issues raised.

Discussion points

● Relationships are often complex, and can involve a number of roles.

● Roles in existing relationships may change as women grow older.

- Relationship changes may be positive or negative (or both, e.g. grand-children may be a delight, but not when they are 'dumped' on you!).

- How can women explore possibilities for new relationships.

Note for tutor

This activity could be a very emotional or stressful activity for women in the group who have difficult relationships with, say, members of their family.

ACTIVITY 8.17

Loss and growing older

Aims

- To introduce a general overview of the nature of loss and grief.

- To encourage women to consider losses related to growing older.

Materials

Paper, pens, flipchart, markers.

Method

1 Introduce the topic of loss and grief as a familiar one for women. For example, the loss of a cherished possession, a much loved pet, a special friend who has moved away – all these may be painful losses because of their emotional overtones or memories, and because they cannot be replaced.

2 Ask women to reflect silently on one such loss they have experienced (allow a minute or so).

3 In pairs, or small groups, ask women to list the sort of losses associated with growing older. Ask women to work quickly in the group without discussion to cover as broad a range of losses as possible.

4 Feed back to the large group. Ask each small group or pair in turn to call out two of the losses they identified, and flipchart them. Continue in turn until all losses are noted.

5 Group the losses into different categories (e.g. physical, economic, role/identity, emotional, social, etc.).

Discussion points

- Losses may relate to:

    - changing bodies – physical attributes of the normal ageing process;
    - changes in health status e.g. flexibility, mobility, eyesight, hearing, memory;
    - illness (debilitating or chronic or necessitating surgery, e.g. hysterectomy, mastectomy);
    - changes in work and social status – issues for own or/and partner's retirement;
    - relationship changes, family upheavals;
    - death of a partner/friend/parent;
    - moving, or family moving away; or
    - income changes.

- Given that in any loss there is opportunity for personal growth, how might women move forward positively?

ACTIVITY 8.18

Dealing with loss

Aim

- To identify and discuss ways of dealing with loss.

Materials

Paper, pens, flipchart, markers, list of local addresses/ resources.

Method

1 In pairs, take three minutes each to share a time of personal loss (it need not be a 'major' loss, but something which caused you to grieve). Remind women to reveal only what they feel is safe. As each woman speaks the other pays attention without interrupting. Change over.

2 In the same pairs, ask women to discuss and write down the things that help us cope during a time of loss.

3 In the large group, feed back and flipchart responses, and discuss.

Discussion points

- Ways of coping may include:

    - physical activity, e.g. exercise, gardening;

- getting angry safely (e.g. hitting a pillow, stamping, shouting in a private space);
- keeping a journal about feelings;
- crying;
- praying;
- massage;
- giving yourself tasks to do;
- seeking counselling; and
- attending a relevant support group.

- Affirm the ways in which women take care of themselves. Raise the issue of being gentle with themselves and not expecting too much of themselves while grieving.

- There is no set pattern or length of time for grieving, only what it takes for each individual woman.

- Destructive ways of dealing with loss and grief include:

  - drinking;
  - tranquillisers;
  - neglecting yourself; and
  - not eating or sleeping.

  Be prepared to acknowledge these, and suggest resources for information, support and counselling.

ACTIVITY *8.19*

Who cares?

Aims

- To explore the types of caring women continue to do throughout their lives.

- To provide an opportunity for women to express feelings about expectations placed upon them.

- To give support and credence to the unpaid work women do for others.

Materials

A copy of Worksheet 8.12 *Who cares?* for each woman, pens.

Method

1 In small groups go through the worksheet and note responses.

2 In the large group, each group reports back.

3 Discuss.

Discussion points

- What needs do women themselves have?

- How are these met?

- How would women like these to be met?

Notes for tutor

- Women who live alone, not through choice, may feel vulnerable with this activity.

- Some women live in difficult situations with little or no respite care.

- It may be useful to have lists of local contacts such as Age Concern, Pensioners Link (see Information Sheets 8.2 and 8.3 *Useful national organisations*).

ACTIVITY *8.20*

Passing the word on

Aim

- To focus upon what is good about becoming older.

Materials

Flipchart paper, markers.

Method

1 In pairs, women brainstorm what is good about becoming older.

2 In fours, they put together points for inclusion in a younger women's magazine.

3 Each group reports what they would say in their article. Discuss.

Discussion points

- What is the breadth of things that come up?

- Are there differences, and what might these be due to?

Notes for tutor

- This is useful for ending a session on a positive note.

- The tutor may have to start the group off with positive examples of growing older.

ACTIVITY *8.21*

The way it should be – a guided fantasy

Aim

- To encourage women to imagine a society that values older women to the fullest extent in whatever their choices.

Materials

None.

Method

Read the following out loud to the group, slowly and in a relaxed manner.

Make yourself as comfortable as possible in your seat. For those who wear glasses, take them off, gently close your eyes. Take a few deep breaths . . . let yourself relax . . .

It is important for the purpose of this fantasy to let your imagination run free. Imagine that you live in a society that values all women whatever their age, colour, sexual preference, race or class . . .

Imagine life – not just the opposite of the way it is now, but the way you really would like it to be . . . A world where the leaders of countries are women, where women are prominent among the law and policy makers . . . and involved in all areas of work . . . where women work co-operatively with each other and are paid on the basis of their ability not their sex . . . a world where women are held in the highest esteem. Let's look now specifically at older women . . . let your imagination go into as many details as possible. Imagine, for example, that there is no question about the right of older women to a decent income – that social security is never put on the block to be whittled away, and older people are not seen as a burden on the economy, that the pension is automatically increased, and the real value of women's income is maintained. To provide less for older women would be unthinkable . . .

Imagine that employers vie for the part time or full time services of older women . . . since everyone knows what richness of experience and dedication older women bring to their jobs . . . Imagine that the choice to work or not is simply made by each individual older woman, with no stigma attached to her choice . . .

In keeping with the special status of older women you are naturally a part of any social circle you choose – young, old, mixed, because you live in a non-segregated society . . . You are attended to in large and small ways . . . Clothes and shoes are designed for the older figure . . . clothes that are beautiful, colourful and comfortable . . . When someone gives you a compliment, they might say 'You look almost good enough to be old' . . . Older women are seen in the media all the time . . . as newsreaders, political figures, women of action, women of ideas and direction, as the beloved or the lovers . . . no one would dream of leaving older women out of any important projects . . . You decide what you choose to participate in and what you want to say no to . . . No one dares to tell you what you are capable or not capable of doing . . .

And since everyone knows that older women, like vintage wines, are the best lovers . . . you are considered especially sexually desirable . . . you never lack for lovers or affectionate friends or comrades. It is your choice . . .

Some of you, as you have always been, are studious, sedentary and contemplative, while others continue to climb mountains and enjoy great physical activity . . . Some of you are in poorer health or just feeling the twinges of your bodies growing older . . . a bit of difficulty hearing, or seeing, or remembering, a twinge of arthritis . . . all simply signs of a long and fruitful life . . . Some of you might become quite frail and need the help of others, and since everyone is honoured to help, the load does not fall to just a few, there are adequate resources to look after you comfortably . . . There is of course no question about your right to full and complete medical care by doctors and health workers who listen to what you have to say – really listen – without dismissing you with a prescription. They treat your older, beautiful bodies with the greatest of care and attention.

Being older or sick would never mean that you would not make decisions about your own care. If your capacities become diminished you are still in charge of making decisions for yourself to the fullest extent of whatever those capacities are. It is unthinkable that any member of the 'helping' professions would dare to presume otherwise . . .

Whatever you are involved in and however you choose to lead your life as an older woman, you will be respected, supported and cared for in a manner that recognises your individual needs, relishes your experience and provides for the continued changes and growing explorations that you need to complete your life, to your satisfaction . . .

Allow these images to settle . . . savour them . . . and when you are ready, slowly stretch your beautiful bodies and open your eyes.
End of fantasy.

Variation: ask each woman to share one positive aspect of her own fantasy.

Source: from *Women Growing Older, a Health and Wellness Manual for Working with Women Around 60 Years and Over*, Southern Women's Health and Community Centre, Australia.

WORKSHEET *8.1*

Who is an older woman?

How would you define an 'older' woman in terms of:

- AGE

- EXPERIENCES

- ATTITUDES

- ANYTHING ELSE

- What do you think is the difference between 'old' and 'older'?

WORKSHEET *8.2*

What is a 'senior citizen'?

A senior citizen is one who was here *before* the Pill, *before* television, frozen food, credit cards and ballpoint pens.

For us time sharing meant togetherness, not apartments in Spain. Computers hadn't been invented: a chip meant a piece of wood, hardware meant hardware, and software wasn't even a word.

Teenagers never wore slacks. We were before panty-hose, drip-dry clothes, dishwashers and electric blankets.

We got married first and then lived together (how quaint can you be?). Girls wore Peter Pan collars and thought cleavage was something butchers did.

We were before Batman, vitamin pills, disposable nappies, ozone, jeeps, pizzas – instant coffee and Kentucky Fried weren't even thought of.

In our day, cigarette smoking was 'fashionable', grass was for mowing, pot was something you cooked in. A 'gay' person was the life and soul of the party and nothing more, while AIDS meant beauty lotions or help for someone in trouble.

We are today's Senior Citizens. A hardy bunch when you think of how the world has changed and consider the adjustments we have had to make . . .

Source: some older women in Blackpool.

WORKSHEET *8.3*

Lifeline

- Put a cross on this lifeline chart to show where you are now.

- Add the main events of your life onto the chart using words or symbols. Below are some suggestions of events you may want to chart, but include any others which are important to you.

- Now try to imagine what the rest of your life will be like. In a different colour pen, fill in future events when you expect them to happen.

Possible significant life events

first period	moving/migration/emigration
leaving school	new job
starting work	the menopause
important romances	children leaving home
new friend/s	retirement from work
getting married	new interest/hobby/education
birth of child/ren	death of parent/s
going to college	death of partner
divorce/end of relationship	

Birth	10	20	30	40	50	60	70	80	90	Years 100

WORKSHEET *8.4*

Issues for older women ('SLOT')

Strengths

Limitations

Opportunities

Threats

WORKSHEET *8.5*

Images of older women 1

Read through the following case study:

> One of the crucial things for me was my image of myself and how I looked was an important part of that image. That affected me more because I'm female. Women are judged more by their looks than are men. I worry about what I want to look like, now that I'm in my forties. I'm afraid of looking ridiculous but I also don't want to look dull. There don't seem to be any attractive images of what a woman over forty should look like.[1]
>
> Margaret

1 Do you agree with what Margaret is saying?

2 How do you feel about getting older?

3 Can you think of any attractive images of older women? Are these images that we can identify with?

4 What other positive images of older women can you think of?

[1] Reprinted with permission from Nairne and Smith, *Dealing with Depression* (1984), Women's Press, £3.95.

WORKSHEET *8.6*

Images of older women 2

Warning

When I am an old woman I shall wear purple
With a red hat which doesn't go, and doesn't suit me.
And I shall spend my pension on brandy and summer gloves
And satin sandals, and say we've no money for butter.
I shall sit down on the pavement when I'm tired
And gobble up samples in shops and press alarm bells
And run my stick along the public railings
And make up for the sobriety of my youth.
I shall go out in my slippers in the rain
And pick the flowers in other people's gardens
And learn to spit.

You can wear terrible shirts and grow more fat
And eat three pounds of sausages at a go
Or only bread and pickle for a week
And hoard pens and pencils and beermats and things in boxes.

But now we must have clothes that keep us dry
And pay our rent and not swear in the street
And set a good example for the children.
We must have friends to dinner and read the papers.

But maybe I ought to practise a little now?
So people who know me are not too shocked and surprised
When suddenly I am old, and start to wear purple.

   1 What are your first impressions of this poem? Do you like it? Does it shock
       you?

   2 Write down words which describe this old woman. Do you think they
       present a positive or a negative picture?

   3 How would you like to be when you are old?

Source: Joseph, Jenny, *Rose in the Afternoon* (1974), Dent (now out of print).
Reprinted with permission from the author.

WORKSHEET *8.7*

Older women and attitudes to sexuality

'In most books, films and plays there seems to be an unwritten rule that older women are less attractive than younger women, and that they do not experience the same feelings of sexuality and desire.'

- Do you agree with this statement?

- Why do you think this attitude is so common?

- Have such attitudes shifted in the last 30 years, and if so in what way?

WORKSHEET *8.8*

Change and sexuality: true or false?

1 As women become older they have a shorter duration of orgasm. TRUE/ FALSE

2 As women become older the fatty tissues in their breasts reduces. TRUE/ FALSE

3 As women get older they are more likely to get vaginal infections. TRUE/ FALSE

4 Only women who have had a bad menopause will experience vaginal dryness during sexual activity. TRUE/FALSE

5 Alcohol reduces sexual interest and desire. TRUE/FALSE

6 Hysterectomy has no negative effect upon women's sexual appetite. TRUE/ FALSE

7 Women who have mastectomies can continue to lead sexually active lives. TRUE/FALSE

8 Women with physical disabilities lead active sexual lives. TRUE/FALSE

WORKSHEET *8.9*

Space invader

Alex Reid on why her husband's retirement fills her with trepidation.

Today is my husband's retirement party. Today he celebrates his 42 years of work and looks forward to a life of leisure. He's had cards. He's had presents, he's had counselling. And I hope the counselling wasn't just about him and his adjustment to a new life.

I know it sounds selfish, but what's really in my mind – the big question that I can't get rid of – is: what happens to me? I mean, I've come to some sort of ease with my life. I've been through all the traumas of being a young mother, of being trapped at home with the children, of feeling inadequate because I wasn't doing anything. Of the menopause. Of the empty nest. Even of going out and finding a job again. And I've got to a stage where things have evened out and I've made some sort of routine for myself that gives me a great deal of pleasure.

I work two mornings a week. Eat lunch if I want to. See my friends. Go for walks. Listen to music. Sit and think. Just sit, if that's all I feel like doing. And all without having to discuss it with anyone else or even consider them. In fact, I've come to regard Monday to Friday as *mine*, and I resent having to give them up.

It's not that I don't want Fred to retire. It's not that we don't get on well or that I don't look forward to our spending more time together. But I look at my friends who have been through this last stage of marriage and I see capable, responsible women suddenly becoming 'junior partners' again and I don't want it to happen to me. I sympathise with the husbands; nothing left to organise but the way the home is run and no one to impress but the wife. But don't they realise that we've been running the homes and organising things for just as many years as they have?

I don't need someone to re-educate my shopping habits or put a new set of values on what I do. And I don't need someone getting at me because I'm not willing to drop everything at a moment's notice. Fred's new life may be a wide open space – but mine isn't, and I don't want it to be.

In a way, I suppose I see Fred as an intruder. I feel guilty about it, but I can't help it. The weekday home has always been my territory. Now it's going to be *ours* and I hope I'll be able to make the adjustment. I want the companionship – but I want a bit of space as well. And recognition – not just for the Saturday/Sunday wife, but for the Monday/Friday person as well. That's not a person Fred's used to. He wasn't around when she was forged and I'm not sure how he'll take to her. She's not 'Andrea's Mother' or 'Fred's Wife', but she's *me* and I don't want to give her up.

Source: *The Guardian*, 29 January 1992. Reprinted with permission.

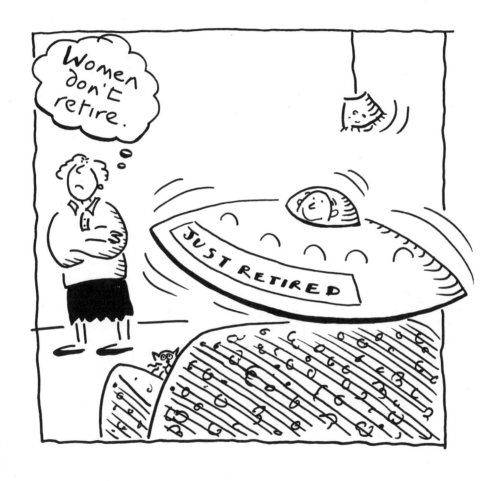

WORKSHEET *8.10*

After retirement

Self

	Monday	Tuesday	Wednesday	Thursday	Friday	Saturday	Sunday
Morning							
Afternoon							
Evening							

Partner

Morning							
Afternoon							
Evening							

WORKSHEET *8.11*

Relationships

- Look through the list below and tick those that apply to you (add any others not listed).
- Go through the list, noting what role you have in each of the relationships you have indicated (roles might be e.g. functional, family, emotional, sexual, financial, dependent, caring, etc. or a combination).
- Indicate which are positive relationships at present, and which are negative.

Relationships with:	*Role I have in relationship*	*Positive or negative relationship (or both)*
my partner		
my parents		
my brothers and sisters		
my children		
my grandchildren		
my friends		
my partner's friends		
my neighbours		
my employer		
my colleagues		
other (please explain)		

- Which relationships may change as you get older?
- How might they change?
- Which relationships do I want to maintain or expand as I get older?
- What new relationships do I see for myself?
- What new relationships would I like?
- How might I pursue these new relationships?

WORKSHEET *8.12*

Who cares?

'Women bear the responsibility for caring for others' well being, and this occurs through all the stages of women's lives. They often care for the physical and emotional needs and feelings of their partner and children. They are expected to look after elderly parents and often need to care for ill partners.'

- How far would you agree with this viewpoint?

- Does it match any of your own experiences? In what way?

- How do caring roles change as women become older?

RESOURCES

For contact details of distributors and organisations listed here, see Chapter 11 *General resources*.

Publications

Alexander, J, et al, *Women and Ageing: an Anthology by Women* (1986), Calyx Books, USA, £8.95, ISBN 0934971 00 5.
A wonderfully powerful collection of photographs, essays, fiction, journals, poetry, profiles, art and reviews – which celebrate growing older.

The Age of Adventure: Health Advice and Leisure Opportunities for Older People with a Visual Impairment (1991), Age Concern England/Royal National Institute for the Blind, £1.50. Available from Royal National Institute for the Blind and from Age Concern England.
Advice on health matters – such as relaxation techniques, and facts on ageing and sight loss; information and encouragement on a wide range of leisure activities and involvement in the community.

Batchelor, M, *Forty Plus* (1988), Lion Paperbacks, £4.99.
Offers helpful, factual information, sympathetic understanding and a basic optimistic approach to dealing with the changes midlife can bring.

Biggs, Simon, *Confronting Ageing: A Groupwork Manual for Helping Professionals*, Central Council for Education and Training in Social Work, £7, ISBN 0 904488 37 3. Available from CCETSW.
This manual explores the barriers to understanding older age and contains exercises which anyone in a training role can use with groups. Can be used in community settings and across professional boundaries.

Boston Women's Health Book Collective, *Ourselves, Growing Older: Women Ageing with Knowledge and Power* (1989), Fontana/Collins, £9.99.
A detailed handbook covering medical, social and emotional matters. Issues covered include sexuality, contraception, body image, the menopause, osteoporosis and others.

Collick, E, *Through Grief: the Bereavement Journey* (1986), Darton, Longman & Todd (in association with CRUSE), £3.95.
A personal experience of death of a partner, taking the reader through the process of grief.

Cooper, Baba, *Over the Hill: Reflections on Ageism Between Women* (1988), Airlift, £5.95.
American feminist view of the subject.

Ford, Janet and Sinclair, Ruth, *Sixty Years On: Women Talk About Old Age* (1987), Women's Press, £4.95.
Interviews with 14 women between the ages of 60 and 90. Useful for starting discussions.

Greengross, S (ed), *Ageing: an Adventure in Living* (1985), Souvenir Press, £4.95.
A positive and informative book which sets out to dispel the notion that old age starts from the day of retirement. The book covers issues of relationships in old age; opportunities for education, leisure and new activities; making decisions about your home; residential care; coping with death and bereavement.

Greengross, W, and Greengross S, *Living, Loving and Ageing* (1989), Age Concern England, £4.95.
Interesting and sensitive book dealing with values and attitudes towards sexuality and older people.

Hemmings, Susan, *A Wealth of Experience: the Lives of Older Women* (1985), Pandora, £4.95.
Eighteen women between the ages of 40 and 50 talk about their personal experiences and lives.

Health Education Authority, *Call for Care: Advice for Asian Carers of Elderly People* (Bengali, Gujarati, Punjabi, Urdu and English), £1.95. Available from the Health Education Authority.

MacDonald, Barbara and Rich, Cynthia, *Look Me in the Eye: Old Women, Ageing and Ageism* (1984), Women's Press, £2.95.
Looks at the ageing of women and the prejudice that permeates even the language used to describe it.

McEwan, Evelyn (ed), *Age: the Unrecognised Discrimination*, (1990), Age Concern England, £9.95. ISBN 0 86242 094 6. Available from booksellers or from Age Concern England.
A series of essays which challenge passive popular acceptance of ageism, examine evidence of age discrimination within particular fields and outline action points for its elimination. Includes a chapter on age discrimination in healthcare.

Nash, Caroline and Carter, Tony, *Age Well Handbook: Step-by-Step Guide to Setting up Local Community Health Initiatives for Older People* (1992), £1.50 plus 50p p&p. Available from Age Concern England.

Planning Retirement Training Pack (undated). Open University study pack £26.00; assessment pack £15.00; course £38.00; tutor video £23.00; discussion pack £8.00.
A pack for those about to retire and who already have retired. Practical activities to help learners draw up their own retirement plans. Discussion pack leaflets focus particularly on health. Not aimed specifically at women.

Patel, N, *A "Race" Against Time? Social Services Provision to Black Elders* (1990), Runnymede Trust, £2.95.
There are almost 100,000 Black elders in Britain; while they share the situation of

elders in general, they have additional concerns generated by experiences and consequences of racism. This book maps out areas for policy development regarding Black elders.

Roberts, Anne, *Keeping Well: a Guide to Health in Retirement* (1991), Faber, £4.99.
A guide to keeping healthy; includes exercise, safety, smoking, sex, common illnesses, medicines and help.

Rule, Jane, *Memory Board* (1987), Pandora, £4.95.
A novel about the struggles and joys of two women ageing together, one with Alzheimer's and one with arthritis.

Shapiro, Jean, *Get the Best Out of the Rest of Your Life: a Woman's Guide to the Second Half of Life* (1990), Thorsons, £4.99.
Questions and answers on health, family, relationships, work, retirement and money.

Smith, M, *The Best is Yet to Come: a Workbook for the Middle Years* (1989), Lifeskills Publishing Group, £12.95.
A workbook which stresses that mid-life transition can be a positive and highly motivational part of our lives. It consists of exercises which explore areas such as work, money, managing change, time management, job search, self-employment, health, and stress management.

Stoppard, Miriam, *The Prime of Your Life* (1986), Penguin, £5.95.
A thorough guide to all aspects of ageing including adapting to your environment and living with long-term ailments.

Videos

Asian Carers: Caring and Sharing (1988), (Hindi and English; booklets available in Bengali, Gujarati, Punjabi, Urdu, English), video £25.00; booklet £1.00 Available from Voluntary Action Leicester.
Explains services that could help those caring for someone at home in the Asian community.

Going Well Over Sixty (undated), 30 minutes, Disabled Living Foundation. Available from Concord.
Video about the different occupations enjoyed by older people; includes exercises. Not specifically aimed at women.

Growing Older, Keeping Well: Chinese Elderly Healthcare, (Cantonese, and Cantonese with English subtitles), £25. Available from Bloomsbury and Islington (Southside) Health Promotion Department, St Pancras Hospital.

Organisations

Age Concern England
Publications, information and policy work on all issues concerning older people. The Age Well Campaign produces resources on health and older people.

Beth Johnson Foundation
Charitable trust. Aims to sponsor and encourage innovative work for the benefit of the over 50s. Publishes books and reports.

Carers National Association
Information and support for people who care for ill, disabled or elderly friends or relatives at home. Leaflets, journal for members. Local groups for self-help.

Centre for Health and Retirement Education, University of Surrey
Consultancy, education and training, research and resources.

Help the Aged
Seniorline is a free information service for senior citizens, their relatives, carers and friends. Produces booklets on a wide range of subjects including gardening, security, food and safety.

Older Feminists Network
Unfunded group of older feminists. Newsletter published every two months, subscription £5.00 per year.

Older Lesbian Network (OLN)

Pensioners Link
London-wide organisation provides information, and services and leaflets.

Older Women's Project
Gives help to older women's groups – administration, help and support for a range of projects. Holds conferences.

9 Sexual health

INTRODUCTION

This chapter contains four sections: *Sexuality, Contraception, Sexually transmitted diseases* and *HIV and AIDS*.

Sexual health is about more than the absence of sexually transmitted diseases and unwanted pregnancies. A positive attitude to sexuality, and fulfilment from sexual activity, may be prevented by:

- fear of unwanted pregnancy;
- fear of contracting disease;
- insecurity and lack of confidence about sex;
- lack of knowledge about basic sexuality;
- difficulties with relationships;
- lack of opportunity to explore one's own sexual preference;
- heterosexism;
- homophobia; and
- guilt and stigma.

In order to achieve good sexual health, women need to feel confident about their sexuality, their sexual preference, and understand their sexual needs. This is not always easy for women faced with conflicting messages and pressures.

Women need a more positive attitude to sexuality to enable greater comfort with sexual issues, to seek out accurate information, to practise safer sex, and achieve good sexual health.

Sexual health involves partnerships, and therefore communication skills are essential. Women need to have the confidence to negotiate both in and out of relationships according to their own sexual and personal needs.

In order to achieve sexual health, women need:

- access to client-centred sexual health services:
  - family planning clinics
  - well-women clinics
  - primary health care services
  - maternal and child health services
  - pre-pregnancy services
  - pre-natal and post-natal services
  - fertility investigation
  - abortion facilities
  - special clinics (sometimes known as GUM, STD or by the old name of VD clinics)
  - menopause clinics and other services for older women
- accurate information in order to make informed choices;
- lack of constraints to making healthy choices about sexual health, which may be caused by fear, guilt, lack of money, political or other factors and pressures.

PRACTICAL POINTS

- Sexual health is an emotive area. Many women may feel uncomfortable talking about sexual and personal matters. On the other hand, women may welcome the opportunity to share knowledge, experiences, fears, and hopes within a safe and supportive environment.

- Ground rules need to be established to facilitate trust between group members. Confidentiality is an important ground rule.

- As a tutor, you will need to be aware of your own attitudes to sexual health.

- In any group there may be women who consider themselves heterosexual, others who consider themselves to be lesbians and some who are bisexual. All activities around sexual health will need to address sexual preference.

- There will also be other differences between women. Age, culture, race, religion, class and ability may be relevant. Building on differences between women can mean more enriching sessions on sexual health.

- Teaching methods are important. Those which do not require women to share personal information may be more appropriate in some situations. Humour is always a useful aid to teaching.

- Aim to provide as much back-up information as possible for women who want it.

Sexuality

BACKGROUND INFORMATION

Sexuality is an important aspect of women's health. We all have a sexuality – a sense of ourselves as a sexual person, capable of giving and receiving physical or emotional pleasure through sexual relationships. We have a right to express that sexuality for ourselves (whether or not we have a partner). Women's sexuality is beginning to be discussed more widely by women themselves. The advent of AIDS has encouraged this.

Sexuality is not just about physical pleasure, but about emotions too – our need to feel loved, valued, cared for. We may stay in an unsatisfactory relationship because we fear we would be unloved without a sexual partner, or because we lack the skills to make positive sexual relationships. It is possible to change sexual expression within an existing sexual relationship, and so express our sexuality. Emotional needs can be met in other ways too, such as good friendships or wider family links. We may also enjoy sensual pleasure in a variety of ways – a lazy bath, or massage.

Definitions of sex and sexuality in our society do not always allow women to explore their own sexual needs. Sex is often seen narrowly as sexual intercourse. There are strong pressures on women to be heterosexual, and a lack of positive images of lesbians. The most acceptable outlet for a woman's sexuality is still seen to be within a permanent male/female relationship leading to sexual intercourse and children.

The 1960s saw a breakthrough in contraception with the Pill. It gave women more freedom to be sexually active without being faced with an unwanted pregnancy and it enabled the emotional and physical side of sex to become separated from the reproductive aspect. But this did not coincide with an acceptability for women to become sexually experienced or explore their own sexuality.

Women need to be able to explore their sexuality, while at the same time be able to protect themselves against unwanted pregnancies, sexually transmitted diseases and HIV. Skills in assertiveness and high self-esteem are vital for this, as well as access to accurate information.

PRACTICAL POINTS

- A tutor needs to be aware of her own attitudes to sexuality, and to decide how much to disclose of her own experiences.

- Many women feel uncomfortable talking about sexual matters. Aim to create an environment where it feels 'safe' to do so. Ground rules, including confidentiality, will be important for this (see p. 18).

- Do not assume all women are heterosexual, or that they have sexual partners of either sex or of only one sex. Some women in the group may have had painful sexual experiences, either as children or adults. Some women may experience sexual violence from partners.

- Be conscious about differences between women as well as similarities. Age, cultural, religious or class differences may be important. Be prepared for differences in tolerance to expressions of sexuality.

- This issue can contain a lot to laugh about – humour may be a good way to dispel nervousness.

- This section can be a useful way for developing a broad awareness and positive attitude to sexuality. You may wish to find out about local agencies and contacts for women who want more individual attention, or information on specific issues.

INFORMATION SHEET *9.1*

Bisexuality

Bisexuality refers to sexual attraction and sexual activity with people of both genders. Some bisexuals are primarily attracted to one gender and only secondarily to the other, some have a series of monogamous relationships regardless of gender, others seek different relationships from different sexes. Bisexuals are not in transition between heterosexuality and homosexuality, but in fact have a sexual identity of their own.

Many bisexuals have identified as such in order to challenge social labelling, positively proclaiming themselves to be different from those who identify as gay, lesbian or heterosexual. The term bisexual has therefore taken on more political significance rather than relating to people who are labelled according to what gender their sexual partners have been.

A common myth is that bisexuality is related to promiscuity. In reality, bisexuals have not necessarily had sex with either an opposite sex or same sex partner. Bisexuality does not necessarily involve having lovers of both sexes at the same time – monogamous relationships are just as likely.

People's sexual preference may lead them to identify as heterosexual, gay or lesbian, or bisexual; or it may be more complex and they may not see themselves as having a clear identity. Coming to terms with your sexuality, and meeting others who share it, can be empowering. Bisexual women remain comparatively invisible but there are a growing number of groups and events being organised by and for bisexuals. The following national contacts may be able to give you information about local activities:

> Bisexual phoneline: 031 557 3620 Thursday 7.30–9.30 pm; 081 569 7500 Tuesday and Wednesday 7.30–9.30 pm
> Bisexual pen-pals: send s.a.e. to pen-pal scheme, EBG, 58a Broughton Street, Edinburgh, EH1 3SA
> Working Class Bisexual Women's Network: write to Kelly, 7 Warlters Road, Islington, London N7 0RZ
> *'Bifrost'* monthly magazine for bisexuals, PO Box 117, Norwich NR1 2SU

Although expression of sexuality is important for personal sexual health, it is sexual behaviour that is related more to prevention of unwanted pregnancy and sexually transmitted infections. It's important to practise safer sex, and the same guidelines apply to everyone (see Information Sheet 9.15 *Safer sex guidelines for women*).

ACTIVITY *9.1*

Attitudes to sexuality

Aim
- To explore the way sexuality may be shaped by early experiences.

Materials

A copy of Worksheet 9.1 *Attitudes to sexuality* for each woman; pens.

Method

1 Ask women to work through the worksheet individually.

2 In small groups, women discuss each of the questions on the worksheet making a note of any points they want to tell the other groups.

3 In the large group, report back and discuss.

Discussion points
- Where did most learning about sex and sexuality take place? Was this at school? At home? Or in other ways?

- What messages did we learn about sexual morality?

- How important was religious upbringing?

ACTIVITY *9.2*

The double standard

Aims
- To evaluate the language we use when talking about sex, and the messages it conveys.

- To investigate sexual 'shoulds' and 'should nots'.

Materials

A copy of Worksheet 9.2 *The double standard* for each woman; pens.

Method

1 Divide into small groups, each one to complete the worksheet together.

2 In the large group, pool ideas and discuss.

Discussion points

- What kinds of messages are conveyed in the words written down in part 1 of the worksheet. How many are positive, how many negative? For men, for women?

- What do the findings in part 2 say about the sexual standards in our society? Are they fair to both men and women?

ACTIVITY 9.3

Physical pleasure

Aims

- To raise awareness of our needs for physical pleasure.

- To look at the different forms it can take.

Materials

A copy of Worksheet 9.3 *Physical pleasure* for each woman; pens, flipchart.

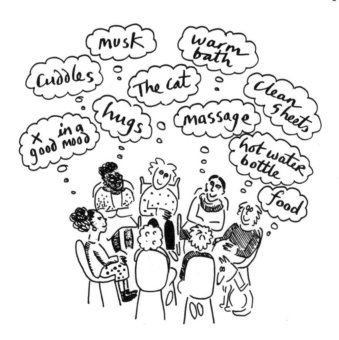

Method

1 Introduce the worksheet, emphasising our right to physical pleasure, and that the activity can help to make us more aware of this.

2 Women work individually with the worksheet to make their own lists.

3 Go round the group. Each woman reads out the main items on her list. Pool the group's ideas on one large list.

Discussion points

- Was this a difficult list to make? How did you feel while making it?

- How often do we find or make time for our favourite physical pleasures? Discuss this together and see what the range of views is in the group.

- How could we make a little more time for physical pleasure in our lives? Would this be easy to do?

ACTIVITY *9.4*

Sensuality and sexuality

Aims

- To consider individual differences in defining 'sexuality' and 'sensuality'.

- To begin discussions on sexuality in general.

Materials

Two flipchart sheets, each with a large outline of a woman's body; thick markers in two different colours, blutack.

Method

1 Divide into two groups and give each group a flipchart sheet with the outline of woman's body, and one set of same colour markers.

2 Ask one group to colour in parts of a woman's body which are 'sexual'. Ask the other group to colour in parts of a woman's body which are 'sensual'.

3 Stick both finished flipchart sheets to the wall and, in the large group, discuss.

Discussion points

- Was this difficult to do? Why?

- What are the differences and similarities?

- How can we define both these terms?

    Penguin English Dictionary definitions:

    > *sexual*: 'associated with, arising from, or based on sex; of, associated with, copulation; reproducing by union of male and female cells'

    > *sexuality*: 'quality of being sexual; emotions, attitudes as determined by sexual impulses; sexual desire'

    > *sensual*: 'of physical pleasures, especially those of sex and food and drink; unduly fond of such pleasures; lustful; voluptuous; of or perceived by the senses'

    > *sensuality*: 'quality of being sensual; proneness to sexual indulgence'

    Do we agree with these definitions?

- How can an understanding of sexuality and sensuality help us in negotiating a safer, healthier sex life?

*ACTIVITY *9.5*

Heterosexism and homophobia

Aims

- To enable heterosexual women to recognise and consider their own heterosexism and homophobia.

- To challenge some myths and misinformation about lesbians.

- To provide women with possible tools for dealing with heterosexism and homophobia in others.

Materials

A copy of Worksheets 9.4A and 9.4B *Heterosexism and homophobia A and B* for each woman; flipchart, pens.

Method

1 Make sure women understand the terms 'heterosexism' and 'homophobia'. It may be useful to have definitions flipcharted for all to see.

Heterosexism: the automatic assumption that every individual has relationships with members of the opposite sex, unless specific information about them is available to the contrary; the belief that heterosexuality is more valid/better/'the norm'/more natural than homosexuality or bisexuality.

Homophobia: the irrational fear, intolerance or hatred of homosexuality.

2 Divide women into small groups, give out copies of Worksheet 9.4A and ask women to discuss heterosexist and homophobic remarks.

3 When discussion appears to have finished, give out copies of Worksheet 9.4B for women to compare comments and discuss further.

ACTIVITY 9.6

Attitudes to lesbians

Aims

- To enable women to recognise and consider any homophobic attitudes they may have.

- To enable women to recognise the difference between liberal tolerance of lesbians and actively challenging attitudes.

Materials

A copy of Worksheet 9.5 *Your attitude to lesbians* for each woman; pens.

Method

Either: when dealing with the subject of sexuality, the worksheet could be given out at the end of one session for women to do at home, with discussion the following session;

or: divide women into small groups; ask them to go through the worksheet on their own, and then discuss with others in their group why they ticked the responses they did.

ACTIVITY 9.7

Sexuality and relationships

Aims

- To look at a range of common sexual and relationship issues.

- To allow women to share their feelings and experiences around sexuality and relationships.

- To consider what is meant by a 'sexual problem' and who defines it.

Materials

Copies of Worksheet 9.6 *Sexuality and relationships – case studies.*

Method

1 Divide into small groups, and give out one or more case studies from the worksheet to each group. Discuss the case studies, making any practical suggestions that seem appropriate.

2 In the large group, report back and discuss.

Option: the case studies could be used as a basis for role play.

Discussion points

- What is a sexual problem? For whom is it a problem?

- Do sexual problems cause problems in relationships, or is it the other way round?

WORKSHEET *9.1*

Attitudes to sexuality

1 How were you told about sex and what were you told?

2 What were your family's attitudes to sex, nakedness and bodily functions?

3 Can you remember any childhood sexual feelings?

4 If you have children, do you feel comfortable talking to them about sex?

WORKSHEET *9.2*

The double standard

1 Terminology

Think of as many words as you can to describe women and men who are:

Not in a long-term relationship or married

Women   Men

Sexually active

Women   Men

2 Sexual standards for women and men

See if you can complete the following sentences, in ways that describe what sexual standards are normally expected of women. Think of as many examples as you can.

'Women should . . .

'Women should not . . .

Then do the same for men:

'Men should . . .

'Men should not . . .

WORKSHEET *9.3*

Physical pleasure

Physical pleasure may sometimes be sexual, but can also take other forms. Three examples are, a long hot bath, lying in the sun and eating.

List your favourite kinds of physical pleasure (as many as you can think of).

We are often preoccupied with catering for other people's needs. When do you find or make time for your own physical pleasures?

WORKSHEET *9.4A*

Heterosexism and homophobia A

- 'After the last session of the course why don't we all ask our husbands and boyfriends along for a bit of a party?'

- 'Protect yourself from AIDS – have safer sex – use a condom.'

- 'She never got married you know; she must have been very lonely.'

- 'I was really surprised when I heard she was a lesbian, she's really rather attractive!'

- 'I don't mind what they do with each other but they shouldn't be allowed to have children.'

- 'Our organisation is an equal opportunities employer – we encourage all applicants regardless of sex, race, colour, nationality, physical ability, marital status or responsibility for dependants.'

WORKSHEET *9.4B*

Heterosexism and homophobia B

After the last session of the course why don't we all ask our husbands and boyfriends along for a bit of a party?

This excludes both women in lesbian relationships and any other women, lesbian or heterosexual, who do not currently have a partner. It also reinforces the idea that women can only have a good time socially if men are present, and disregards the positive choice some women will have made to be in a women-only environment.

Protect yourself from AIDS – have safer sex – use a condom.

These messages are targeting those who have penetrative sex, which are generally gay men, and heterosexual partners. Different sexual health messages are needed for lesbians and others with specific information needs. But if there are no safer sex messages other than condom use, then lesbians may feel invisible and unimportant.

Furthermore, the message to heterosexual women is that sex involves penetration by the penis. There has been less promotion of the many other ways of relating sexually. In this way the idea is reinforced that lesbian sex is somehow 'inferior' or not 'real sex' because it does not involve sexual intercourse.

However, lesbian sex is a safer sexual practice, since HIV transmission from woman to woman is extremely rare, although lesbians may get HIV infected in other ways (e.g. through sharing needles and other drug injecting equipment, by self-insemination using infected semen or through sex with men). Two out of three lesbians have had sexual relations with men, many are still married, some are sex workers and some women are bisexual. There is also a theoretical risk from menstrual blood, and care during menstruation to avoid exchange of blood is also important for lesbians.

She never got married you know, she must have been very lonely.

This reinforces the idea that marriage is the key to happiness for all women, and the only way to sexual/interpersonal relationships. It disregards the fact that many women can have fulfilling lives without a partner, that women may be in relationships with men but not married, and that many women have relationships

$\triangleright$

▷ 9.4b cont.

with other women but these are simply invisible because their lesbian or bisexual relationship is not disclosed or recognised by others.

I was really surprised when I heard she was a lesbian – she's really rather attractive!

It is a surprise because 'she' clearly doesn't fit how the person 'expects' lesbians to be, look or behave – the stereotype being of women too unattractive to get a man, or that lesbians are themselves butch women who want to be men. In fact it is precisely because there is as much diversity in looks, dress style and behaviour among lesbians as among heterosexual women, that most lesbians go unrecognised unless they choose to make their sexuality known to others. Since at least one in ten women are lesbians it should really come as no surprise to find that many female friends, neighbours, colleagues and relatives are lesbians.

I don't mind what they do with each other but they shouldn't be allowed to have children.

The first part of this remark still implies that there is something odd or unnatural about lesbian sexuality, but in any case this attempt to demonstrate liberalism is totally negated by the proviso. Nor is there any recognition that women may be bisexual. There is no evidence to prove that lesbians do not make mothers as good as heterosexual mothers. Nor is there any evidence to show that children need the presence of both a man and a woman, only that they need love, care and security, and the sexuality of the parents does not influence this. Yet lesbian mothers often face having their children taken into care, losing their children in custody cases for no reason other than their sexuality. There are moves to outlaw donor insemination of lesbians, and to prevent lesbians adopting or fostering.

Our organisation is an equal opportunities employer – we encourage all applicants regardless of sex, race, colour, nationality, physical ability, marital status or responsibility for dependants.

A lot of equal opportunities policies, while appearing comprehensive in other respects, exclude any commitment not to discriminate on the grounds of sexuality or sexual orientation. This makes lesbians and gay men feel even more excluded from the rest of society, when other minority groups are being included. However the need for protection is particularly important because in many jobs, such as teaching, youth work or health work, lesbians and gay men are particularly vulnerable due to incorrect and irrational homophobic beliefs that they are likely to assault, seduce, molest or harass other people, particularly children.

WORKSHEET *9.5*

Your attitude to lesbians

Answer each question by circling your choice of the four options. Then turn to the end and add up your score to find out how 'broad-minded' you are about lesbians.

1 If your teenage daughter came home and said she was in love with her best (female) friend, would you:

   (a) ban her from seeing her friend again;

   (b) ask her to invite her friend to stay for the weekend;

   (c) take your daughter to a psychiatrist; or

   (d) try to stay calm and console yourself with the idea that it's just a phase lots of girls go through?

2 Your mother has just told you she is having a lesbian relationship. Do you:

   (a) say nothing to her but blame it on the menopause – she's been acting very strangely for a while . . .;

   (b) don't let her look after your children (her grandchildren) any more;

   (c) find the address of the nearest older lesbians group for her and her friend; or

   (d) disown her as your mother?

3 A woman at work has just told you she feels very attracted to you. Do you:

   (a) try to avoid her as much as possible and hope that she gets over it quickly, but know that you will never be able to feel relaxed in her company again;

   (b) explain that you don't feel the same way but offer to go with her to the local women's disco so that she can get to meet other lesbians;

   (c) tell her that you don't feel the same for her and hope it won't spoil your friendship; or

   (d) report her to the boss and refuse to work with her any more?

4 Your young daughter's class teacher has told the Parent Teacher Association that she is bisexual. Do you:

   (a) keep your daughter away from school;

   $\triangleright$

▷ 9.5 cont.

    (b) congratulate the teacher for her courage in 'coming out' and publicly offer your support both to her and any other teachers who want to 'come out' about their sexual orientation but fear reprisals;

    (c) tell the other parents that lots of good teachers are bisexual or lesbians, but secretly be quite relieved that your daughter moves into another class at the end of this term; or

    (d) demand her immediate dismissal?

5 Your best friend has told you that she thinks she is a lesbian. Do you:

    (a) talk with her at length if she wishes, reaffirm your friendship and support and give her the number of the nearest Lesbian Line;

    (b) hope you are never left in a room on your own with her;

    (c) refuse to see her anymore and think that you never really liked her much anyway; or

    (d) try to reassure her that it won't change your friendship, but be worried that it will?

6 Your teenage daughter comes home from school and says that in her sex education lesson the teacher told them that lesbians were nasty perverts who do unnatural things with other women. Do you:

    (a) discuss this with your daughter and explain that lesbians are neither sick nor nasty, but simply prefer to have sexual and emotional relationships with other women;

    (b) fear that the mention of lesbianism may make your daughter want to find out more about it;

    (c) be pleased that the school is upholding such good moral standards; or

    (d) go straight to the Head Teacher, point out that about 1 in 10 of the pupils are or will become lesbians, and many more will have lesbian experiences at some time, and insist that someone from Lesbian Line is invited not only to speak to the class to provide accurate information and put the record straight, but also to do an in-service training session for all the teachers?

7 You notice that a documentary on lesbian mothers is due to be screened on television. Do you:

    (a) think that might be interesting and try to remember to watch it;

    (b) make sure you watch it and then write an angry letter of complaint to the

▷

▷ 9.5 cont.

TV station protesting about the disgusting and immoral programmes they show on TV;

(c) tell all your friends that it's coming on and ask one to video it in case any of the others miss it. Watch it yourself and then write to the TV station congratulating them on showing a programme on this subject and asking for more programmes about, or including positive images of, lesbians; or

(d) make absolutely sure that the whole family is out that night so there's no chance of you or any of them seeing any of it?

8 You are in a group with some friends and one of them tells a joke about lesbians. Do you:

(a) laugh loudly and tell some more anti-lesbian jokes that you know yourself;

(b) laugh loudly and make sure everyone has seen that you are laughing;

(c) think how sad it is that people find humour at the expense of oppressed groups, and do not laugh;

(d) tell the group that you think it is offensive and upsetting that they should find lesbianism amusing and explain why?

9 Your child comes home from junior school with yet another book about Jim and Jane and their mother and father. Do you:

(a) wish that the reading material did not always give such white hetero-sexual nuclear family images and make sure that you provide books at home which show single-parent families and people of different colours (but never realise that you haven't made sure to include some with lesbians/lesbian mothers in!);

(b) not notice or think anything in particular about it;

(c) search the shops for a list of anti-sexist and multicultural books, espec-ially ones which include lesbian and gay families, take them to the school and insist that they portray a realistic picture of society in their reading material; or

(d) add it to the stack of very similar books you've already bought for the children at home?

Please turn over now to calculate your score.

▷

▷ 9.5 cont.

1.	a = 1	b = 5	c = 0	d = 3
2.	a = 3	b = 1	c = 5	d = 0
3.	a = 1	b = 5	c = 3	d = 0
4.	a = 1	b = 5	c = 3	d = 0
5.	a = 5	b = 1	c = 0	d = 3
6.	a = 3	b = 1	c = 0	d = 5
7.	a = 3	b = 0	c = 5	d = 1
8.	a = 0	b = 1	c = 3	d = 5
9.	a = 3	b = 1	c = 5	d = 0

Your score

0–3   You are rather bigoted and it looks like it will be a difficult job discussing the issue with you as you seem so convinced that your views and beliefs are right.

4–13   Your fear of lesbians is probably based largely on ignorance, myth and misinformation. Although you appear very prejudiced, if you could allow yourself to consider finding out more about lesbians and bisexuals you might find some of your opinions do change. (On the other hand some women's fears might also be because they fear their own sexuality might be concealing a lesbian or bisexual potential!)

14–32   You probably think you are very liberal, tolerant and broad-minded, and by most standards you probably are. But being 'tolerant' is not enough to change other people's attitudes. Lesbians need assumptions about them to be challenged all the time. Don't keep your views to yourself, actively do something to help them combat the misinformation and prejudice most people have against them. Some women scoring in this range will be lesbians who are 'in the closet', bisexual or women who are not quite sure of their own sexuality.

33–45   Well either you are an 'out' lesbian or you are the sort of friend we need! Whether you are lesbian, bisexual or heterosexual, it is this sort of positive challenging of people's prejudices and stereotypes about lesbians which will help towards creating a society in which women will be more able to choose their sexuality freely.

WORKSHEET *9.6*

Sexuality and relationships – case studies

1 Mehrain has been living with John for a year and has a new baby. She is very wrapped up with her son and also tired and does not feel like making love. Her partner is impatient to resume their sex life, jealous of the baby and keeps demanding sex. There are a lot of rows.

2 When Margaret was growing up, sex or even bodily functions were never talked about at home. Now she has her own children she finds it hard to talk to them about sex.

3 Phyllis's husband Frank has been under a lot of stress and for some time has been unable to get an erection. Phyllis does not miss intercourse but she is missing the cuddling, caressing and kissing that was an important part of love-making for her. Frank feels a failure and that his 'impotence' means he cannot make love at all. Whenever Phyllis begins to kiss or cuddle him he withdraws, because he feels it will lead to failure again.

4 Clare had an accident and is now paralysed from the waist down. She is still aware of her sexual needs but other people seem to assume that someone in a wheel-chair is non-sexual. Clare wonders if she will ever have a sexual relationship again.

5 Kathy isn't sure what to do about her three-year-old daughter who masturbates a lot.

6 Josie is a widow and does not want to marry again. She does not believe in sex outside marriage but misses the physical warmth and comfort she had with her husband.

7 Maya is a single parent with a daughter of nine and a thirteen-year-old son. She has recently begun a relationship with Anil who is very caring, and fond of the children. They seem to get very jealous when Maya and Anil hug or kiss. Maya wants Anil to stay the night openly but is worried about how the children will react.

8 Rose is going through the menopause and is well except for vaginal dryness. She does not want hormonal treatment because it is not suitable for her. Intercourse is painful for her so she wants to explore other ways of making love, but her partner is not very imaginative.

RESOURCES

For contact details of distributors and organisations listed here, see Chapter 11 *General resources*.

Publications

Armstrong, Ewan McKay and Gordon, Peter, *Sexualities: an Advanced Training Resource* (1992), Family Planning Association, £14.99.
Discussions and exercises.

Bell, R, *Changing Bodies, Changing Lives: A Book for Teenage Sex and Relationships* (1988), Vintage Books, New York, £10.95, ISBN 0 394 75441 3. Available from women's or radical bookshops.
A valuable book for teenagers by authors of *Our Bodies, Ourselves*, which focuses on sexuality, and taking care of yourself emotionally and physically. Usefully illustrated, and laid out in a user-friendly way.

Brown, Paul and Faulder, Carolyn, *Treat Yourself to Sex: a Guide to Good Loving* (1988), Penguin, £3.99.
Suggests exercises for dealing with common sexual problems.

Comfort, Alex, *The New Joy of Sex* (1991), Mitchell Beazley, £17.99.
Ideas for increasing sensuality and imagination in sexual relationships.

Coward, Rosalind, *Female Desire: Women's Sexuality Today* (1984), Granada, £3.99.
A collection of essays about women's sexuality and what it means to women themselves.

Delacoste, Frederique and Alexander, Priscilla, *Sex Work: Writings by Women in the Sex Industry* (1988), Virago, £5.50.
Women in the sex industry write on a range of topics – the work, organising and many more.

Dickson, Anne, *The Mirror Within: a New Look at Sexuality* (1991, c1985), Quartet, £3.95.
For women wanting to develop their sexuality. Includes many activities for individual or group work.

Friday, Nancy, *My Secret Garden: Women's Sexual Fantasies* (1988), Quartet, £5.95.
Women describe their own sexual fantasies.

Friday, Nancy, *Women on Top: How Real Life has Changed Women's Fantasies* (1991), Hutchinson, £8.99.
A collection of sexual fantasies, sent in by women of all ages and conditions, which represent a collection of female sexuality – angry, tender, lustful, guilt-ridden and powerful.

Heather, Beryl, *Sharing: a Handbook for Those Involved in Training in Personal Relationships and Sexuality* (1987), Family Planning Association, £9.99.
Exercises, helping strategies, action plans and relationship building.

Heiman, Julia and Lo Piccolo, Joseph, *Becoming Orgasmic: a Sexual Growth Program for Women* (1988), Piatkus, £8.95.
A practical series of self-help exercises for all women who want to enhance their sexual pleasure.

Hooper, Anne, *The Body Electric: a Unique Account of Sex Therapy for Women* (1992), Pandora, £6.99.
A personal look by six women on a course about sexuality.

Loulan, Joanne, *Lesbian Sex* (1985), Spinsters Ink, £8.95.
Covers sex, long-term relationships, disability, motherhood and ageing. Includes exercises for self-help.

Phillips, Angela and Rakusen, Jill (eds), *The New Our Bodies, Ourselves* (1989), Penguin, £15.99.
Has useful chapters on sexuality, relationships and lesbians.

Sandford, Christine E, *Enjoy Sex in the Middle Years* (1990), Optima/Relate, £5.99.
Discusses overcoming sexual changes and problems in the middle years.

Trenchard, Lorraine, *Being Lesbian* (1989), GMP Publishing, £4.95.
A guide to help lesbians enhance their sexuality.

Videos

Talking About: Sexuality – Understanding and Helping (1986), 43 minutes, Concord.
Looks at sexuality in a broad sense. Considers the needs of the elderly, disabled and unemployed. Emphasises that sex is not simply equated with sexual intercourse. Accompanied by notes for course leaders. Not aimed particularly at women.

Women Like Us (1989), 50 minutes, Clio (Concord).
Sixteen lesbians aged 50 to 80 talk about their lives.

Organisations

Discern
Counselling for people with disability who are experiencing sexual difficulties.

Lesbian Line
Information and support for women who are or think they might be lesbians. Has details of local Lesbian Line services throughout the country.
See also Resources listed under the other sections in this chapter.

Contraception

BACKGROUND INFORMATION

- Women have always sought to control their own fertility. They make different choices about contraceptive methods dependent on their age and specific circumstances. Throughout their fertile lives they may make different choices for different reasons.

- Contraception has a role in prevention of pregnancy, and barrier methods have a role in preventing transmission of infections. There is still no contraceptive method which is 100% safe and 100% effective. All methods have risks and benefits. It is important that women are enabled to make informed choices about methods through objective and up to date information.

- Women of different ages, culture, religion, class require access to information about, and supplies of, all contraceptive methods.

- In some cultural communities where it is perceived to be the responsibility of the man to provide for his wife and children, contraception decisions may be made mainly by the husband.

- Certain communities (e.g. Roman Catholic, Jewish, Muslim) may in some cases consider artificial contraceptive methods as contrary to their religion.

- Contraception has obvious links with sexuality for women who are sexually active with men.

- Choices of contraceptive methods today need to recognise not just the prevention of unplanned pregnancies but also the importance of protection against STDs and HIV.

PRACTICAL POINTS

- Women may welcome the opportunity to exchange information, work through issues, consider contraceptive options and evaluate their specific needs.

- Some women may not wish to participate in a session on contraception. Lesbians may feel the issue is not relevant to them.

- Have back-up information available, including useful local contacts.

- Successful use of a particular contraceptive method may require assertiveness skills on the part of women.

INFORMATION SHEET *9.2*

Family planning services

Who can get contraceptives and advice?

Anyone! You can go to a family planning clinic to get contraceptives and advice if you are: single or married, young or older, a woman or a man. If you would like to take along a partner, they will be made welcome too.

Where to go for contraceptives and advice

You can go to any of the following for contraceptive help and advice:

- your family doctor;
- another family doctor who gives contraceptive advice;
- a family planning clinic;
- a Brook Advisory Centre (for young people);
- a fee-paying clinic;
- a chemist or pharmacy.

Contraceptives and advice are free

If you usually live in this country, you can get contraceptives and advice free on the National Health Service. You do not have to pay. But you can go to a private clinic where you pay for contraceptives and advice if you want to.

Going to a family doctor

You can get contraceptives and advice from your own family doctor. If for some reason you do not want to talk to your own family doctor about contraception, you can go to any other family doctor who gives contraceptive advice. The other doctor does not have to be in the same practice as your own family doctor.

Finding a doctor who gives contraceptive advice

Lists of family doctors are kept in the places in the list below. The family doctors who give contraceptive advice have the letter 'C' after their names.

▷

▷ 9.2 cont.

You can find lists of family doctors:

- in libraries;

- in post offices;

- from Family Health Services Authorities – the address and phone number is in the phone book;

- from advice centres like a Citizens' Advice Bureau or Community Health Council.

Family doctors will give you a prescription to get the contraceptives from chemists or pharmacies. You will not have to pay for the contraceptives, they are free. You cannot get contraceptive sponges from family doctors.

Going to a family planning clinic

You can find out where your nearest family planning clinic is, and the times it is open from:

- the phone book – just look under family planning clinic;

- the District Health Authority – look for their address and phone number in the phone book;

- a health centre;

- your midwife or health visitor;

- a hospital;

- the Family Planning Association;

- a GP.

At a family planning clinic you will get contraceptive advice and you will get your contraceptives free.

Going to a Brook Advisory Centre

Brook Advisory Centres provide a contraceptive and counselling service for young people (under 25 years old). People who are under 16 are welcome. Phone 071 708 1234 to find out where your nearest Brook Advisory Centre is.

Going to a fee-paying clinic

If you want to, you can go to a family planning clinic where you pay for the advice

▷

▷ 9.2 cont.

and the contraceptives. Just write to the Family Planning Association to find out about your nearest fee-paying clinic.

Going to chemists or pharmacies

Chemists or pharmacies sell condoms, diaphragms, caps, spermicides and sponges. And the pharmacist there is highly trained. You can ask them for information about any contraceptives, how other drugs might affect the Pill, and where to go for free contraceptives and advice.

Source: based on the Family Planning Association leaflet *Your choices*, March 1992. Information in this area changes rapidly and readers are advised to update their information as it becomes available.

INFORMATION SHEET *9.3*

Methods of contraception

Combined pill
How it works

This is usually just called 'the Pill'. It contains two hormones: oestrogen and progestogen. The pill stops ovulation, which is when an egg is released each month in a woman. So there is no egg for the sperm to fertilise. But you will get bleeding that is like a period every month, a few days after you have stopped the Pill (during the break between packets).

Reliability

Careful use – less than 1 woman in 100 will get pregnant.

Less careful use – up to 7 women in 100 will get pregnant.

Where you can get it

Family doctor or family planning clinic.

Advantages

- Easy and convenient to use.
- You often get less bleeding with your period, less pain and less premenstrual tension.
- Protects against cancer of the ovary and cancer of the womb.
- Does not interrupt love-making.
- Reduces pelvic infections.

Disadvantages

- Some women have minor side-effects. But these usually disappear after a few months.
- Not suitable for smokers over 35.

▷

© Health Education Authority, 1993

▷ 9.3 cont.

- May not be suitable for women with health problems such as raised blood-pressure, or who have blood relatives who got heart disease or thrombosis at an early age.

Other information

The Pill may not work:

- if it is taken over 12 hours late;

- if you have sickness or severe diarrhoea;

- with certain other tablets – always discuss with your GP.

  So you must use another contraceptive method in any of these cases.

Progestogen-only pill

How it works

People used to call this the 'mini-pill'. It has a type of hormone in it called progestogen. Women take the progestogen-only pill at the same time every day. The hormone causes changes in the cervical mucus, which is the fluid at the entrance to the womb. These changes make it very difficult for the sperm to enter the womb. In some women the progestogen-only pill may stop ovulation.

Reliability

Careful use – less than 1 woman in 100 will get pregnant. But you must take it at the same time every day. (And if you weigh more than 11 stone (70kg), this may make the progestogen-only pill less effective.)

Less careful use – 1 to 4 women in 100 will get pregnant.

Where you can get it

Family doctor or family planning clinic.

Advantages

- Easy and convenient to use.

- Useful for older women who smoke.

- You can use it when you are breast-feeding.

- Does not interrupt love-making.   ▷

▷ 9.3 cont.

Disadvantages

- Some women have side-effects. But these usually last only two or three months.

- Your periods might not be regular. You might get some bleeding between periods.

- Sometimes you might miss a period, but this is not harmful.

Other information

The progestogen-only pill may not work:

- if you take it more than three hours late; or

- if you have sickness or severe diarrhoea.

So you must use another contraceptive method if either of these happens.

Intra-uterine device (IUD)

How it works

A small plastic and copper device put into a woman's womb by a doctor. It works mainly by stopping the sperm and the egg meeting. It might also slow down the egg coming towards the womb. And it might stop a fertilised egg from settling in the womb. IUDs used to be called coils or loops.

Reliability

1 to 3 women in 100 will get pregnant.

Where you can get it

Family doctor or family planning clinic.

Advantages

- Works as soon as it is put in.

- Very suitable for a woman who wants a space between having her children or has decided she does not want any more children.

- You do not have to think about it every day.

- Does not interrupt love-making.

▷ 9.3 cont.

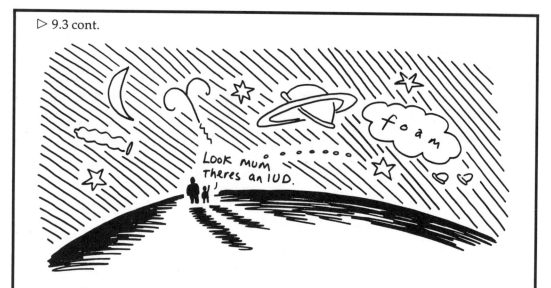

Disadvantages

- Some women find that their periods are heavier and longer at first, and their periods might be more painful.

- Not suitable for women who have heavy and painful periods.

- Some women get a little bleeding before and after their periods. This is called spotting.

- Sometimes the IUD might come out.

- Some women get a pelvic infection.

- There are other rare complications.

- Not a first choice for young women who have never been pregnant.

Other information

- IUDs are usually changed every five years.

- You can check an IUD is still in place by feeling for the threads that are attached to it. You can feel these high in your vagina and you will be taught how to do this.

- You can use tampons if you have an IUD.   ▷

▷ 9.3 cont.

Diaphragm or cap with spermicide

How they work

A woman puts the diaphragm or cap into her vagina with some spermicide before intercourse. And it must stay in for six hours after intercourse. A diaphragm is a soft rubber dome. It covers the entrance to the womb which is called the cervix. A cap is smaller and fits neatly over the cervix. They work by stopping the sperm getting into the womb to meet the egg. You need to get one specially fitted to make sure it is the right size for you.

Reliability

Careful use – 2 women in 100 will get pregnant.

Less careful use – 2 to 15 women in 100 will get pregnant.

Where you can get them

Family doctor or family planning clinic. They can also be bought from chemists or pharmacies if you know your size.

Advantages

- You can put a diaphragm or cap in at any time before intercourse, so it does not interrupt love-making. But if you put the diaphragm or cap in more than three hours before you have intercourse, you do need to use some more spermicide.

- May help to protect you from cancer of the cervix.

Disadvantages

- Need to plan ahead and put your diaphragm or cap and spermicide in before love-making.

- Your diaphragm or cap should be checked every six months to see if it still fits properly. It also needs to be checked if you gain or lose more than 7lb (3kg), or if you have a baby, miscarriage or abortion.

- Some women and men are allergic to spermicide.

▷

▷ 9.3 cont.

Vaginal ring

How it works

It is a soft rubber ring which is put into the vagina. You leave it in your vagina all the time. It releases a type of hormone called progestogen. Progestogen causes changes in the cervical mucus, which is fluid at the entrance to the womb. These changes make it very difficult for the sperm to enter the womb and meet the egg. In some women the vaginal ring stops ovulation. One vaginal ring works for three months before you need a new one.

Reliability

Careful use – 4 to 5 women in 100 will get pregnant.

Less careful use – No test results available.

Where you can get it

Family doctor or family planning clinic.

Advantages

- Easy and convenient to use.
- Useful for women who cannot take oestrogen.
- Useful for women who do not like taking a pill every day or find it difficult to remember.
- Does not interrupt love-making.
- You can use it when you are breast-feeding.

Disadvantages

- You may get bleeding between periods.
- Sometimes you might miss a period or the time between each period might be different.
- A few women get vaginal irritation or discharge.
- Very occasionally a vaginal ring comes out when you go to the toilet or when you take a tampon out.

▷

▷ 9.3 cont.

Other information

You should leave the vaginal ring in during intercourse and when you have a period.

Natural methods

How they work

Natural methods of birth control work by helping a woman to know when she is most likely to get pregnant. This is called the fertile time and is about 12 to 16 days before a period starts. You do not have intercourse around this fertile time. Or you use a barrier method of contraception, such as a diaphragm or condom, at this time.

Natural methods of birth control need the co-operation and support of your partner.

There are different methods of natural birth control. The most reliable is the sympto-thermal method which means that:

- you take your temperature every day;
- you notice the changes in your vaginal fluids; and
- you notice other signs of ovulation.

Reliability

Careful use – 2 women in 100 will get pregnant.

Less careful use – 2 to 20 women in 100 will get pregnant.

Where to find out about them

Learned from a specially trained teacher. Ask where to find one at a family planning clinic, or at the Family Planning Association (for address see Resources).

Advantages

- No mechanical devices or hormones are used.
- Couples share responsibility for birth control.
- No side-effects.
- Natural birth control can help you to plan to get pregnant as well, because you will know when you are at your fertile time.

▷

© Health Education Authority, 1993

▷ 9.3 cont.

Disadvantages

- You need to keep careful records every day.

- Women who do not have regular periods may need to be extra careful. This particularly applies to women who have just had a baby and older women.

Sterilisation for women

How it works

This is a permanent method of birth control. A woman's fallopian tubes are cut or blocked by an operation so that the eggs cannot travel down to meet the sperm. Sterilisation does not affect your sex drive.

Reliability

1 to 3 women in 1,000 will get pregnant.

Where you can get it

Family doctor or family planning clinic who refers you to hospital, or a private clinic or hospital if you want to pay.

Advantages

- It is permanent.

- Effective immediately after the operation.

Disadvantages

- Very occasionally the tubes join together again and then the woman is fertile again.

- A few women have heavier periods.

Other information

Sterilisation is only for people who have decided they do not want any children in the future. You should not have it done if you or your partner have any doubts. Make sure you discuss this fully before you have the operation. The operation can be done under local anaesthetic which means the area that is cut is numbed. You will be awake during the operation. Or it can be done under general anaesthetic

▷

▷ 9.3 cont.

which means you are asleep during the operation. The operation can only be done in a hospital or private clinic. Many women have this operation and go home on the same day. Others need to stay in the hospital for a day or two.

Vasectomy for men

How it works

This is a permanent method of birth control. The man has a small operation in which tubes in his testicles are cut. These are the vas deferens tubes that the sperm travels through to get to the penis. When they are cut there are no sperm in the semen, which is the fluid that comes out of the penis when a man comes or ejaculates. Vasectomy does not affect your sex drive.

Reliability

1 in 1,000 failure rate.

Where you can get it

Family doctor or family planning clinic, or a private clinic or hospital if you want to pay.

Advantage

It is permanent.

Disadvantages

- It can take some time for all the sperm to disappear from the semen. You must use another contraceptive method until two tests, one after the other, show that there are no sperm left.

- Occasionally the tubes join together again and then the man is fertile again.

Other information

Vasectomy is only for people who have decided they do not want any children in the future. Men should not have it done if they or their partners have any doubts. He should discuss this fully before he has the operation.

The operation can be done while he is awake. He has an injection to numb the area that will be cut. The operation takes only about 15 minutes and can be done at a

© Health Education Authority, 1993

▷ 9.3 cont.

doctor's surgery or clinic. He can have a general anaesthetic in a hospital or private clinic. This means he is asleep during the operation and it takes longer.

Condoms for men

How they work

The male condom is made of very thin rubber. It is put onto the man's penis when it is erect and stops the sperm from getting into the woman's vagina. Some male condoms are lubricated with spermicide which kills sperm.

Reliability

Careful use – 2 women in 100 will get pregnant. Careful use means putting on a male condom every time you have intercourse. Put it on before the penis touches the woman's vaginal area. The penis should not touch the woman's vaginal area when the condom is taken off.

Less careful use – 2 to 15 women in 100 will get pregnant.

Where you can get them

Free from some family doctors. Ask yours. Free from family planning clinics. They can be bought from chemists or pharmacies, garages, many shops, supermarkets, barbers, some clothes shops, slot machines, mail order, adverts in magazines.

Advantages

- Easy to get and to use.
- Can help to protect both the man and the woman against sexually transmitted infections including HIV.
- May protect women against cancer of the cervix.

Disadvantages

- May slip off during intercourse if not put on properly. Also need to be careful when the man pulls out of the woman's vagina to make sure it does not slip off. But when he is used to doing this it should not be a problem.
- Very occasionally a male condom splits during intercourse.

▷

▷ 9.3 cont.

Other information

Condoms that have a kitemark like this 𝅏 on the pack have been properly tested. Condoms also have a date on the pack which is the last date they should be used.

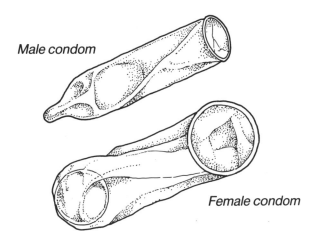

Male condom

Female condom

Condoms for women

How they work

The female condom is made of soft polyurethane – which is like plastic. It is a sheath which you put inside the vagina.

The inner ring, which is at the closed end of the sheath, is used to insert the sheath. The lower half of the inner ring is squeezed between thumb, index and middle finger to give a confident and secure grip. The squeezed ring is inserted into the vagina as far as possible. A finger is then inserted into the sheath until it touches the bottom of the inner ring, and pushed upwards until it is just past the symphisis pubis. There is no requirement for the inner ring to lie over the cervix.

The outer ring and a small part of the sheath lie outside the vagina. The partner's penis should be guided into the sheath and the outer ring will lie flat against the vulva during intercourse. After withdrawal, the outer ring is twisted to retain the ejaculate and the sheath is gently pulled out of the vagina. Put the condom back in the packet after use. This should be resealed and put in a bin.

Insertion may be awkward at first, but becomes easier after practising. Make sure you use an alternative form of contraception as well until you feel confident.

▷

▷ 9.3 cont.

Reliability

At the moment there are no large scale studies to tell us how reliable the female condom is. Such information can only be available after wider use and further research, but it is expected to be as reliable as the male condom.

Where you can get them

Free from a very few family planning clinics; or on sale at chemists or pharmacies.

Advantages

- Easy to obtain.
- Women can take responsibility for a contraceptive method that also protects against sexually transmitted infections.
- You can put it in before love-making starts, so it does not interrupt love-making.
- Can help to protect both the man and the woman against sexually transmitted infections including HIV – the virus which can lead to AIDS.
- Covers a larger area around the vagina – therefore more protection.
- May help to protect women from cancer of the cervix.

Disadvantages

- Expensive.
- May get pushed into the vagina during intercourse or may slip off. If it does you must stop and put it back in the right place.
- The penis may slide between the condom and the vaginal wall.

Other information

A female condom can only be used once.

Contraceptive injections

How they work

Women have an injection once every two or three months. The injection is the hormone progestogen, which is absorbed into the body very slowly. It works in the same way as the combined pill, so it stops ovulation. ▷

▷ 9.3 cont.

Reliability

Less than 1 woman in 100 will get pregnant.

Where you can get them

Family doctor or family planning clinic.

Advantages

- You need only one injection every two or three months.

- Very effective.

- Does not interrupt love-making.

Disadvantages

- You may miss periods – but this is not harmful.

- If you stop the injections it may take up to a year for your periods to start again regularly. This means you may not be able to get pregnant for up to a year.

Other information

There are two different injections. One is called Depo-Provera and the other is called Noristerat. Contraceptive injections are usually only recommended for women who cannot use other contraceptive methods for medical or other reasons. Some women find them convenient. You choose whether to use them or not. Make sure you get full information from your doctor to help decide.

Sponge

How it works

It is a soft round sponge which contains spermicide, that a woman puts into her vagina at any time before intercourse. You should not leave it in for more than 30 hours. And you must leave it in for 6 hours after the last intercourse.

▷

▷ 9.3 cont.

Reliability

Careful use – 9 women in 100 will get pregnant.

Less careful use – 9 to 25 women in 100 will get pregnant.

Do not use a sponge if it is important to you to avoid getting pregnant.

Where you can get it

Some family planning clinics (free), or on sale at chemists or pharmacies.

Advantages

- Easy to get.

- Works for 24 hours after you put it in. You can have intercourse more than once without using extra spermicide.

- You do not need to get a special size for you. One size fits everybody.

Disadvantages

- Expensive and not very reliable.

- Should not be used during a period.

- Some people are allergic to spermicide.

Other information

Read the instructions in the packet carefully to make sure you put it in the right position, over the entrance to your womb or cervix.

Source: based on Family Planning Association leaflet *Your choices*, March 1992. Information in this area changes quickly and readers are advised to update their information as it becomes available.

INFORMATION SHEET *9.4*

Emergency contraception

Emergency contraception was previously known as the 'morning after' pill.

If you want emergency contraception it is important to see a doctor as soon as possible. You can get emergency contraception:

- if you have intercourse and make a mistake with contraception, or your contraceptive method fails for any reason; or

- if you have intercourse and do not use any contraception.

But it is for emergencies only – it is not a regular method. It is important to use a contraceptive method every time you have intercourse.

Occasionally people make a mistake with contraception. For example:

- a condom may slip off or split while you are having intercourse;

- you take out your diaphragm too soon after intercourse;

- you forget a Pill.

Where you can get emergency contraception

Family doctor, family planning clinic, or casualty department. If your family doctor will not give you emergency contraception or you do not want to go to them – you can go to another family doctor who gives contraceptive advice.

What is emergency contraception?

- Either two special doses of the combined pill – you must start to take these within three days of intercourse, so you must see a doctor within three days (less than 4 women in 100 will get pregnant);

- or putting in an IUD – you must have this done within five days of intercourse, so you must see a doctor within five days (less than 1 woman in 100 will get pregnant).

After five days it is too late to have emergency contraception.

Occasionally a woman cannot use either of these methods.

Source: based on Family Planning Association leaflet *Your choices*, March 1992.

INFORMATION SHEET *9.5*

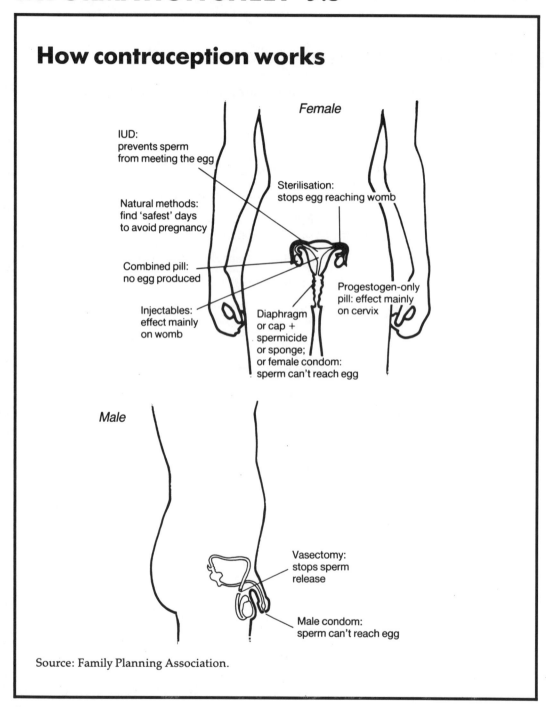

How contraception works

Female

IUD:
prevents sperm
from meeting the egg

Sterilisation:
stops egg reaching womb

Natural methods:
find 'safest' days
to avoid pregnancy

Combined pill:
no egg produced

Progestogen-only
pill: effect mainly
on cervix

Injectables:
effect mainly
on womb

Diaphragm
or cap +
spermicide
or sponge;
or female condom:
sperm can't reach egg

Male

Vasectomy:
stops sperm
release

Male condom:
sperm can't reach egg

Source: Family Planning Association.

INFORMATION SHEET *9.6*

Factors which can affect choice of contraceptive method

- knowledge of different methods
- availability of different methods (some GPs don't issue condoms, for example)
- cost
- accessible services
- number of sexual partners
- whether in a steady relationship or not
- whether or not you mind getting pregnant
- whether contraception is seen as a joint responsibility between you and your partner
- partner's attitude to different contraceptive methods
- how methods work (e.g. believing that life begins at conception)
- cultural/religious acceptability of method
- family and social traditions and pressures
- disability
- prevention against STDs, including HIV
- if you've had a miscarriage/abortion/just had a baby
- if you are breast-feeding
- whether or not you've already had a baby
- if you are going through the menopause
- whether or not you smoke
- age
- benefits or costs of children
- income and economic circumstances
- body's response to different methods.

INFORMATION SHEET *9.7*

A short history of contraception

Throughout history people have always sought to control their fertility. This has included abortion, infanticide, and crude measures which have damaged women's health and threatened their lives. The history of the struggle for decent contraception has been full of moral righteousness, racism, classism, and eugenics (the science of race improvement). Both the Church and the State have played a key role.

The earliest known references to contraceptive methods were the Egyptians' use of barrier methods and 'withdrawal'. In the eighteenth century, the vaginal sponge was mentioned. In the nineteenth century condoms made from animal membranes began to be sold. The first cervical cap was invented. Annie Besant began campaigning. Medical opinion was strongly against contraception. By the late nineteenth century contraceptive options were: withdrawal, condoms, douching, vaginal sponge, pessaries, rubber cervical caps.

The First World War marked a turning point in public opinion in Britain regarding contraception. Medical opinion began slowly to change.

1916   Margaret Sanger opened the first birth control clinic in the USA.

1918   Marie Stopes' *Married Love* was published.

1921   The first birth control clinic in Britain (The Mothers' Clinic for Constructive Birth Control) opened in London. Unfortunately Marie Stopes – for all her good work – believed in eugenics and the sterilisation of those she saw as "unfit".

1920s   Eugenics began to give way to feminist ideas; women began to argue that women had a right to control their reproduction.

1926   Dora Russell established at a Labour Party Conference that birth control was a party political issue.

1930s   Development of the first latex condom.

        The Ministry of Health agreed that mother and baby clinics could give contraceptive advice to married women whose health was at risk from further pregnancies.

        National Birth Control Association founded (changed its name to Family Planning Association (FPA) in 1939) – to give advice to married women who wanted to limit the number of children they had.

▷

▷ 9.7 cont.

1946   The NHS empowered local Health Authorities to open clinics for advice to mothers on medical grounds.

1961   The contraceptive Pill became available for the first time.

1960s   New IUDs became available.

1967   The Abortion Act was passed (legalising abortion under certain conditions).

The NHS Family Planning Act was passed (enabling advice and supplies to people wanting contraception – single as well as married).

1973   NHS Reorganisation Act passed, which set up free family planning services in clinics and hospitals.

1975   GPs allowed to provide free contraceptive services.

1976   The FPA completed the transfer of its clinics to the NHS.

1990s   Free contraception is available from: hospital clinics, family planning clinics/well-women clinics, GPs, voluntary sector clinics (e.g. Brook) and private clinics.

Abortions (under the terms of the 1967 Act) are available from NHS provision, the voluntary sector (e.g. British Pregnancy Advisory Service) and private clinics.

ACTIVITY *9.8*

Family planning services

Aim
- To clarify with women what family planning services are available.

Materials
A copy of Worksheet 9.7 and Information Sheet 9.2 *Family planning services* for each woman.

Method
1 Give each woman a copy of the worksheet.
2 Ask women to discuss the questions in small groups, and pool their knowledge.
3 Feed back to the large group.
4 Hand out the information sheet to check out where to go for contraceptives and advice.

Discussion points
- How appropriate are the available services for women?
- What are women's experiences of using different agencies for contraceptive services?
- Do women feel that they always get enough information to make informed choices?
- Have you ever felt a particular contraceptive method has been promoted? Why might this be so?

ACTIVITY *9.9*

Contraceptive methods

Aims
- To enable women to learn about the range of methods available, in order to make informed choices.

- To consider advantages and disadvantages of particular methods.

Materials

Flipchart and pens; a copy of Information Sheets 9.3 *Methods of contraception* and 9.4 *Emergency contraception* for each woman.

Method

1 Brainstorm all possible methods of contraception, and flipchart them.

2 Consider advantages and disadvantages of each method.

3 Give out information sheets to check out information.

Discussion points

- What factors affect our choice of contraceptive methods?

- Are all methods available from your family planning services?

- Whose responsibility is the choice of contraceptive method? Why?

ACTIVITY *9.10*

How contraceptive methods work

Aims

- To help women understand how each contraceptive method works.

- To enable women to make informed choices.

This activity follows on well from Activity 9.9.

Materials

A list of different contraceptive methods on a flipchart, copies of Information Sheets 9.3 *Methods of contraception* and 9.5 *How contraception works* for each woman.

Method

1 In the large group, go through each method, asking women to explain how they work (you will probably need to give additional information).

2 Divide methods on the flipchart into different categories under the following headings:

- barrier (e.g. diaphragms and caps, condoms (male and female);

- hormonal (e.g. combined pill, progestogen only pill, injectables (e.g. Depo-Provera), emergency contraception (pill));

- Chemical (sponge, spermicides);

- other (IUDs, sterilisation, withdrawal, natural methods).

3 Give out information sheets to back up and extend information.

Discussion points

- Why is it important to understand how different contraceptive methods work?

- Does this affect women's choice of different methods?

ACTIVITY *9.11*

Choosing a contraceptive method 1

Aim

- To enable women to clarify acceptability of different contraceptive methods.

Materials

A copy of Worksheet 9.8 *Choosing a contraceptive method* for each woman; pens.

Method

1 Give a copy of worksheet to each woman.

2 Ask women to go through questions on the worksheet in small groups.

3 Feed back to the large group.

Discussion points

- Why did women use a particular contraceptive method at any one time?

- What affected women's choice of different contraceptive methods?

- Should contraception be the woman's, her partner's, or joint responsibility?

Note for tutor

This activity is useful for a group where you *know* women are heterosexual and have used/do use contraception. Otherwise, use Activity 9.12 *Choosing a contraceptive method 2 – case studies.*

ACTIVITY *9.12*

Choosing a contraceptive method 2 – case studies

Aim

- To consider what factors affect women's choice of contraceptive methods.

Materials

Copies of Worksheet 9.9 *Contraceptive methods – case studies* and Information Sheet 9.6 *Factors which can affect choice of contraceptive method* for each woman; flipchart, pens.

Method

1 Divide into small groups, and give each group different case studies to look at and discuss.

2 Feed back to the large group, so that women have a chance to hear about case studies different from theirs.

3 Give out the information sheet and discuss.

ACTIVITY *9.13*

Contraception game

Aims

- To facilitate discussion among women about different methods of contraception.

- To identify factors which affect choice of contraceptive method.

Materials

Small cards with different contraceptive methods written on (see Worksheet 9.10 *Contraception game*); carrier bag, flipchart and pen.

Space is needed for women to stand in one long line.

Have back-up information leaflets available on each contraceptive method.

Method

1 Put small cards with different methods in a carrier bag and ask each woman to take one.

2 Flipchart the question 'What is the best contraceptive for women?'

3 Ask women to stand in a line depending on the method on their card with the *best* method at one end and the *worst* at the other.

4 When women are finally in a line, ask them to read out what is on their card, starting from the best method along a spectrum to the worst.

5 In the large group, discuss issues which this activity has raised.

Discussion points

● What does *best* mean? Best in terms of low failure rate, or best for women's bodies?

● Where does contraception end, and abortion start?

● How much did women's individual experience enter in to the activity?

● How much 'choice' do we actually have over contraceptive methods? What might affect that choice?

● Should the male pill ever become a reality? Would women like their partners to use it? Why? Why not?

ACTIVITY *9.14*

Contraceptive methods through the ages

Aims

● To enable women to consider current contraceptive methods within a historical framework.

● To realise the social and political struggle for family planning.

Materials

A copy of Information Sheet 9.7 *A short history of contraception* for each woman; paper, pens, access to reference books.

Method

Project work

1 Ask women, before the next session, to ask sisters, mothers, grand-

mothers, older women they know about contraceptive methods they have known or used – and factors which affected their choice of method.

2 Ask women to check in the local library for old magazines or books with adverts for various contraceptive methods.

3 Bring collected information to the next session, and share it in the large group.

4 Give out the information sheet, discuss, and write up as a group project.

5 Give out a booklist for further reading (see Resources).

Variation

1 In pairs, ask women to share their knowledge of contraceptive methods used in the past. (If your group has a wide age-range, pair up younger women with older women).

2 Share findings in the large group.

3 Give out the information sheet and discuss milestones in the struggle for the right of women to determine their fertility.

4 Give out a booklist for further reading (see Resources).

Discussion points

- Older women may have graphic tales to tell of lack of access to contraception, life before the 1967 Abortion Act etc.

- If the group includes women from different cultures, religions, classes, or women with a disability, compare their experiences. Are there similarities? What are the differences?

- It has been said that there was not a single contraceptive method in existence in Britain in the early 1960s (apart from the Pill) which had not been available and in a greater variety in 1890 (see Leathard, *The Fight for Family Planning*). Did this surprise women? Why was this?

- Do women think there is a wide range of safe, reliable contraceptive methods today?

- If men got pregnant, what might be the situation regarding contraceptive methods?

WORKSHEET *9.7*

Family planning services

1 Who provides family planning services?

2 How can I find out where services are?

3 Who is entitled to family planning services?

4 What can my GP provide?

5 What should routine family planning clinic services provide?

6 Where can I get *emergency* (which used to be called 'morning after') contraception?

WORKSHEET *9.8*

Choosing a contraceptive method

1 List contraceptive methods you have used.

2 Why did you use a particular method?

3 Why did you change from one method to another?

© Health Education Authority, 1993

WORKSHEET *9.9*

Contraceptive methods – case studies

Carol is 37 and single. She has several close male friends, but at present does not have a sexual relationship with any. She anticipates only occasional sexual activity, and because of this does not want to use the Pill or IUD which provide protection all the time. She thinks that in the unlikely event of spontaneous intercourse taking place she would use emergency contraception, or if faced with an unwanted pregnancy she would request a medical method of abortion such as mifegynl (the abortion pill).

If you were in Carol's position, might you choose the same? What other steps could Carol take?

Kath believes firmly that life begins when sperm meets the egg – at conception. She would never agree to an abortion, whatever the reason. She enjoys sexual intercourse, though is not in a steady relationship. She is clear that she does not want children within the next few years.

What might her contraceptive options be?

Sharon is about to go abroad to work for three years, and is unsure of the range of contraceptive methods available to her in the new country.

What might she do?

Imtiaz has been to her GP for contraceptive advice. He wasn't very helpful, offering her only 'the jab' (long acting injectable contraceptive such as Depo-Provera) as he felt it would be the best method for her. Imtiaz feels she would like to get more information on contraceptive methods generally to help her choose.

What could she do?

Jenny is 41, smokes about ten cigarettes a day, and has several male partners. She already has three children, all delivered by caesarian section – she can have no more.

What do you think her options could be for contraception? Should protection from HIV enter into this decision?

▷

> 9.9 cont.

Louise is 15 years old and wants to make love with her steady boyfriend. Her doctor will not prescribe the Pill for her as she is only 15. The cost of condoms seems too much for her small allowance.

What can she do to get adequate protection? Do you think she should be able to get contraception given her age?

Hilda is 53 and has been experiencing the menopause for several years. She feels that there is little chance of her getting pregnant, but wants to make quite sure she doesn't. Her husband and herself have always attempted to take joint responsibility for contraception.

What would be the best option for Hilda? What can be her husband's role in this?

Helen feels she is stuck in a violent relationship where sexual violence is not uncommon. She has had two abortions and cannot face any more of these. She does not want to get pregnant as her two children are quite enough for her in her current situation. Her husband is a strict Catholic and will not condone any form of contraception – he does not know about the abortions.

What can she do?

Jasmine has just had her first baby and is breast-feeding her. Her mother and her mother-in-law have given her contradictory advice about the need for contraception during this time. She feels very confused and her husband is no help – he does not see contraception as part of his responsibility.

What advice would you give to Jasmine? Where could she go for support and advice?

WORKSHEET *9.10*

Contraception game

MALE PILL

'NATURAL'
METHODS
(reliably taught)

INTRA-
UTERINE
DEVICE
(IUD)

CONDOM

VASECTOMY

STERILISATION

ABORTION

EMERGENCY
CONTRACEPTION

SPERMICIDES,
e.g. THE
CONTRACEPTIVE
SPONGE

'WITHDRAWAL'
METHOD

NO SEX
WITH
MEN

THE PILL

PILL WITH
CONDOM

NON-
PENETRATIVE
SEX

FEMALE
CONDOM

CELIBACY

IUD
and CONDOM

NEW ABORTION
PILL

DIAPHRAGM OR
CAP AND
SPERMICIDE

LONG-ACTING
INJECTABLES
(e.g. Depo
Provera)

RESOURCES

For contact details of distributors and organisations listed here, see the list of organisations in Chapter 11 *General resources.*

Publications

Bromwich, Peter and Parsons, Tony, *Contraception: The Facts* (1990), Oxford University Press, £5.95.
Second expanded edition covers all currently available methods of contraception. FPA approved.

Brook Advisory Centres, *Abortion: an Introduction to the Facts about Abortion* (1990), £1.95.
Brief, impartial guide to facts and figures about abortion – useful to stimulate discussion.

Christopher, Elphis, *Sexuality and Birth Control in Community Work* (1987), Tavistock, £15.99.
Resource for health and social workers with information on sexuality and contraception. FPA approved.

Cowper, Ann and Young, Cyril, *Family Planning: Fundamentals for Health Professionals* (1989), Chapman and Hall, £11.50.
Illustrated introduction to anatomy, physiology, contraception, interviewing techniques and related areas.

Davies, Vanessa, *Abortion and Afterwards* (1991), Ashgrove Press, £6.99.
Comprehensive information on legal, medical and practical aspects of abortion from confirmation of pregnancy, decision-making and emotional aftermath.

Estaugh, V, and Wheatley, J, *Family Planning and Family Well-Being* (1990), Family Policy Studies Centre occasional paper No. 12. £5.50. Available from Family Planning Association.
Includes brief history of family planning; use of contraception; fertility trends; teenage pregnancy; changing family patterns; work and the family; health and family planning.

Flynn, Anna M, and Brooks, Melissa, *A Manual of Natural Family Planning* (1990), Unwin, £4.99.
Second edition of the guide to a full range of natural contraceptive methods; includes special situations such as during the climacteric and breast feeding. FPA approved.

Fried, Marlene Gerber, *From Abortion to Reproductive Freedom: Transforming a Movement* (1990), South End Press.
Thorough guide to reproductive rights issues. American.

Goulds, Sharon, *Making History: Birth Control* (1988), Channel 4, £1.50.
Clear brief introduction to the history of birth control.

Guillebaud, John, *Contraception: Your Questions Answered* (1989), Churchill Livingstone, £8.95.
Answers to questions asked by health professionals, women and their partners about all reversible methods of contraception. FPA approved.

Leathard, A, *The Fight for Family Planning* (1980), Macmillan, £14.95 (hardback).
The development of family planning services in Britain. Highlights birth control battles and controversies, hostility to contraception, developments to provide services and changing public attitudes to birth control. Provides a history of the Family Planning Association.

Mosse, Julia and Heaton, Josephine, *The Fertility and Contraception Book* (1990), Faber, £7.99.
Covers history, function and pros and cons of each method of contraception along with advice on the best methods at different times of life.

Sapire, K Esther, *Contraception and Sexuality in Health and Disease* (1989), (UK edition revised by Toni Belfield and John Guillebaud), McGraw-Hill, £25.00.
Covers all aspects of family planning, men's and women's sexuality, and reproductive health care. Aimed at professionals. FPA approved.

Shapiro, Rose, *Contraception: a Practical and Political Guide* (1987), Virago, £5.99.
A historical review, followed by a practical guide to contraception including reliability.

Szarewski, Anne, *Hormonal Contraception: a Woman's Guide* (1991), Optima, £6.99.
Basic guide. Includes a fairly positive view of Depo Provera.

Williams, Cerys (ed), *The 'Abortion Pill': (mifepristone/RU486): Widening the Choice for Women* (1990), Birth Control Trust, £4.95.
Looks at how the drug works, results of trials, legal and political ramifications.

Winn, Denise, *Experiences of Abortion* (1988), Optima, £4.99.
Women talk about their experiences of abortion.

Organisations

Birth Control Trust
Aims to advance medical and sociological research and public education. Newsletter (*Abortion Review*). Booklist available.

British Pregnancy Advisory Service
Advice, counselling and treatment for women; 24 branches and 6 nursing homes nationwide.

Brook Advisory Centres
Advice, support and counselling for under 25s. Contraception, post-coital, sex

education, HIV/AIDS, referral for antenatal care or abortion. Wide range of publications, newsletter (*Newsprint*), educational materials, videos, teaching packs.

Family Planning Association
Wide range of leaflets, educational materials, pamphlets, videos and other publications. Healthwise (see Chapter 11 *General resources*) is the bookstore attached to the London branch. Family planning leaflets available in Bengali, Gujarati, Hindi, Punjabi and Urdu. Quarterly journal (*Family Planning Today*) covers sexual health, contraception and relationships, £10.00 p.a.

International Planned Parenthood Federation (IPPF)
Works to promote and support family planning internationally. Bulletins, leaflets, other publications.

National Association of Natural Family Planning Teachers
Publishes a wide range of books, a newsletter, list of NFP teachers in England and Wales, information on technological aids for NFP. Send s.a.e.

Sexually transmitted diseases

BACKGROUND INFORMATION

Sex is a very normal and healthy part of our lives. It's a way of sharing affection and tenderness, excitement and enjoyment. Some women have sex without being in a steady relationship, while for others sex is part of a long-term relationship. Sexual activity is today more readily accepted as a normal part of our lives, and more infections are known to be passed on during sex. These are known as **sexually transmitted diseases (STDs)**, or **genito-urinary (GU) infections**. They are so-called because they can affect the genital area as well as the parts that your urine passes through – the bladder and the urethra. GU infections are usually (though not always) spread through sexual contact.

There are at least 25 different infections. What they all have in common is that they can be spread during sexual activity. Some infections are spread not only by vaginal intercourse but also during oral sex (where partners kiss or stimulate each other's genitals or anus with their tongue), and anal sex (where the penis enters the anus).

When spread through oral sex, these infections can also affect the mouth and throat.

We all get infections of some kind at some time in our lives. STDs may not be worse than the many other kinds of diseases such as flu or measles. Every year over half a million new cases of STDs are seen at clinics in the UK. What is special about STDs is that some of them can cause serious and permanent damage to your health *if left untreated*. And some can make women infertile. So it is especially important that all STDs are diagnosed by a doctor and treated promptly.

Just about anyone who is having sexual activity can get an infection. If you have sex with someone who has already got an infection, then you may get it too. You don't have to be 'sleeping around' to either pass on or get an infection. Even if you and your partner have been having sex only with each other for a long time, it is possible that one of you might suddenly discover an infection. This can happen because some infections lie dormant in the body and often don't cause any symptoms for several months or more. An infection could have been passed on from a previous sexual relationship and become apparent only later.

This section aims to put STDs into perspective, as infections which usually respond well to early treatment, and shows that women can do something to protect themselves and their partners.

PRACTICAL POINTS

- There may be stigma surrounding 'VD'. Previously, venereal diseases (usually meaning syphilis or gonorrhoea) were seen as 'dirty' and the result of 'immoral' behaviour. While we may live in more enlightened times, some people may have difficulty shaking off out-of-date attitudes.

- STD remains an area which requires sensitivity, compassion and tact in group discussion.

- Do not assume that all women in the group have sexual relationships with men.

- Be aware that in any group of women, it is likely that more than one will at some point in her life have had an STD. Women may not want to share personal experience. If the tutor discloses personal information this may open up the group to share their experiences.

- Do not assume wide medical knowledge. Women may be confused about medical terms. Try and stick with the language women themselves use in discussions.

- There may be anxieties among women in the group as to whether they have an STD infection. It is useful to have back-up literature on the different kinds of infections, and information on where to go for help locally.

- End on a positive note, such as a short discussion on how safer sex practices can enrich our sex lives (see sections on *Sexuality* and *HIV and AIDS*)

- Be prepared for discussion about the possibility that an infection could be passed on without sexual contact. Some infections, e.g. wart virus, can be passed on without sexual contact but this is extremely rare. As far as is known, thrush is the only genital infection which may occur without prior transmission from another person.

INFORMATION SHEET *9.8*

Areas of the body where genito-urinary infection occurs

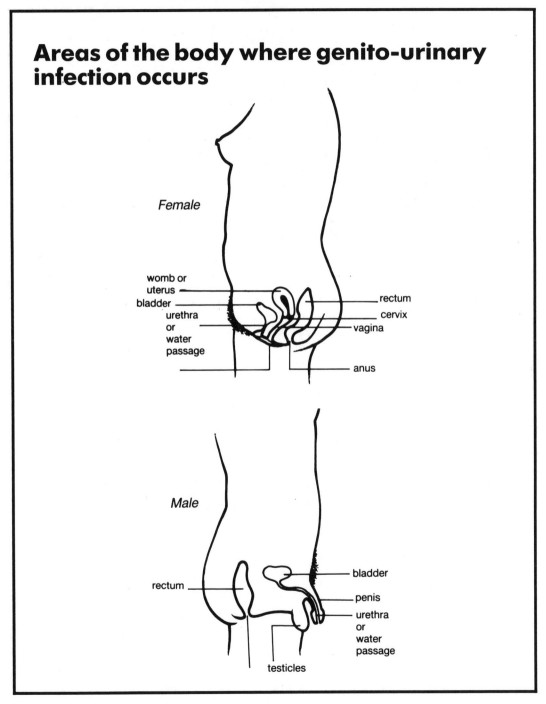

Female

womb or uterus
bladder
urethra or water passage

rectum
cervix
vagina
anus

Male

rectum

bladder
penis
urethra or water passage

testicles

INFORMATION SHEET *9.9*

Infections

Cystitis, vaginitis, urethritis

These infections are inflammations of the bladder, vagina and urethra, respectively. They can be symptoms of non-specific genital infections. They can be spread through sexual contact, but can also occur in other ways.

Chlamydia

A bacterium which infects the genitals (and occasionally throat or eye). It needs early treatment to prevent infertility. Chlamydia infection can be transmitted only through sexual contact (vaginal/anal/oral).

Gonorrhoea

A bacterium which can infect the cervix, male and female urethra, the rectum or the throat. It can be treated with antibiotics. Gonorrhoea can be transmitted only through sexual contact (vaginal/anal/oral).

Thrush

An infection caused by a yeast-like fungus (*Candida albicans*) which is found naturally on the skin, in the mouth and the bowel. Under certain conditions, particularly when the balance of the body's natural organisms is upset, the yeast multiplies in the vagina and causes discomfort. Thrush responds to treatment, but can often recur.

While thrush can be transmitted sexually, it can often also be caused by:

- continual wearing of tight clothes (especially nylon);
- pregnancy;
- ill health, or times when your resistance is lowered;
- diabetes; and
- antibiotics.

▷

▷ 9.9 cont.

Genital warts

These are caused by types of the human papilloma virus (HPV) – different from the types causing ordinary skin warts. Genital warts can be removed. Warts caused by HPV occurring on the genitals are always sexually transmitted (except in rare cases, when it is possible for ordinary skin warts to occur on the genitals).

Women who carry the wart virus HPV should have regular cervical smears as it appears they are at increased risk of cervical cancer.

Genital herpes

Caused by the *Herpes simplex* virus (HSV). There are two types of HSV: HSV1 usually causes cold sores around the mouth; HSV2 usually causes cold sores (or ulcers) on the genitals. Crossover can occur through oral/genital contact. Treatment is available to ease the discomfort of genital herpes, but there may be a recurrence of ulcers.

Genital herpes is usually sexually transmitted, but in rare cases can also be acquired by touching open cold sores on the mouth, and inadvertently transferring the virus to the genitals.

Trichomoniasis (TV)

Caused by a parasite (*Trichomonas vaginalis*) which may be found in the vagina and urethra. Responds to medication. TV is always sexually transmitted.

Pubic lice

Small lice which live in pubic hair. Pubic lice are spread by close bodily contact, including during sexual activity between two people. Occasionally they may be transferred from infested bedding or towels.

Syphilis

Caused by a treponema organism present in the blood and other body fluids of an infected person. Responds to antibiotics. Syphilis is transmitted sexually. Babies may contract syphilis from a mother infected during pregnancy.

▷

▷ 9.9 cont.

Hepatitis B

Caused by a virus (HBV) which infects body fluids (blood, saliva and urine). The only treatment for hepatitis B is plenty of rest and nutritious food. Hepatitis B may be transmitted from an infected partner during sexual intercourse, but may also be transmitted in other ways.

HIV

Human immunodeficiency virus (HIV) can damage the body's defence system so that it cannot fight certain infections. HIV causes AIDS. HIV survives in body fluids such as blood, semen and vaginal fluids. (see page 463). While treatment is available for the various infections caused by HIV, there is nothing known to destroy the virus in the body.

HIV can be transmitted through sexual intercourse. It can also be transmitted through:

- getting infected blood into your bloodstream (e.g. through sharing syringes and needles and other drug injecting equipment, or by blood transfusion with infected blood. Note: all blood for transfusion in the UK is screened for antibodies to HIV); or

- pregnancy and childbirth from a mother with the virus to her child, and rarely through breast milk.

Gardnerella (bacterial vaginosis)

Occurs when bacteria that normally grow in small numbers in your vagina multiply. It seems that men don't get gardnerella but can pass on the infection. It can be treated with antibiotics.

INFORMATION SHEET *9.10*

How to protect yourself from infection

You need to protect yourself and your partner from passing on infection to each other. If there is any chance that either of you could pass on a sexually transmitted infection you should talk about it together, and see a doctor for a sexual health check if necessary.

You should always practise 'safer sex' with a new partner, just in case either of you has an infection and doesn't know. Safer sex means giving and getting sexual pleasure in ways that don't put you or your partner at risk of STDs. It's important to talk to each other about sex – what you feel and what you like to do. The small inconvenience is worth it if you can avoid getting an STD which may affect you in the future.

For safer sex

- Always use a condom for vaginal and anal sex. Getting used to putting one on may take some practice, but once you've got the knack, you may find condoms are not the 'passion killers' you may have been led to believe. Read the instructions on the packet carefully.

- Enjoy sex without penetration – by kissing, masturbation, stroking or sensual massage. Oral shields (or dental dams) can also be used as a barrier against infection.

- You can use sex toys such as vibrators, but don't share them with each other unless protected with a condom, and always clean them afterwards.

Pass urine and wash your genital area as soon as possible after making love. This may not always be convenient, but it may help you to avoid cystitis and urethritis.

Tell your partner if you know you have an infection so that they can also have a sexual health check. This may not always be an easy thing to do. But it may be that your partner has passed the infection on to you in the first place, and may be reinfecting you without knowing.

© Health Education Authority, 1993

INFORMATION SHEET *9.11*

Signs and symptoms of infection

If you notice any of the warning signs listed below, go to your nearest GUM clinic (sometimes called 'STD', 'special' or 'VD' clinic) or see your family doctor right away. Remember, the sooner you recognise early symptoms and go for treatment, the quicker and easier it will be for the doctor to cure you.

Possible signs of an infection

- Unusual change in the amount or type of moisture in the vagina. It is normal for the vagina to be moist to keep the genital area clean and healthy. So don't worry unless:

  - there is more discharge than you would normally expect;

  - it looks different, especially if the colour is unusual;

  - it feels different;

  - it has a strong, unpleasant or unfamiliar smell;

  - it makes your vagina itch.

- Discharge (or leakage) from the penis.

- Sore or blister near the vagina, penis or anus.

- Rash or irritation around the vagina, penis or anus.

- Pain or burning feeling when you pass urine.

- Passing urine very frequently or more often than usual.

- Pain when you have intercourse.

No symptoms

Some people can have an infection without noticing any symptoms at all. In fact, 9 out of 10 women with gonorrhoea do not get any symptoms; and a large proportion of people with herpes don't get sores. This can happen either because no symptoms appear at all or because symptoms may be inside your body where you cannot see or feel them. So, if you have a reason to think that you might have caught an infection (for instance, if you've had sex with someone who might have had an infection), go for a check-up anyway. You won't be wasting anyone's time.

INFORMATION SHEET *9.12*

Getting help for infections

Where to get help

If you think you might have caught an infection, whether you've got symptoms or not, go either to a clinic which specialises in genito-urinary infection, or to your GP.

Why a clinic?

Clinics are special centres designed to treat people of all ages who have genito-urinary infections. Often attached to main hospitals, clinics give free, confidential advice and treatment – and you don't need a letter from your GP.

Many clinics are open at certain times during the day and you can turn up without an appointment. However, some clinics prefer you to make an appointment first. So it's a good idea to ring them first to check on their arrangements.

How to find your nearest clinic

Depending on the area you live in, the clinic might be called a:

- genito-urinary medicine (GUM) clinic;
- sexually transmitted disease (STD) clinic;
- special clinic; or
- special treatment centre.

For the address and phone number of your nearest clinic look in the phone book under genito-urinary medicine, STD, or VD, or phone:

- your local family planning clinic;
- your local hospital (and ask for the 'special' or GUM clinic);
- the Family Planning Information Association (tel: 071-636 7866) and ask for their Clinic Enquiries Service; or the National AIDS Helpline (0800-567-123), a free, confidential, 24-hour phone line that can tell you where your local clinic is.

▷

▷ 9.12 cont.

What happens at a clinic?

The staff at the clinic are trained to treat sexual infections efficiently and confidentially. They are helpful and understanding, so you don't need to feel embarrassed about going.

When you see the doctor you will be asked about any symptoms you've had and about your general health. You might also be asked about the kind of sex you've been having. These questions are to help the doctor find out which infection you have.

You will then be given a thorough check-up. The doctor will ask you to:

- have an examination of the genital area;

- give a sample of urine;

- have a sample of any discharge taken;

- have a blood test (routine syphilis test); and

- women will also have an internal examination. This enables the doctor to take a 'swab' or sample from the vagina and the cervix (neck of the womb). This test will show whether there is any infection or abnormality. It is not painful but may be a bit uncomfortable. If you feel uneasy about being examined internally by a male doctor, you can always ask to be seen by a female doctor. Or you can have the nurse with you when you're examined.

Tell the doctor at the clinic if you are pregnant. This is because some treatments may affect the unborn child.

Sometimes the doctor will be able to tell you straight away which infection you have, and will give you some treatment or a prescription there and then. Usually, however, you will be asked to return for another appointment in a few days' time for the results of your tests.

It is extremely important that you attend for all the appointments the doctor asks you to make so that you can be sure that the treatment has worked.

Telling your partner

After receiving some treatment, you will be asked to advise any partners you've had over the previous few months to attend the clinic. This is because they are probably infected too and will need to be seen and treated as soon as possible.

Sometimes couples attend the clinic together. This can be very helpful because you can give each other emotional support and also be sure that you won't be reinfecting each other.

▷

▷ 9.12 cont.

If you are not in a steady relationship and your contact was a brief relationship, it's just as important that he or she is encouraged to attend the clinic. They may well be infected without knowing and may be infecting other people too. So, even an anonymous letter is better than nothing.

Specially trained staff at the clinic, called health advisors, will help you decide how you would prefer your partner to be contacted.

Remember: any information you give at the clinic is treated in the strictest confidence.

ACTIVITY *9.15*

Infections

Aims

- To increase women's knowledge of sexually transmitted diseases and vaginal infections.

- To discuss signs and symptoms of infections.

- To share information on where to go for help.

Materials

A copy of Worksheet 9.11 and Information Sheet 9.9 *Infections* for each woman; flipchart, markers.

Method

1 Give a copy of worksheet to each woman. In pairs or small groups discuss the questions.

2 Discuss in the large group.

3 Give out the information sheets and check out information.

Discussion points

- Chlamydia, genital herpes (HSV) and genital warts (HPV) are the most common STDs.

- HIV is increasing.

- There is a low incidence of gonorrhoea and syphilis. Gonorrhoea and syphilis are more common in the USA than in Europe. Both are declining in the UK (except there is possibly an increase in gonorrhoea in some parts of the UK).

- Vaginal infections are very common. Thrush is not caused by sexual transmission, but can be sexually transmitted once a woman has it.

- Often, one STD masks another.

- Many infections have no symptoms. It can be difficult to know if you have an infection – sometimes not until a sexual partner develops symptoms.

- If you or your sexual partner suspect you have an infection, have a sexual health check at your local GUM clinic (sometimes called 'STD', 'special' or 'VD' clinics). The service and treatment they offer are free and confidential – that means they won't let anyone know you have been to them, except those helping with your treatment. And they won't judge you about anything, or about anyone you may have been with.

- If you suspect an infection, you should tell your sexual partner. It is preferable if your partner also has a sexual health check at a special clinic. It is no use if you alone get treated if you have contracted the infection from your partner; you could continue to re-infect each other.

- See Information Sheets 9.10 *How to protect yourself from infection*, 9.11 *Signs and symptoms of infection*, and 9.12 *Getting help for infections*.

*ACTIVITY 9.16

Telling a partner

Aim

- To enable women to feel more confident about raising the issue of infections with sexual partners.

Materials

Flipchart, markers.

Method

1 Write a list of infections on the flipchart (use the list on Worksheet 9.11 *Infections* as a prompt).

2 Divide women into pairs and ask each pair to choose one of the infections – try to ensure that there is an equal mix of STDs and vaginal infections.

3 Each pair role-plays – one woman takes the role of having the infection, the other takes the role of her partner.

4 Change over, so that both women have a chance to practise telling the other.

5 Large group discussion on issues raised by the role play.

Discussion points

- Was it hard to tell a partner? Why might this be so?

- Are there more useful ways than saying 'I have a sexually transmitted disease'? Is 'infection' a better word? Would it be better to say, for example: 'you know some people get cold sores on their mouths? Well, I have that virus too, but the sores occur on my genitals'.

- Was it more difficult to tell a partner about a serious STD (e.g. HIV) than a vaginal infection?

- Is there a best time to tell a sexual partner? Is during sexual activity a good time?

- How did the partner react to the information? Supportive? Angry? Accusing? Scared? Wanting to share responsibility?

- How might telling a partner be made easier? Would having all the relevant information for you to go through together make it more helpful?

- Where might you get hold of the relevant information you need?

- Where could you go for help for such infections? How can you encourage a reluctant partner to go for a sexual health check?

WORKSHEET *9.11*

Infections

Consider the following infections

Cystitis	Genital herpes
Vaginitis	Trichomoniasis (TV)
Urethritis	Pubic lice
Chlamydia	Syphilis
Gonorrhoea	Hepatitis B
Thrush	HIV
Genital warts	Gardnerella (bacterial vaginosis)

1 Which of the above infections can *only* be transmitted sexually?

2 How common are the above infections?

3 Can you have more than one infection at a time?

4 What are the symptoms of the infections?

5 Which of the above infections can be cured?

6 Where can you go for help for such infections?

7 Should you tell a sexual partner if you have an infection?

8 How can you protect yourself from infection?

RESOURCES

For contact details of distributors and organisations listed here, see the list of organisations in Chapter 11 *General resources*.

Publications

Adler Michael (ed), *The ABC of Sexually Transmitted Diseases* (1990), British Medical Journal, £11.95.
Covers diagnosis and control of STDs. Detailed, medical language.

Blanks, Sue and Woddis, Carole, *The Herpes Manual: the Book for Everyone Concerned about Herpes* (1983), Settle and Bendall, £3.99.
A useful guide to the subject.

Kilmartin, Angela, *Sexual Cystitis* (1988), Arrow, £3.99.
Specific attention to the sexual causes of cystitis. Covers psychological issues with practical suggestions.

Llewellyn-Jones, Derek, *Sexually Transmitted Diseases* (1990), Faber, £4.99.
Clear descriptions, illustrated. Covers a range of STDs including AIDS.

Mindel, Adrian and Carney, Orla, *Herpes: What it is and How to Cope* (1991), Optima, £6.99.
Information includes transmission, diagnosis, treatment, prevention and self-help.

Winn, Denise, *Below the Belt: a Woman's Guide to Genito-urinary Infections* (1987), Optima, £3.95.
Briefly covers a full range of women's STDs.

Organisations

Herpes Association
Provides information for those who have herpes.

HIV and AIDS

BACKGROUND INFORMATION

HIV infection is the greatest new public health challenge this century.

Since January 1992 about half the one million newly infected adults in the world have been women – which also means that more children will be born to women with the virus. Most people with HIV will eventually develop AIDS, and about half will do so within ten years. No cure for AIDS is yet available and so the only way of controlling the epidemic is through a change in sexual and drug injecting behaviour.

Although the number of women with AIDS in the UK is only a small proportion of the total (6.5%), it has been steadily increasing since reporting began in 1982. During the past year the number of women with AIDS has increased by 34%. The number of HIV reports among women (2,128 up to June 1992) represents 12% of the total but many more women have the virus without knowing it. Anonymous antenatal screening has shown a rate of 1 in 200 women in some London clinics. Women are also infected at a much younger age than men.

The major route of HIV transmission among women is through hetero-sexual intercourse and as heterosexual spread increases women are more vulnerable than their male partners, particularly as a result of their unequal position in society which sometimes prevents them from making healthy choices. There is a need to focus on removing the barriers to choice for women. However, women with relatively powerful positions in the family or community, have an important educational role to play in HIV pre-vention.

Today, partly because of HIV and AIDS, it is more acceptable to discuss intimate matters openly. And while AIDS may have the potential to lead to further restrictions on women's reproductive rights, it may also lead to new understandings of sexuality that are not based solely on heterosexual intercourse.

The following issues around HIV and AIDS may have particular relevance for women:

- women who are sexually active, need to protect themselves;
- parenting;
- HIV testing;
- sexual violence against women;
- women's paid and unpaid work (in the sex industry, in the health services, caring for others at home);
- discrimination, marginalisation, racism;
- lifestyle and risk-taking;
- effects of alcohol and drugs in decision making;
- significance of greater travel opportunities;
- assertiveness and negotiating skills;
- women's communicator role in families;
- lesbians affected as part of lesbian and gay community;
- women as non-injecting sexual partners of men who inject drugs.

This section includes activities to enable women to work through some of their concerns, to learn some facts, dispel some myths and find out more about safer sex practices.

PRACTICAL POINTS

- All issues related to sexual health are emotive, sensitive and need careful facilitation. This is particularly so for HIV and AIDS.

- There is a wealth of information on the subject of HIV and AIDS (see Resources). What women often want is an opportunity to discuss facts, their concerns, and look at how to make choices.

- This can best be done in a safe, supportive atmosphere. Ground rules are very important, for women may wish to disclose very personal experiences.

- The tutor needs to be aware of her own attitudes, assumptions and prejudices. She will need to be clear about her role in the group.

- Confidentiality with regard to HIV antibody status will be important in any discussions on HIV and AIDS. There may be women in the group who will not wish to disclose their HIV status.

- Within any group there will be women with different sexual preferences – which they may wish to disclose, or not. Whatever your own sexual preference, remember when facilitating activities that some women consider themselves heterosexual, some bisexual, some lesbian (even if they have sexual relationships with men).

- Teaching methods which get issues into the open (e.g. using small cards, case studies) without needing women to disclose personal information may be most successful. Articles or letters from newspapers can also be a useful trigger. Humour is a useful tool.

- In enabling women to recognise and discuss their possible unequal power relationships with men there is a danger of sessions moving into 'man-bashing'. This is sometimes not helpful, and the discussions might better be directed towards questioning why male attitudes are as they are, and what can be done to help men understand women's needs better.

- It is important to end any session on a positive note, and to have allowed time for women to consider what else they need to know or do, and how they might go about it. Local information should be available as a back-up.

INFORMATION SHEET *9.13*

Definitions of HIV and AIDS

What is HIV?

Human	only affecting humans (cannot be passed from animals to humans)
Immunodeficiency	damage to the body's 'defence-system' so that it cannot fight certain infections and diseases
Virus	smallest known organism. Can only multiply within body cells

HIV interferes with the very cells which protect us against infection, hence someone who is HIV antibody positive is poorly protected against specific infections and diseases.

What is AIDS?

Acquired	contracted (rather than, for example, genetic)
Immune	able to resist infection
Deficiency	malfunctioning
Syndrome	specific group of diseases (not a single disease)
	opportunistic infections: PCP – a kind of pneumonia; Kaposi's sarcoma – a form of skin cancer (these are rare in women); other bacterial, fungal and viral infections.

AIDS is diagnosed by the presence of one or more of the opportunistic infections, in the *absence* of all other possible causes of immune deficiency.

People with HIV are asymptomatic (without any symptoms of any illness) for many years, but may develop at any time symptoms such as PGL (persistently swollen glands), herpes zoster, night sweats, persistent diarrhoea or general weakness. They may shift from being symptomatic to asymptomatic, and vice versa, but on current knowledge most people with HIV will develop AIDS within 20 years of becoming infected.

INFORMATION SHEET *9.14*

HIV and AIDS issues for women

- The percentage of women with HIV and AIDS is increasing.

- Black and minority ethnic women are disproportionately affected.

- Transmission from men to women is more efficient than vice versa.

- Anonymous HIV antibody testing is carried out in some antenatal and GUM clinics as part of a national survey. Some women may be concerned about HIV testing and screening, particularly in pregnancy. They can phone the National AIDS Helpline (page 626) for confidential advice.

- Some of the clinical manifestations of HIV disease among women are different from those in men or children. (However, the lack of data makes it difficult to determine whether these differences are due to a variety of underlying health and social factors – such as discrimination, drug use, poor nutrition, poverty and lack of access to care.) Studies are needed to assess the nature and frequency of various clinical conditions such as vaginal thrush, pelvic inflammatory disease and cervical cancer in women with HIV. The progression of HIV disease in women needs further study.

- Women with HIV may be misdiagnosed during the early stages of their disease.

- Health and social services often do not recognise that many women with HIV infection also need services and care for their children.

INFORMATION SHEET *9.15*

Safer sex guidelines for women

How is HIV transmitted?

There are three main ways in which HIV can pass from one person to another.

- Through unprotected sexual intercourse (anal or vaginal). Unprotected penetrative sex – vaginal and anal sex – carries risks when one partner is infected. Condoms can reduce the risk. Oral sex (mouth or tongue touching the genitals) also carries some risk, and therefore to make oral sex safer a condom or an oral shield, sometimes known as a dental dam, should be used.

- Through blood. In the UK this occurs mainly through drug injectors sharing contaminated injecting equipment (needles and syringes). If you have a blood transfusion (receive blood) in the UK, it will have been screened for antibodies to HIV, so the risk of being infected is almost negligible. Similarly, blood plasma products (e.g. Factor Eight) are made safe using special treatments. In the UK you cannot become infected by HIV when donating blood because all equipment is sterile and only used once.

- From an infected mother to child. A mother may pass the virus to her child, either during pregnancy, at birth or during breast-feeding.

Specific guidelines for sexual activity

Safer sex means practising sexual activities which prevent the exchange of body fluids i.e. blood, semen and vaginal secretions.

Safe

- massage
- hugging
- body-to-body rubbing
- voyeurism, exhibitionism, fantasy
- touching your own genitals (masturbation)

▷

▷ 9.15 cont.

Safer Sex

- vaginal and anal intercourse with a condom

- fellatio/blow jobs with a condom

- cunnilingus with a latex barrier

- hand/finger-to-genital contact (mutual masturbation, hand jobs, locals, vaginal or anal penetration with fingers).
  This can be made safer by using a latex glove.

High risk activities

- cunnilingus without a latex barrier (particularly during menstruation)

- fellatio/blow jobs without a condom

- semen in the mouth

- vaginal or anal intercourse without a condom

- rimming (oral–anal contact). There is no evidence that you can contract HIV by rimming but both partners are at a risk from other infections including hepatitis.

- sharing sex toys that have contact with blood and body fluids

In any situation, sexual or otherwise, sharing needles is unsafe.

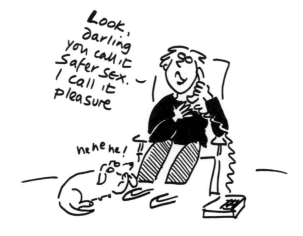

INFORMATION SHEET *9.16*

Preventative measures

Condoms

Condoms are known to be effective in preventing sexually transmitted diseases such as gonorrhoea, syphilis, herpes, chlamydia and HIV.

If you want to use extra lubricant, it is very important that you use a water-based lubricant like KY Jelly. Oil-based lubricants damage the rubber. Never use petroleum jelly (Vaseline), massage oil, body lotions, baby oil, moisturisers or cooking oil for lubrication.

Never re-use condoms. Wrap them in a tissue and put them in a bin. Do not flush them down the toilet as they cannot be broken down in the sewage system.

Spermicides

Nonoxynol-9, the active ingredient in most spermicides (foams, creams and jellies), has been found to kill HIV in the laboratory (although we don't know if it will kill the virus in the body). Many researchers believe, however, that it is a good idea to use a spermicide containing nonoxynol-9 in case a condom breaks or slips. Some lubricants on condoms also contain nonoxynol-9.

Caution: some people experience irritation with nonoxynol-9. If you do experience irritation it is important that you try another brand or avoid using nonoxynol-9.

Disposable latex gloves

If you have cuts on your fingers or hands, disposable latex or rubber gloves will prevent contact with HIV during hand–genital or hand–anal contact. Gloves can be bought at chemists.

Latex barriers (oral shields or dental dams)

Cunnilingus may be safer if done using a latex barrier between the tongue and vulva. Oral shields, sometimes known as dental dams, come in various sizes, colours and flavours and are about the same thickness as a doctor's disposable latex glove. They are available from some chemists, and by mail order.

INFORMATION SHEET *9.17*

Safer sex for lesbians

Most lesbians with HIV appear to have become infected either from sharing needles or other drug injecting equipment, or by heterosexual intercourse. Lesbian sex generally appears to carry little risk of HIV infection. There are almost no reports of women becoming infected with HIV through lesbian sex.

There is no need to worry about becoming infected with HIV through:

- hugging or massaging;
- touching your own genitals;
- kissing (there is no evidence of transmission of HIV solely through saliva);
- body-to-body rubbing;
- body kissing;
- sharing sexual fantasies;
- using vibrators or other sex toys *providing* that they are not shared. Or a condom may be used over them, but again this must not be shared.

But, to be on the safe side, take care with:

- oral sex – there are few reports of HIV infection through oral sex (mouth or tongue touching genitals). To make oral sex safer an oral shield (or dental dam) should be used;
- finger-to-genital contact, if you have cuts, scratches or sores on your fingers; and
- unprotected oral sex during menstruation.

It is not safe to share vibrators or other sex toys that have come into contact with blood or vaginal secretions.

INFORMATION SHEET *9.18*

Communication towards safer sex

Six point plan

1 Knowing what you want and like: this is important for you.

2 Knowing or asking what your partner wants and likes.

3 Knowing your own boundaries and limitations.

4 Being clear of your messages (body language and other forms of communication may be far more important than words themselves).

5 Practising ways of feeling comfortable in asking for what you need.

6 Being realistic.

Language and assertiveness

1 Use 'I' statements, not 'we' or 'you'. It is empowering to own what is important to you.

2 Use 'could' instead of 'should' or 'must'. This implies options and choices instead of rules and judgements.

3 Use 'and' not 'but' when seeking to change behaviour; 'but' wipes out what went before and acts as a warning sign to the other person . . . something bad is coming. However, 'and' implies an equality and balance to discussions.

ACTIVITY *9.17*

Concerns about HIV and AIDS

Aims
- To enable women to express their concerns in a 'safe' way.
- To enable women to see that others share similar concerns.
- To help identify an agenda for a particular group.
- To enable women to evaluate their own learning over a session, day or course.

Materials
Small cards, pens, carrier bag, flipchart, markers.

Method
1 Give a small card to each woman. Ask her to write down her greatest concern about the issue of HIV and AIDS. Stress that what she writes will be anonymous, though the information will be shared among the group. (Variation: give women more than one card, one concern to be written on each card.)

2 Women place completed card(s) in the carrier bag. Each woman takes out a card (if she takes her own, she should replace it and take another).

3 Women read out, in turn, what is on the card they are holding.

4 Write up concerns on the flipchart and display them in the room (the tutor may do this during the following activity).

5 At the end of the session (or course), refer back to the flipchart. Ask women to consider whether their concerns have been lessened now. What else do they need to know? How might they take the next step?

Discussion points
Concerns may fall into the following areas:
- being HIV+ and not knowing it;
- how to get (safely) pregnant;
- lack of knowledge as to how the virus is transmitted;
- illness affecting people you love (partner, friends or children);
- children growing older and becoming sexually active;
- facts about HIV and AIDS constantly changing – 'how can I keep up?';

- how to enjoy sex these days;
- stigma/discrimination/marginalisation;
- trust in a sexual relationship;
- being lesbian and not wishing to disclose sexual preference;
- lesbian women feeling that their sexual health has not been considered because of widespread assumptions of heterosexuality in our society.

*ACTIVITY 9.18

Personal stories

Aims

- To personalise the issues around HIV and AIDS.
- To acknowledge that HIV has affected us all in some way.

Materials
Blank paper and coloured pens.

Method
1 Working individually, women draw a visual representation of how HIV and AIDS has affected their life, using colours or drawings.

2 In small groups, women share what they feel comfortable with and draw out the main points for feedback to the main group.

3 In the large group, flipchart the main responses, drawing out like and unlike.

Variation: use collage instead of colours/drawing. Bring lots of magazines to cut up.

Note for tutor
Confidentiality is vital. Disclosure of HIV antibody status is on a 'need to know' basis only i.e. how essential is it for someone to know HIV status in any given situation?; what risk is there of transmission? Usually the answer is 'no need'. Confidentiality of HIV status is paramount because of stigma, discrimination, and implications of positive status. There may be difficulties with this activity if someone has or knows of a partner or friend with HIV.

ACTIVITY *9.19*

Information line-up

Aims

- To explore what women feel they need to know.
- To start discussion around the issues involved in HIV and AIDS.
- To create an agenda of issues for the session.

Material

Flipchart paper and pens, blutack.

Method

1 Designate one end of the room 'a lot of knowledge about HIV and AIDS', and the opposite end 'very little knowledge'.

2 Ask women to place themselves along this continuum representing their own feelings.

3 Each woman discusses with those next to her why she put herself there.

4 In small groups with flipchart paper, each woman gives two issues or facts she wants clarifying. Display the lists on a wall for everyone to see.

Discussion points

- This activity can be used as an agenda-setting or needs-assessment tool.
- It can lead into discussion about adequacy of information, especially when scientific 'facts' are changing rapidly.
- It can raise the issue of what type of information is trustworthy . . . what is the ideology or politics of the organisation giving the information?
- It can raise issues of confidentiality and 'need to know' basis for HIV status disclosure (e.g. children with HIV at school).

ACTIVITY *9.20*

Rumours, myths and information

Aims

- To explore rumours about HIV and AIDS.
- To practise responding to rumours and myths about HIV and AIDS.

Materials

Flipchart paper and pens.

Method

1 In groups of four, two women relate common myths and rumours about HIV and AIDS, and the other two women respond to these as best they can.

2 Swap roles at half time.

3 In the large group, flipchart the first reactions/feelings in responding to these rumours.

4 Discuss what women feel they need to know more about, in terms of both issues and information. Flipchart these perceived needs.

Discussion point

This could set the basis for an information exchange or give ideas for future sessions, or the need for specific handouts.

ACTIVITY *9.21*

Knowledge about HIV and AIDS

Aims

- To dispel some of the myths surrounding AIDS.
- To enable women to evaluate their own learning from an information-giving session.

Materials

Post-it notes, pens, markers, blutack; a flipchart sheet for each small group, each sheet divided into three columns, headed 'Agree', 'Disagree', 'Don't know'; copies of information sheets from this section.

Method

1 Give three post-it notes to each woman. Ask them to write down three things they have heard about HIV and AIDS, one on each post-it.

2 Shuffle the post-its and share them between two or more small groups.

3 In small groups, women discuss each post-it and negotiate in which column each statement should go.

4 Display the completed flipchart sheets around the room.

5 Follow by providing information sheets about HIV and AIDS.

6 At the end of the session, divide women into the same number of small groups as before (it doesn't have to be the same women in each group), and give each group a completed flipchart sheet with post-its.

7 In the light of what they have learned, ask women if they are still satisfied with the placings of the post-its? Alter them if necessary.

Discussion points

- What kinds of statements did women write on each post-it? Were they 'facts' from the media or information from colleagues or friends? Where do we get most of our information from about HIV and AIDS? Do we feel we have adequate information, given our concerns?

- By the end of the session, are there still some post-its in 'don't know' columns? If so, is this because we really don't know at this stage? If so, how might women find out?

- Do women feel that during this session they have learned things they didn't know? Did the session confirm what you were already thinking or believing? Was it useful to have confirmation?

ACTIVITY *9.22*

Body positive

Aims

- To enable women to be clear about how HIV is transmitted.

- To confirm women's existing knowledge, or provide women with knowledge that will enable them to consider wider issues more relevantly.

Materials

Six flipchart sheets, glued together (two sheets across, three sheets down) – or enough to provide a total paper area large enough to draw round a woman's body; marker pens.

Method

1 Ask for a volunteer to lie on the paper on the floor (if no volunteer is forthcoming, lie down yourself and ask for a volunteer to draw round you).

2 Add to the outline of body, drawing on facial features (eyes, nose, mouth, ears), breasts, and female and male genitals.

3 Ask women to brainstorm all the body fluids in a human, starting from the head and working down to the feet, and write them down by appropriate part of the body (you may need to prompt if important body fluids aren't mentioned, see the diagram on next page). Make sure all the women understand language used by others – some women will use medical terms, others will use common terms.

4 Once all body fluids are listed around the body, go through each and ask 'has it been demonstrated that this body fluid can contain HIV?'. If yes, ask whether this is under laboratory conditions, or if the body fluid has been known to have been the route of transmission in specific cases. Can you envisage a situation whereby this body fluid can get into the bloodstream of another person?

5 Go through all body fluids, until the group itself has decided that the crucial body fluids for HIV transmission are blood, semen and vaginal and cervical secretions.

Note: this activity can take as long as two hours, depending on the existing knowledge of women in the group. Some may have more knowledge than others, so women will learn from each other. If you allow whatever time is needed for a particular group, you are more likely to make better use of subsequent activities you choose to do.

Discussion points

● The body fluids which may cause disquiet are those that have been demonstrated under laboratory conditions to contain HIV (e.g. urine, sweat, breastmilk). Also, since faeces and vomit may contain blood, there is often concern about these.

● If women are concerned about these fluids, you may need to talk about the concentration of the virus in them; there must be an adequate quantity of the virus to cause infection. In the examples given here, the quantity of HIV is known to be poor.

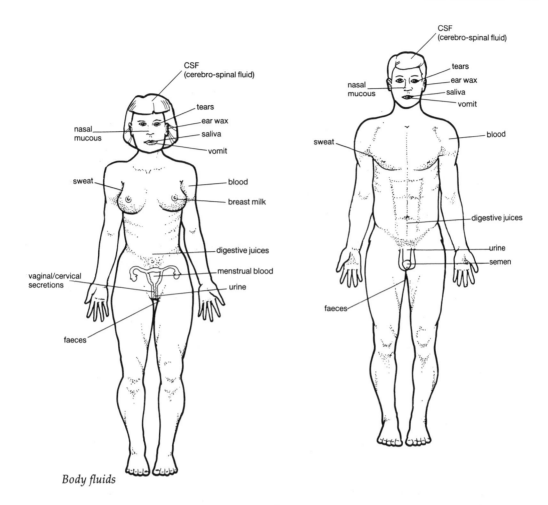

Body fluids

- HIV must also be of suitable quality to cause infection (i.e. undamaged by chemicals, bleach or heat).

- You could use specific instances or particular concerns of women over transmission. A common worry is 'catching' the virus from someone bleeding on you:
  - reiterate that any infected blood has to get into your bloodstream to be dangerous;
  - point out that the skin is an excellent barrier;
  - even if you have wounds in your skin, unless wounds are open (which is unlikely?) how could infected blood get into yours? If you are bleeding yourself, your blood is coming out.

By the end of the activity women should be really clear about potentially dangerous body fluids. Highlight that it is what you do i.e. unsafe sex, sharing drug injecting equipment, that is crucial for the transmission of HIV.

ACTIVITY *9.23*

Statements

Aims

- To examine risks of contracting HIV associated with different activities or situations.

- To identify areas where there is a lack of knowledge in this field.

Materials

Statements on small cards (see next page); a set of five envelopes for each small group, labelled: 'no risk', 'low risk', 'high risk' 'don't know' and 'it depends'.

Method

1 Give equal numbers of statement cards to each woman.

2 In small groups ask women to place their cards in the appropriate envelopes.

3 In the large group report back the contents of the different envelopes.

4 Discuss any differences in classifications. Are there any right answers?

Discussion points

- This could lead into a discussion of credibility of information and perceived risks.

- It is useful to highlight the differences between high risk groups and high risk behaviours.

Statements for cards

prostitute using condoms with customers

heterosexual relationships

injecting drugs with shared needles

lots of sexual partners

using drugs for the first time

using someone else's toothbrush

vaginal sex when on the Pill

sex with a lover

sex with a husband

ear piercing

oral sex with a condom

oral sex with an oral shield (dental dam)

public swimming pools

'french kissing'

sex with a drug user

lesbianism

HIV positive child in a class or playgroup

sharing cups and cutlery

nursing people with AIDS

caring for a person with HIV

being bisexual

the 'kiss of life'

blood transfusions in this country

donating blood

using a public loo

love bites

tattoos

'petting'

anal sex with a condom

helping someone with a nosebleed

someone with HIV in your house

head lice

sex in another country

anal sex

being gay

oral sex with women only

being married and 'faithful'

having haemophilia

*ACTIVITY *9.24*

Safer sex

Aims
- To consider how much importance is given to safer sex.
- To generate discussion about the realities of women's lives, safer sex and choices that are made.

Materials
Small cards, a bag and pens.

Method
1 Each woman has a small card, and writes down sexual activities which she practises (if she is currently in a sexual relationship), or would be prepared to, which she believes are safer. Stress that although answers will be shared with the group, they will be anonymous.

2 Place all cards in a bag, and ask women to take one at random. Go round the circle reading the contents of each card, with no interruptions.

3 Discuss, allowing ownership of statements if women choose.

Discussion points
- Are women clear which sexual activities really *are* safer? (You cannot assume that having sex only with one partner is safe, without knowing if the partner is involved in other sexual activities).
- Is it possible to have absolutely *safe* sex? Why not?
- How do we make choices about risks involved in sexual activities?
- While there may be agreement that safer sex is a good ideal, the reality of applying it can be difficult.

Notes for tutor
- This activity could be stressful if the group is not working well together. It may need careful facilitation.
- This activity can be particularly useful when working with professionals who are trying to influence others' behaviour.
- It might be useful to follow up this activity with other activities around safer sex, such as those in this section.

ACTIVITY *9.25*

Safer sex game

Aims

- To facilitate discussion and group interaction among women.
- To clarify relative risks of various sexual practices.

Materials

Small cards with various sexual activities written on them, a bag, copies of Information Sheets 9.15 *Safer sex guidelines for women* and 9.17 *Safer sex for lesbians* for reference.

Activities to write on cards

- solo masturbation
- using vibrators
- oral sex between two women
- massage
- mutual masturbation (two women)
- sex without touching
- oral sex between a man and a woman
- french (wet) kissing
- body-to-body rubbing
- sex involving fantasy
- oral sex between a man and a menstruating woman
- anal sex between a man and a woman, with a condom
- vaginal sex between a man and a menstruating woman
- mutual masturbation (man and woman)
- vaginal sex between a man and a woman without a condom
- sexual activity not involving penetration
- anal sex between a man and a woman without a condom
- vaginal sex between a man and a woman with a condom

Method

1 Put the sexual activity cards in a bag, and invite women to take one each.

2 Ask the women to put themselves in a line depending on the card they are holding, with the most risky sexual activity at one end, and the least risky at the other (the discussions and negotiations may take 15 minutes).

3 When women are all in line, ask them to read out their activity, from the most risky along the spectrum to the least risky.

4 Allow time for discussion in the large group afterwards.

Discussion points

• Make sure women are clear about the meaning of various sexual practices on the cards.

• This focuses attention on *high risk activities* rather than *high risk groups*.

• Some women may question whether some of the activities are indeed 'sexual', or frequently practised, which could lead into a useful discussion about sexuality.

• This may lead into discussion about how to negotiate safer sexual activity with a partner (see Activity 9.27 *Negotiating safer sex*).

• Women may ask (particularly if they are interested in becoming pregnant) when it is safe to stop using safer sex practices. This is a difficult issue.

• Make sure you don't end on a negative note – practising safer sex can enrich your sex life!

ACTIVITY 9.26

Creative safer sex

Aims

• To explore creative ways of developing safer sexual activity.

• To lighten a possibly difficult subject!

Materials

Pens, four flipchart sheets, each with one of the following headings: 'Sex using condoms', 'Sex without penetration', 'Sex involving touching' and 'Sex involving fantasy'.

Method

1 Divide the women into four groups.

2 Give each group one of the headed flipchart sheets, and ask them to discuss and write down as many ways as they can of enjoying sex under that heading. Give them a time limit.

3 *Either*: when each group has finished, pass each flipchart on to a different group. Read what others have written and add to it if possible. Continue until everyone has had a chance to contribute to all four flipcharts.
Or: one woman from each group feeds back ideas to the large group and extra ideas are added.

Note: if any of the groups appears 'stuck' initially, go round and prompt.

Discussion points

- Some creative sexual practices may be challenged by others as not being 'sexual'. This could lead to useful discussion about sexuality.

- Have women learned during this activity a 'bank' of creative sexual activities? Would they feel able to use these with partners? If not, why not? This may lead to discussion on how to negotiate safer sex (see the information sheets and other activities on safer sex).

- Are women used to taking the initiative in sexual activity with a partner? What might inhibit us?

Note for tutor

Be aware of possible different sexual preferences within your group. Lesbian women may find 'sex using condoms' and 'sex without penetration' irrelevant to them. They may say so, or they may choose not to . . .

Source: adapted from Dixon, H, and Gordon, P, *Working with Uncertainty* (1991), FPA.

ACTIVITY 9.27

Negotiating safer sex

Aims

- To enable women to practise negotiating safer sex, in a safe environment.

- To enable women to become aware of possible difficulties or responses in raising certain issues.

Materials

A flipchart and marker (maybe), small cards, pens, a bag, Information Sheet 9.18 *Communication towards safer sex* for each pair of women.

Method

1 *Either*: ask women to brainstorm scenarios they would like to consider; these could be relevant to their own situations or hypothetical ones.
Or: give women small cards and ask them to write scenarios they would like to consider. Place these in a bag. Read out the cards and link like with like to make a set of different scenarios.

2 Divide women into pairs. Give each pair one scenario to negotiate, and the information sheet to refer to.

3 Feed back in the large group.

Discussion points

- What helped in the negotiation? What got in the way?
- Did women find obstacles in the partner that they hadn't envisaged?
- Was it easier than they thought?
- Was using certain words a problem?
- What else do women need in order to negotiate with an actual partner?
- What is the best time to negotiate safer sex? In bed or sitting around the kitchen table, and why?

Note for tutor

This may be a difficult role play for some women – make sure the group feels comfortable with the activity.

*ACTIVITY 9.28

HIV antibody positive or not? – issues for women

Aims

- To explore the differences and similarities between HIV antibody positive women and women who think they are not HIV antibody positive.

- To highlight specific needs for HIV antibody positive women.

Materials

Flipchart, pens, blutack.

Method

1 Divide into two groups, each with flipchart paper and pens.

2 One group brainstorms issues for women who are antibody positive; the other group brainstorms issues for women who do not perceive themselves to be HIV antibody positive.

3 Put the flipchart sheets on the wall, and look at both sets of flipcharts.

4 In the large group, flipchart the differences and similarities between the two groups and discuss.

Discussion points

HIV ANTIBODY POSITIVE WOMEN

- being pregnant
- isolation
- celibacy?
- no spontaneity in sex
- people judging you
- responsibility for educating others
- illness and children
- lack of emotional and economic support

WOMEN NOT HIV ANTIBODY POSITIVE

- getting pregnant
- celibacy?
- practising safer sex
- consequences of testing
- trusting sexual partners
- responsible for others
- false sense of security

Notes for tutor

- Some women in the group may be, or know of women who are, HIV antibody positive – this may be emotional and prevent their full participation in the activity.

- Care is needed with confidentiality if women choose to disclose HIV status.

- Some women may display judgemental attitudes.

*ACTIVITY 9.29

Who gets a cure?

Aims

- To explore assumptions around concepts of 'innocent' and 'guilty'.

- To acknowledge that we all have prejudices and assumptions.

Materials

Three small cards with the following groups written on:

Card 1: babies with HIV
Black Africans with HIV
Card 2: gay men with HIV
injecting drug users with HIV
Card 3: people with haemophilia and HIV
female partners of bisexual men with HIV

Method

1 Divide women into three small groups, and give each group a card.

2 Tell the groups that a cure for HIV has been found, but that there is only enough treatment for *one* of the two groups on their card. Which group should get the cure? Why?
STRESS THAT ACTUAL DISCUSSION WILL NOT BE FED BACK TO THE LARGE GROUP.

3 Feed back *issues* which arose in the small groups, to the large group.

Discussion points

- Some women may object to this activity on the grounds that it is impossible to make such a choice. You could acknowledge their objections as valid, but reiterate the aim of the activity.

- What do women feel about this activity? Did they learn anything about themselves by doing the activity? Did women hold back any thoughts or feelings, for fear of rejection by others in the group? Did women manage to voice and 'own' any prejudices?

- Prejudices and assumptions may interfere with the way we interact with others. Being aware of our prejudices and assumptions may help us in the future.

Source: adapted from Dixon, H, and Gordon, P, *Working with Uncertainty* (1991), FPA.

ACTIVITY *9.30*

HIV and AIDS issues for women

Aims
- To encourage discussion about women's responses to HIV and AIDS.
- To look at choices and options open to women regarding HIV and AIDS.
- To appreciate some of the difficulties and challenges women face in asserting their needs.

Materials
Case studies (see Worksheet 9.12 *HIV and AIDS issues for women – case studies*); flipchart, paper and pens.

Method
1 Divide into small groups, and share out a number of case studies per group, ensuring that each case study will be considered by more than one group.
2 Discuss the case studies in small groups, noting responses on flipchart paper.
3 In the large group, feed back responses and discuss.

Discussion points
- Encourage women to feed back to the large group the case study they had most difficulty with – others may be able to come up with different ideas.
- Are there any 'right' answers? How do we make choices?
- Are there differences between us in the amount of risk-taking we are prepared to engage in? Why might this be so?
- Many of these case studies highlight the need for women to be assertive, especially in dealing with health professionals, sexual relationships with men and choice of contraceptive methods.
- A woman may detail another 'case study' or scenario which is of particular relevance to herself, about which she would like feedback from the group. Encourage this.

WORKSHEET *9.12*

HIV and AIDS issues for women – case studies

1 Sarah is very close to her daughter, who still lives at home. Her daughter has a new boyfriend whom Sarah likes very much. The two seem well suited and are 'going steady'. In the course of conversation the daughter casually mentions that her boyfriend has haemophilia.

What is your reaction?
What could Sarah do?

2 June is pregnant and attending a London antenatal clinic. She has heard that 1 in 200 women in some London clinics have HIV.
   - She doesn't know whether she is one of those who has tested positive or not
   - She wonders if she should ask for a named HIV antibody test
   - She wonders if she could become infected through vaginal examination by the medical staff or inadequate infection control measures in the clinic.

What could June do about these anxieties?

3 Yasmine has been on the Pill for years. She hasn't been particularly happy with it but her partner has been reluctant for her to use any other method of contraception. Now, with HIV around, Yasmine really wants him to start taking responsibility and use condoms when they make love.

What is your reaction?
What could Yasmine do?

4 Hazel adopted a baby at birth, whose biological mother was an IV drug user. Now the baby is settled, Hazel wishes her to go to a childminder where her elder child goes. In passing, Hazel has mentioned the baby's background to the childminder. The childminder is now saying that she couldn't possibly take the baby – for the sake of all the other children she childminds; it wouldn't be fair on them or their parents . . .

What is your reaction?
What could Hazel do?

5 Andrea was raped by a man she did not know four weeks ago. She wishes to have the HIV antibody test. But she does not want to explain why she wants the test to the male social worker at the Special Clinic.

What is your reaction?
What could Andrea do?

▷

▷ 9.12 cont.

6 Your lover who is a nurse has recently been given the chance of working on a ward where people with AIDS are nursed. It would mean promotion.

What is your reaction?
What do you do?

7 Your friend Annabel wants a child, and is thinking of artificial insemination. She says she knows of a sympathetic man who would be willing to donate sperm.

What is your reaction?
What would you do?

8 Your sister Christine tells you in confidence that she has discovered that her lover injects drugs.

What is your reaction?
What do you do?

9 Sue and Bob have been married for fifteen years, each having had lovers during that time. Due to increased awareness of HIV they decide to practice safer sex. For Bob this means using a condom, but Sue feels that this is too narrow and limits their relationship.

Do you think men and women have different ideas about what they want from sexual relationships?
What could Sue do in this situation?

10 Margaret is divorced and is 45 years old. Recently she met a man and their relationship has developed a sexual side to it . . . however he is married and has had many affairs. After reading about HIV and AIDS, Margaret suggests they use a condom when they have sex. He refuses to, saying AIDS is a 'gay disease' and using a condom takes away the pleasure.

Do you think this is a common attitude among men?
What can Margaret do and what could be the consequences for her?

11 Liz and Sarah are lovers and they feel lesbians are in a low risk group. Sarah hears through mutual friends that her ex-husband has been tested positive for HIV antibodies.

Are lesbians a low risk group? Are Liz and Sarah now at risk?
What behaviour could be potentially risky for either Liz or Sarah . . . or has been?
Is it useful to think in terms of risk groups or risk activities?

12 Lucy is seventeen and is having a relationship with Mark who is four years older. He told her that he once had a sexual relationship with another man. After seeing adverts about AIDS, Lucy bought some condoms and meant to

▷

▷ 9.12 cont.

talk to Mark . . . but Mark found them in her bag and left, calling her a slag. Now he won't talk to her.

Do you think Lucy should have bought them?
Did the information about AIDS help Lucy at all?
If she had been older would she have been treated any differently?

13 Pratima is pregnant, and has just learned through the antenatal clinic that she is HIV antibody positive. Her pregnancy was planned, and she has always felt she would never have an abortion. She has heard alarming stories about the incidence of HIV in babies born to women who are HIV antibody positive.

What could Pratima do?

RESOURCES

For contact details of distributors and organisations listed here, see Chapter 11 *General resources*.

Publications

Act Up, *AIDS, Women and Activism* (1990), South End Press, £6.95.
The American activist organisation's position on women and AIDS.

Adler, Michael (ed), *The ABC of AIDS* (1990), British Medical Journal, £11.95.
Articles from BMJ. Discusses symptoms, treatment, counselling and nursing and the control of infection. Detailed, medical, second revised edition.

Asistent, Niro Markoff, *Why I Survive AIDS* (1991), Fireside, £7.99.
A woman's story of dealing with AIDS – issues include children, facing fear and shame, meditation, nutrition and exercise. American.

Batty, D (ed), *The Implications of AIDS for Children in Care* (1987), British Agencies for Adoption and Fostering (BAAF), £5.95.
Looks particularly at the implications for fostering and adoption, and placement of children generally.

Dixon, Hilary and Gordon, Peter, *Working with Uncertainty: a Handbook for Those Involved in Training on HIV and AIDS* (1990), Family Planning Association, £12.99.
Second edition. Contains training exercises that explore feelings and attitudes and develop communication skills.

Gordon, Peter and Mitchell, Louise, *Safer Sex: a New Look at Sexual Pleasure* (1988), Faber, £4.99.
Discusses attitudes towards sex and sexuality in the context of HIV and AIDS.

Green, J, and McCreaner, A, *Counselling in HIV Infection and AIDS* (1989), £15.95.
For those involved in counselling. Useful for pregnant women and families of infected children.

Health Education Authority, *Multi-Lingual AIDS: HIV Information for Black and Minority Ethnic Communities*, Free. Available from the Health Education Authority.

Health Education Authority, *HIV & AIDS: the Facts You Need to Know* (leaflet) Available in nine languages with equivalent English translations: Afro-Caribbean, Arabic, Bengali, Cantonese, Gujarati, Hindi, Punjabi, Swahili, Urdu. Available from the Health Education Authority.

Henderson, S (ed), *Women, HIV, Drugs: Practical Issues* (1990), Institute for the Study of Drug Dependence (ISDD), £4.95, ISBN 0 948830 80 8. Available from booksellers or from ISDD.
Examines the risk to women of HIV infection and the ways in which health,

welfare and criminal justice systems are responding. It also looks at the role of self-help and community based responses.

Hockings, Jacqueline, *Walking the Tightrope: Living Positively with AIDS, ARC and HIV* (1988), Gale, £7.95.
The emotional and psychological effects of diagnosis of HIV or AIDS. Personal experiences and practical suggestions.

Honigsbaum, Naomi, *HIV, AIDS and Children: a Cause for Concern* (1991), National Children's Bureau, £13.95.
Discusses issues for women and children.

Women's Health, *It's not Who you are, it's What you do: a Guide to Answering Women's Questions on HIV and AIDS* (1992), £2.00. Available from Women's Health.
A general overview of the issues of concern to women. Aimed at health workers, counsellors, etc.

Liverpool Health Promotion Unit, Sefton General Hospital, *HIV and AIDS Training Pack for Young People (16–19 years)*, £3 (payable to Liverpool Health Authority).
A valuable training tool for AIDS workers and trainers, and youth workers. Includes issues around death and bereavement, stereotypes and prejudices, communication as well as information, safer sex and counselling. Participatory exercises.

Macourt, Malcolm, *How Can We Help You?: Information, Advice and Counselling for Gay Men and Lesbians* (1989), Bedford Square Press, £6.95, ISBN 0 7199 1229 6. Available from booksellers or Plymbridge Distributors Ltd.
Details of where lesbians and gay men can get advice and support, how gay helplines can help with a whole range of personal problems; examines the role of the helpline workers themselves, how they cope with the many demands made of them, and assesses the quality of their work.

McCarthy, Michelle, *Directory of Women Working with Women with Learning Difficulties* (1991), Free. Available from Aids Awareness/Sex Education Project, Harperbury Hospital.
Contains 50 entries arranged by geographical area, in England only. Women working in Scotland, Wales or Ireland are strongly encouraged to get in touch with the author. Women with learning difficulties, individually or in groups, are also welcome to send in entries.

Network of Voluntary Organisations in AIDS/HIV (NOVOAH), *Training and Resource Directory*. Available from NOVOAH.
Lists organisations working on AIDS/HIV issues in the UK and Ireland. Includes information on trainers and training organisations; covers counselling, fundraising, therapy, bereavement, carers, outreach with women and Black communities, and welfare rights.

Patton, C, *Sex and Germs: the Politics of AIDS* (1985), South End Press, Boston, £6.95.
Attempts to locate AIDS within a history of changing sexuality, medicine and attitudes. Explores the culture of the gay and lesbian communities and the character of their response.

Richardson, D, *Safer Sex: the Guide for Women Today* (1990), Pandora, £7.99.
A positive and practical guide for every woman who is sexually active. Covers the widest variety of sexual feelings and expressions, and shows how you can explore for yourself your own needs and desires – safely.

Richardson, D, *Women and AIDS* (1988), Methuen, £7.95.
A wide-ranging book which considers all aspects of AIDS, including safer sex, sexual preference, living with AIDS, caring for people with AIDS, policies and prevention.

Richardson, D, *Women and the AIDS Crisis* (1989), Pandora, £4.95.
Explores issues of concern to women.

Rieder, Ines and Ruppelt, Patricia, *Matters of Life and Death: Women Speak About AIDS* (1989), Virago, £6.50.
Women who have been affected by HIV and AIDS write about their feelings. Women include activists, nurses, women with AIDS, carers and others.

Women's Health Information Mobile, *Great Safer Sex for Grown-ups*, (1991). Available from: Women's Health Information Mobile or from Aidsline Health Promotion Services, Enfield Health Authority.
A frank, comprehensive and interesting booklet which looks at safer heterosexual sex, giving advice on unsafe practices plus lots of suggestions for having more fun, exploring fantasies and being more open.

Videos and audio tapes

AIDS/HIV: a Woman's Issue, 34 minute video, £32.91 inclusive. Available from Metro Pictures.

Badelte Riste, Changing Relationships (1990) (Urdu with English subtitles), 28 minute video. £70.00 plus VAT and p&p. Available from Healthwise Productions. Targeted at Muslim population – shows transmission of virus by blood transfusion.

Hasina's Story: a Drama about HIV and AIDS (1991), 32 minute video, £16.17. No English subtitles – an English script accompanies and a bilingual leaflet which gives extra information in some key issues raised in the video. Available from Video Production Unit, Tower Hamlets Health Promotion Service.

Letters Out: a Drama about Women and HIV, 50 minute video, £70 plus VAT, Second Sight with Women and Theatre. Available from Second Sight Productions.
Raises all the issues around women and HIV and AIDS by following the lives of four women (Black and white, middle-class and working class). Accompanied by a 48 page manual containing warm-up sessions, workshop outlines, factual information and resource lists.

Mouthing Off: Women Speak Out About Safer Sex (1990), 35 minute video, Women's Action on AIDS. Available from Concord films.
Aims to raise issues of safer sex to enable women watching to discuss their own fears, successes and experiences.

Women and HIV and AIDS (1990), video of ten short trigger films for use by a facilitator, Humingbird Films for North East Thames Regional Health Authority. Guide included.

Organisations

Black HIV/AIDS Network (BHAN)
Set up to meet the needs of Black people and Black communities affected by HIV and AIDS. Provides community and home care, buddies, support groups, information, education and training courses. Multilingual resources.

Immunity Publications
Produce a range of leaflets on women and HIV; topics include prevention; HIV: the facts for women who sell sex; women, drugs and HIV; HIV, pregnancy and children; and positive result.

London Black Women's Health Action Group
Provides information on Black women's health issues including sexuality, mental health, HIV and AIDS. Aims to provide a national network.

National AIDS Helpline
Leaflets available by phone. Lists local organisations and support groups. Different languages at certain times – see Chapter 11 *General resources*.

National HIV Prevention Information Service
A free service to provide information to those working in the field of HIV education and prevention. Produces information sheets, statistical information, referral and networking services.

Oasis AIDS Resource Project
Resource centre, information and publications for those working in education or training, and for interested individuals.

Positively Women
Support and advice for women who are HIV positive, or have AIDS or associated conditions. Produce a number of useful leaflets.

Terence Higgins Trust
Services include a helpline, counselling, health education and the publication of a wide range of useful posters and leaflets, including many for women.

Women and HIV and AIDS Network
Produces a newsletter.

Women's Action on AIDS
Develop resources on women and AIDS.

Women's Health
Has a resource centre, phone and postal advice services, publications on contraception, abortion, HIV/AIDS and women's health in general.

10 *Staying healthy*

INTRODUCTION

This chapter consists of seven sections: *Complementary medicine; Vaginal health; Premenstrual syndrome; Cancer; Smoking; Drinking;* and *Coronary heart disease.*

Complementary medicine has been included because of the contribution it may offer to the promotion of health for women, and because of the interest which many women have in a variety of remedies and therapies which can be used to complement orthodox medicine.

The different health topics have been selected because of the particular impact they have on women's health and the potential they offer women to help themselves to stay healthy.

The sections on vaginal health and premenstrual syndrome cover issues which, although not life-threatening, affect a huge number of women and cause much suffering and discomfort. The information offered will enable women to understand more about these health concerns and provide suggestions to help prevent or cope with them.

Cancer and coronary heart disease are the major causes of premature death for women. Smoking and drinking play a significant role in both of them and in other health problems affecting women.

Complementary medicine

The HEA does not necessarily recommend any of the following remedies, nor does it know whether they have any side-effects and/or benefits.

BACKGROUND INFORMATION

- Complementary medicine offers a wide range of treatments, remedies and therapies, some of which have been used for centuries in various parts of the world. It uses a 'holistic' approach, which looks at the physical, emotional and spiritual aspects of an individual and considers their whole lifestyle.

- Complementary medicine has a large following in this country, and its credibility has been steadily increasing for several years. There is a growing recognition that orthodox medicine does not have all the answers for our health.

- As complementary medicine gains respect from the medical establishment, some therapies are being offered through the NHS. However, most are not available this way, and must be paid for, although many practitioners offer a sliding scale of charges.

- Traditionally, women developed knowledge and skills to treat ailments, and passed on information about cures and remedies from generation to generation. The male-dominated medical profession is a comparatively modern institution which now dominates health and health care.

- Traditional remedies and treatments have developed and are used within different cultures. Information Sheet 10.1 *Some traditional remedies* has been compiled from the experiences of some African-Caribbean and Asian women, and does not represent *all* traditional remedies available.

- It is important to be well informed about complementary medicine and new developments available, and to demand professionalism from the practitioners we consult.

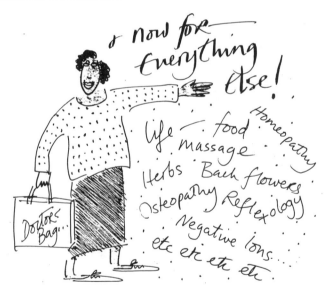

PRACTICAL POINTS

- A woman's health course cannot cover all types of remedies or therapies, but it is possible to outline the issues and to explore specific remedies which are relevant to the group.

- It may be useful to invite practitioners to give demonstrations and information about particular therapies. After they have left, the group can discuss their impressions of that therapy, and issues raised.

- Members of the group may have used particular therapies or remedies and may be willing to share this experience.

- The group could bring in herbal teas to drink, or essential oils to have simple massage (see the *Relaxation and massage* section of Chapter 4).

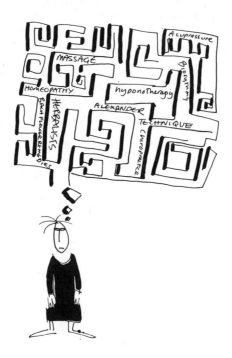

INFORMATION SHEET *10.1*

Some traditional remedies

The HEA does not necessarily recommend any of these remedies, nor does it know whether they have any side effects and/or benefits.

Herbal medicine is used in every country by people of all social classes. Many African-Caribbean and Asian people living in Britain have continued to use these remedies, subject to their availability. The following are some examples of remedies and are not representative of those used by all African-Caribbean and Asian cultures in Britain.

Most herbal remedies are best taken over weeks for healing to take effect. They are not 'cure alls' and if symptoms persist a doctor should be consulted.

Note: Use enamel or stainless steel vessels – never aluminium.

Decotation (hot tea)

Mineral salts and bitter principles of plants extracted by boiling

- ½oz plant material (usually hard matter) to 1 cup of water.
- Boil together for 30 minutes.
- Strain thoroughly and store in the fridge.
- Adult dose: one wine-glass per day.

Infusion (cooling teas)

Green plants or flowers boiled and taken as hot or cold tea

- Steep 2 to 3 teaspoons of leaf or flower in a cup of boiling water for 10 minutes.
- Adult dose: – green herbs: ½ to 1 oz herb to 1 pint of water.
  – dried herbs: 1 teaspoon to 1 cup of water.

Tincture

Alcohol used to extract the active ingredient

- Soak 2 oz herb in 1 pint of alcohol (usually vodka).
- Shake daily.

▷

▷ 10.1 cont.

- Strain and take with water.

- Adult dose: 1 teaspoon 3 times daily.

Remedies for different complaints

Arthritis

- Soak a cup of Methi seeds and leave them overnight. Fry onions and garlic in ghee and cook the seeds in it. Eat with chapatti every day.

- Basil infusion.

Asthma

- Ginger boiled in 1 pint water till reduced by half. Add sugar.

Athlete's foot

- Rub with garlic mixture twice a day (recipe at the end of this information sheet).

Blood cleanser

- Cerassee or bitter bush infusion.

- Nettle infusion.

Colds and catarrh

- One teaspoon of honey and a pinch of ground black pepper before bed.

- Take heeng with a piece of gur (raw sugar).

- Turmeric powder and gur in warm milk.

- Infusion of basil.

- Cerassee leaves (bitter bush) infusion. Not to be taken by diabetics as it conceals sugar content in blood or urine.

- Garlic taken raw.

- Lemon grass/fever grass decotation.

▷

▷ 10.1 cont.

Coughs

- Eucalyptus sweets.
- Basil infusion.
- Ginger infusion.
- Orange peel (dried) infusion.

Cuts and bruises

- Aloe juice.
- Garlic (raw) is an antiseptic.
- Nettle leaves stop bleeding and are antiseptic.

Diabetes

- Squeeze the water from a bitter melon-karola, and drink it.
- Chapatti made from millet flour, and eaten with yoghurt.

Diarrhoea

- Boiled water with salt and sugar prevents dehydration.
- Arrowroot – 2 or 3 teaspoons of arrowroot boiled in a pint of milk or water. Take a cup several times daily.
- Basil infusion.

Earache

- Warm mustard oil – 2 drops in the ear.
- Garlic taken raw.
- 2 drops of garlic mixture (recipe at the end of this information sheet).

Hair tonic

- Nettle infusion rinsed on the hair.

▷

▷ 10.1 cont.

Insomnia

- A cup of hot milk before bed.

Indigestion

- Take ajwain and a pinch of salt.
- Eat small meals, and after meals drink green tea.
- Cinnamon infusion.
- Basil infusion.
- Ginger infusion.

Jaundice

- Juice of sugar cane.
- Roasted chickpeas.
- Sweet marjoram infusion.

Mouth ulcers

- Apply glycerine to the ulcer.
- Cerassee leaves or bitter bush infusion.

Period pains

- Warm milk with 1 teaspoon sugar and 1 egg yolk mixed in before bed.
- Foods containing vitamins A and E.

Sore eyes

- Honey on the eye.
- Bathe with pure rose water.
- Fresh aloe juice – dissolve half teaspoon of juice in boiled water.

▷

▷ 10.1 cont.

Spots and pimples

- Rub with garlic mixture twice daily (recipe at the end of this information sheet).

- Cerassee leaves or bitter bush leaves infusion as a face wash.

Sprains

- Apply pounded saffron to the injured part and bandage, after washing with antiseptic soap.

Stomach ache

- Peppermint oil.

- Liquorice and dry mint tea.

- Cinnamon infusion.

- Peppermint infusion.

- Fennel infusion.

Sunburn

- Aloe juice.

Toothache

- Clove oil rubbed on the affected tooth.

- Cerassee or bitter bush leaves infusion.

Garlic mixture

- 8 oz peeled minced garlic covered with 4 oz warm olive oil. Stand in a warm place for three days. Strain and bottle and keep in a cool place.

INFORMATION SHEET *10.2*

Some complementary therapies

The HEA does not necessarily recommend any of these therapies, nor does it know whether they have any side-effects and/or benefits

ACUPUNCTURE

Origin	China
Equipment/Medium	Fine acupuncture needles
Basic philosophy	There are two opposing forces in the body – Yin and Yang. An imbalance in these can result in ill health. There are about 1000 acupuncture points on the body, and stimulating these with a needle can redress this imbalance and result in the relief of symptoms and stimulate energy forces in the body, so promoting good health.
Practice	The acupuncturist takes a detailed case history and feels various points to find tenderness, or focuses on those parts linked with patients' symptoms.
Particular uses	Almost all chronic and acute conditions, including headaches, acute lung disease, acute rheumatic conditions, menstrual, digestive and nervous problems. No harmful side-effects. Good for children, and during pregnancy.

ALEXANDER TECHNIQUE

Origin	F. Mathias Alexander, Tasmania 1869–1955
Equipment/Medium	Patient practises different postures and co-ordination with the guidance of a practitioner.
Basic philosophy	Posture is the cause of many ailments. Posture regulates breathing and blood circulation. Good breathing and blood circulation is developed through proper body movements and posture.
Practice	Relaxation; the practising of various bodily movements and posturing – especially between the neck, head, back and co-ordination of the body.

▷

▷ 10.2 cont.

Particular uses Rheumatic, spinal, breathing, chronic back and neck problems.

AROMATHERAPY

Origin Ancient Egyptians; term coined by a French chemist

Equipment/Medium Essential oils from flowers, plants, trees and resins. Essence of plants used, picked at different times of the day and night for different uses, and aromatic oil made.

Basic philosophy Belief that aromatic oils can have a therapeutic, balancing effect on mental and emotional state, skin ailments and infections. A sample of blood or aradiesthesia (dowsing with a pendulum) is used.

Practice Oils are taken through massage, inhalation or in the bath. Some contra-indications for pregnant women.

Particular uses Depression, stress, skin conditions, insomnia (and many other claims).

AUTOGENICS

Origin Dr Johannes Schultz, Berlin, 1930s

Equipment/Medium A teacher is necessary.

Basic philosophy Health is promoted by deep relaxation and stimulation of the body's self-healing mechanisms.

Practice Exercise and meditations, taught singly or in groups. Learning to focus attention inwardly by repeating standard phrases.

Particular uses Stress-related problems.

BIOFEEDBACK

Origin Pioneered in USA

Equipment/Medium Biofeedback machines (various sorts with differing functions e.g. mind-mirror, electric skin response meter).

Basic philosophy Electrical activity on the surface of the skin can measure muscle tension, blood-pressure and cortisone levels. These are frequently causes of various ailments. People can reduce/change their levels based on biofeedback.

▷

▷ 10.2 cont.

Practice	Machine attached to the person. Individual works on changing her/his own level.
Particular uses	Used to treat a number of illnesses related to high blood-pressure, muscle tension and blood circulation.

BACH FLOWER REMEDIES

Origin	Dr Edward Bach, Wales 1886–1936
Equipment/Medium	Flowers – 38 identified. Infusion made by boiling flowers.
Basic philosophy	Emphasises the emotional state of the patient. Sees emotional states underlying physical symptoms. Certain plants can alter one's emotional state (positive and negative).
Practice	Flowers are used for seven emotional categories. Each category will use a combination of the 38 flowers.
Particular uses	Used to treat the following categories of emotional states: fear, uncertainty; lack of interest in life; loneliness; over-sensitivity to influence; despondency/despair; over-caring for the welfare of others.

CHIROPRACTIC

Origin	Ancient origins, practised by Greeks, Romans, Egyptians, Chinese. Greek name 'cherio' and 'prakticos' meaning done by hand
Equipment/Medium	Manipulation.
Basic philosophy	If vertebral misalignments occur through accidents, poor posture, etc. the nerve supply to organs will be interfered with. Bones of the skull, thorax, spine, pelvis and limbs are checked and subtly adjusted.
Practice	Chiropractic manipulates joints, especially spinal joints, and helps to correct posture. Used in conjunction with other therapies.
Particular uses	Relief from migraine, back and shoulder pains, sciatica, lumbago, menstrual problems, muscular disorders.

▷

▷ 10.2 cont.

HERBALISM

Origin	As old as history itself; herbs always used to restore good health
Equipment/Medium	Herbs – derived from a vast variety of plant species. Many are the base for modern pharmacy today. Preparation will include teas, ointments, etc.
Basic philosophy	Plant substances can be used to treat ailments, prevent ill health and generally promote good health, through strengthening natural functions of the body.
Practice	Herbalist will select appropriate herbs for individual needs. Many people use herbs on their own without a practitioner. Nutrition and diet need to be considered.
Particular uses	Wide range of usages, for example, acne, asthma, colds, burns, wounds, stomach complaints, nervous complaints, menstrual problems.

HOMEOPATHY

Origin	Samuel Hahnemann, Germany 1755–1843. Greek words homoios – like and pathos – suffering
Equipment/Medium	Medicinal remedies.
Basic philosophy	Based on the belief of treating 'like with like'. Symptoms are treated with the very substance which causes the illness. Substance is diluted. The more it's diluted, the stronger the effect. This mobilises the body's own defences to fight the cause of ill health.
Practice	Homeopath examines patient, diet etc., and actual symptoms. Treatment is highly individualised.
Particular uses	Most illnesses.

HYDROTHERAPY

Origin	Has been used since ancient Greeks. Means 'water healing'
Equipment/Medium	Special baths, hot springs, saunas, water and ice packs. Pure mineral water from wells and springs.

▷

▷ 10.2 cont.

Basic philosophy	Benefits of water to warm or cool us, to relieve fatigue and to prevent stiffness. Taken internally as mineral spa waters, or for bathing in – where buoyancy allows for greater freedom of movement.
Practice	Special exercises prescribed by hydrotherapist in a warm pool, or hot and cold compresses may be advised. Simple self-help of hot and cold water to treat common ailments.
Particular uses	To relieve pain from respiratory problems, backaches, arthritis and rheumatism, bad circulation, urino-genital complaints.

HYPNOTHERAPY

Origin	Promoted by Meseur, Freud and Erickson; Induction of trance-like states used in many civilisations
Equipment/Medium	Reputable hypnotherapist for one-to-one sessions.
Basic philosophy	When the conscious mind is sufficiently relaxed, suggestions can be communicated to the subject without opposition.
Practice	Discussion of problem, then physical relaxation followed by use of pendulum, voice or indirect suggestions to attain trance. Lasts about 1 hour.
Particular uses	Useful for fears, phobias, tension, speech disorders. Useful to stop smoking or other dependent behaviour.

IRIDOLOGY

Origin	Not known
Equipment/Medium	A 'reading' is taken of irises of both eyes as a diagnostic tool.
Basic philosophy	Each area of the iris corresponds to specific part of the body. Studying lines, flecks, and pigmentations allows diagnosis of specific disorders.
Practice	Iridologists will diagnose and refer on to appropriate treatments.
Particular uses	As a diagnostic tool.

▷

▷ 10.2 cont.

NATUROPATHY

Origin	Natural healing used in different forms throughout history
Equipment/Medium	Not one particular remedy – draws from many other alternative approaches.
Basic philosophy	Belief that symptoms are a reflection of the person being out of balance. Focuses on causes of symptoms rather than symptoms themselves. Causes related to poor eating habits, bad posture, stress and tension, emotional state of being – an imbalance in one can cause an imbalance in the others.
Practice	A highly individualised programme is devised with the patient. Involves change in diet, relaxation and massage, vitamin and mineral therapy and draws on other types of alternative therapy.
Particular uses	All illnesses can be treated in conjunction with a naturopathic approach.

NEGATIVE IONS

Origin	Studied by Father Gian Baccaria in Italy, 1775
Equipment/Medium	Certain atmospheric conditions e.g. high rainfall areas, next to the seaside and waterfalls can produce negative ions. Also commercially produced by negative ion generators.
Basic philosophy	Belief that the atmosphere is filled with electrical discharges called ions, which can affect people's moods and health, while an excess of negative ions can restore a sense of well-being and eliminate certain symptoms. Some common modern producers of positive ions include central heating, air conditioning, electrical pylons, pollution and certain weather.
Practice	Negative ionisers can be bought and used by anyone.
Particular uses	Besides general therapeutic value, particularly useful for breathing and respiratory problems, migraines and sleeplessness, fatigue and lethargy, hay-fever and catarrh.

▷

▷ 10.2 cont.

OSTEOPATHY

Origin	Based on ancient Greek and Roman practice; Dr Andrew Taylor Still, USA, 1828–1917 pioneered its modern practice; from Greek words – osteo (a bone) and pathos (disease)
Equipment/Medium	Sometimes X-rays. Manipulation and massage.
Basic philosophy	Many illnesses are related to spinal disorders and minor malpositioning of joints and bones. Emphasis placed on healthy blood circulation which maintains the body's in-built immune and defence systems. Many illnesses related to muscles and bones which restrict blood flow.
Practice	Osteopath will diagnose using X-ray and/or feeling changes in bones, joints and muscles. Lifestyle of patient also taken into account. Manipulates affected parts of body. Often used in conjunction with vitamin therapy, massage and Alexander technique to improve posture.
Particular uses	Back and neck weaknesses, spinal and joint disorders.

RADIONICS AND RADIESTHESIA

Origin	Since Egyptian times, and in this century in France, USA and UK
Equipment/Medium	Blood or hair strand is diagnosed with use of pendulum, analysis chart, colour treatment by skilled and sensitive practitioner.
Basic philosophy	All life forms are connected to energy fields. Illness is a disharmony or distortion in that field. It can be corrected, often by distant healing.
Practice	Filling in a questionnaire, giving case history and symptoms. Giving a sample of hair. Asking a series of mental questions with aid of pendulum.
Particular uses	Longstanding illnesses such as asthma, hay fever, allergies and toxin accumulations. As an aid to diagnosis.

REBIRTHING

Origin	Based on 'pranhyama'; yoga science of breathing
Equipment/Medium	One-to-one sessions or in groups.

▷

▷ 10.2 cont.

Basic philosophy	Using guided, deep, easy connected breathing to discover 'where' in our bodies we 'hold onto' emotional feelings or physical symptoms; then to gradually and safely let them go.
Practice	Breathing sessions lasting 1½ hours. More sessions may be needed.
Particular uses	Emotional and mental problems. Drug dependence, including smoking, anorexia, skin disorders.

REFLEXOLOGY

Origin	Ancient and Chinese medicine
Equipment/Medium	Foot massage.
Basic philosophy	There are thousands of nerve endings in each foot which are connected to various parts of the body. Imbalances in the body leave crystalline deposits on the nerve endings which in turn hinder the energy flow through various meridians. This can result in illness. Massaging appropriate points on the feet releases these deposits, mobilises and stimulates organs and glands to function as they should, and clears the path for the energy flow needed for health and vitality.
Practice	Massage applied primarily by the thumb, pressure is applied to each part, working its way in a rhythmical movement, first the left foot then the right.
Particular uses	Varied, depending on the needs of the individual. Especially for stress-related and immune system disorders.

SHIATSU

Origin	Means 'finger pressure'; therapy related to acupuncture
Equipment/Medium	Loose clothes and somewhere to lie down. One-to-one sessions.
Basic philosophy	Works with the 'Chi' energy along meridian lines. Blockages of energy are dispersed by gentle pressure. Practitioner uses hands, knees, elbows.
Practice	Lasts about 1 hour. Case history is taken, diagnosis made through touch, sound and observation. ▷

▷ 10.2 cont.

Particular uses   Menstrual and menopausal problems. Stress-related conditions. Head and shoulder aches.

SPIRITUAL HEALING

Origin   As old as humankind

Equipment/Medium   A healer – not necessarily religious – who may 'lay' on hands, or who may work from a distance.

Basic philosophy   Healers tune into and can channel their own energy to interact and replenish others' low energy.

Practice   Wide variety of methods – hands-on, using body aura, self-help in form of prayer, affirmations and visualisations. Attitude is critical.

Particular uses   All ailments.

T'AI CHI CHUAN

Origin   From Qi Gong Chinese practitioner of simple exercises

Equipment/Medium   Loose clothing, learning, often from a teacher, usually in a group. Daily practice alone.

Basic philosophy   Moving meditation. A slow and gentle martial art which nurtures 'Chi' energy – similar to acupuncture.

Practice   Daily exercise and learning a 'form' of T'ai Chi.

Particular uses   To improve circulation, peace of mind, self-awareness.

YOGA

Origin   Ancient India

Equipment/Medium   Non-slip mat and loose comfortable clothing.

Basic philosophy   Mind, body, spirit and emotions are integrated through practice of physical postures (asanas), breathing exercises (pranayama), and relaxation and meditation.

Practice   After 'warm-ups' body is taken through a range of postures to stretch and strengthen muscles and when combined with breathing, the mind is ready for relaxation and meditation.

Particular uses   Adaptable to all levels of ability or disability. Increases suppleness, relieves tension, develops body awareness and self-confidence.

INFORMATION SHEET *10.3*

Aromatherapy

The HEA does not necessarily recommend any of these therapies, nor does it know whether they have any side-effects and/or benefits.

A short history

In 3500 BC Egyptians were using principles of aromatherapy in magic, healing, cosmetics and embalment. Roman and Greek empires brought this knowledge further abroad, and there are records of their use in warding off the Black Death, cholera and other diseases.

The nineteenth century saw chemists producing synthetic copies of essential oils as perfumes rather than treatments. The twentieth century saw a move back to the use of natural essential oils for prevention and treatment of illnesses, since synthetic oils had side effects from impurities. Several physicians in this century have pioneered work in this field and have given credibility to aromatherapy.

In Britain today, aromatherapy is part of the complementary health movement and is based upon treating the person as a whole. During treatment, a patient is encouraged to talk about her feelings, and these are taken into account. For example, if she feels anger or resentment at her condition then oils are chosen which help with these feelings.

Aromatherapy oils and how they are used

It is advisable to consult a qualified practitioner if you are interested in using aromatherapy for specific illness treatment. But it can be a simple and pleasant self-help technique for reducing stress and promoting relaxation.

Essential oils are the concentrated organic essences of a wide variety of plants. (It takes, for example, several kilos of lavender to produce a small bottle of essential oil.) Each oil contains unique healing properties and fragrances and may contain over 100 different natural chemicals. It is possible to use combinations of oils to promote healing on different levels – physical, emotional and mental.

The skin absorbs minute quantities of oil from massage, bathing or compresses. Oil can also be absorbed by inhalation. Essential oils should never be taken orally. All essences are antiseptic and some have anti-viral and anti-inflammatory properties as well. The oils work by promoting natural healing through stimulating and reinforcing the body's own defence mechanisms and strengthening immune systems.   ▷

▷ 10.3 cont.

Essential oils are very volatile, that is they evaporate on contact with the air. Some are more volatile than others.

Essential oils to avoid

Sassafras should *never* be used, as it can cause cancer.

Avoid pennyroyal, thuja, wintergreen, thyme and sage.

Essential oils to avoid in some situations

- Do not apply to skin (use only as room perfumes): cinnamon bark and leaf, cloves.

- Not before sunbathing: bergamot, lemon, orange, mandarin, grapefruit, lime and verbena.

- Not during pregnancy: basil, myrrh and sweet marjoram.

Application

Essential oils *should not* be used undiluted.

Baths: 10–15 drops per bath
Compresses: 10 drops per cup of water
Inhalants: 10 drops on a paper towel, *or* 10 drops in basin of hot water
Massage: 15–30 drops in 50 ml of carrier oil.

Carrier oil can be either sweet almond oil, grapeseed oil, peach or apricot kernel. Almond and grapeseed are the least expensive.

Up to four oils can be mixed together in different proportions to give the most desirable aroma, but the total number of drops detailed above must not be exceeded.

▷

▷ 10.3 cont.

Aromatherapy table

Relaxing	*Balancing*	*Stimulating*
cedarwood B	geranium M	coriander T
camomile M	frankincense B	eucalyptus T
clary sage M		ginger M
neroli M		peppermint T
sandalwood B		rosemary M
ylang-ylang M		tea-tree T

Key
T is top note: highly volatile and does not last long
M is middle note: lasts a little longer
B is base note: long-lasting effect

Anti-depressants	camomile, geranium, neroli
Anxiety	sandalwood, ylang-ylang, geranium
Arthritis	lemon, rosemary, ginger
Asthma	lemon, rosemary
Bruises	fennel, marjoram
Burns and scalds	lavender
Chilblains	lavender or lemon
Colds	lavender, tea-tree, lemon
Dandruff	juniper, lavender, tea-tree
Eczema	camomile or lavender
High blood-pressure	lavender, ylang-ylang
Indigestion	basil or lavender
Insect stings	lavender or tea-tree
Insomnia	camomile or lavender
Menstrual problems	geranium, lavender, rosemary
Menopause	clary-sage, geranium, fennel
Migraine	camomile, lavender, peppermint
Muscular pain/aching muscles	lavender, rosemary, cypress
Poor circulation	ginger, lemon, lavender
PMS	geranium, lavender, sandalwood
Rheumatism	rosemary, coriander, lavender

ACTIVITY *10.1*

Traditional remedies

Aims

- To share existing knowledge about traditional remedies, and gather further information.

- To identify natural remedies in everyday use.

Materials

Copies of Worksheets 10.1 and 10.2 *Traditional remedies 1* and *2* for each woman; pens, flipchart, markers, supply of books and leaflets on traditional remedies.

Methods

1 In small groups, work through Worksheet 10.1, noting responses.

2 Using the books available and knowledge of women in the group, complete Worksheet 10.2.

3 In the large group, share information and flipchart the main points.

Variation: women could produce the information in the form of a handout for reference and use by other women.

Discussion points

- Traditional remedies work very differently from orthodox medicine. Generally, orthodox medicine brings speedy cures, whereas many alternative remedies require prolonged use in conjunction with other treatment such as relaxation or particular diet.

- Natural remedies are being marketed in much the same way as other pharmaceutical products, which pushes up the price. Products without a brand-name or fancy packaging are just as effective.

- Different cultures have developed and use different types of remedies (see Information Sheet 10.1 *Some traditional remedies*).

Note for tutor

This activity uses a transcript from white working class history, which may not be relevant for some Black women. However, it may be useful.

ACTIVITY *10.2*

Complementary medicine and the NHS

Aims

- To think critically about the issues surrounding orthodox and complementary medicine.

- To consider the advantages and disadvantages of bringing complementary medicine within the control of the National Health Service.

- To highlight some of the basic philosophies underlying orthodox and complementary medicine.

Materials

A copy of Worksheet 10.3 *Complementary medicine and the NHS* for each woman.

Method

1 Set the scene for the activity. A fictitious Royal Commission of Inquiry has been set up to investigate the value of offering complementary medicine through the NHS. A number of groups have been invited to give their opinions and present their arguments. The worksheet provides a sample of possible arguments from different perspectives.

2 Divide into three groups: *Group A* represents a group of doctors, *Group B* a group of complementary practitioners and *Group C* a group of patients.

3 Give the appropriate section of the worksheet to each group, and ask them to discuss the arguments and/or develop their own. Conflicting views may be expressed by the same interest group. Each group elects a spokeswoman to report to the Inquiry.

4 In the large group, act out the Inquiry. One woman chairs the meeting, and each group presents its views, followed by a general discussion. You may want to conclude the meeting by a vote to see who is in favour of/against complementary medicine being available on the NHS.

5 Feed back how women found the activity, the issues it raised, and whether opinion has changed during the course of the session.

Discussion points

- There are no simple answers – there are complicated arguments for and against providing complementary medicine on the NHS.

- This activity poses some fundamental questions as to the kind of health service to strive for. The ideal may be to develop a health service which offers both orthodox and complementary medicine for prevention, treatment and promotion of physical and emotional well-being.

ACTIVITY *10.3*

Food as medicine and as cosmetics

Aims

- To explore connections between food, health and cosmetics.
- To share knowledge of different remedies.

Materials

A copy of Worksheet 10.4 *Food as medicine and as cosmetics* for each woman; pens, flipchart paper, markers, books/information about natural remedies and cosmetics.

Additional materials for the variation: flipchart paper, magazines, scissors, glue.

Method

1 In small groups, go through the worksheet and note responses.

2 In the large group, feed back and flipchart responses.

Variation: use magazines to make collages about food as medicine and food as cosmetics.

Discussion points

- How surprising are the responses?
- Do the group members use foods in any of the ways identified?
- Does any food appear both as a medicine and as a cosmetic?
- Where has the information about using foods in these ways come from?

Note for tutor

It may be useful to bring in books about natural remedies and cosmetics.

WORKSHEET *10.1*

Traditional remedies 1

Read through the following:

> Well, you didn't call the doctor in unless it was really serious. You did a lot of your own – there was a chemist on Robert Hall Street, and you used to go there. Your mother would write out what you had to have and this man would mix that up. God knows what would be in it. But it was some old remedy . . . We used to go to this little chemist and he would make anything up and there would be a queue, always a queue. And it would cost perhaps 3d or 4d for this bottle of medicine. Camphorated oil was used an awful lot for rubbing chests. Camphorated oil and mustard was the remedy. And you got quite a bottle like that for 2d or 3d. And you rubbed it in, it stunk rotten. But it did a lot of good. My mother, she had bronchitis and asthma which all her family did. Funnily enough they all have except me . . . If you had dirty hair, mother used to bring the children in if the nit nurse was coming, she'd bring the children in and she'd do it. But if there was anybody really ill – I'm trying to think of one, old Mrs Wilkes that lived next door to us, old Mrs Radcliffe was on one side and old Mrs Wilkes on the other. And old Mrs Wilkes she was very ill, but there was never much said about her because I found out later that she died of cancer and you didn't speak of cancer. It's – she's not very well, you know, and that meant anything. So I was sent errands 'Go for this, that and the other'. And she had all sorts of concoctions. My mother used to poultice her with linseed, well really linseed oil. She used to buy the linseed and boil it in a bag and strain it.[1]

Medicines are becoming a big part of our lives, with a cure for every symptom. However, there are now many known side-effects of commonly used medicines, for example, aspirin. Alternative remedies have few known side-effects, and we are more in control of how and when we use them.

What is the place for alternative remedies and conventional Western medicine in our health care?

▷

[1] Excerpt from oral history tape transcript: Reprinted by courtesy of Audrey Linkman, Manchester Polytechnic.

▷ 10.1 cont.

List all the plant/herb-based medicines you can think of which used to appear in home medicine chests and discuss their uses.

Lotions:

Creams:

Liquids:

Inhalations:

Beverages:

How many of these do you use today?

Which foods do you believe to have specific medicinal value?

WORKSHEET *10.2*

Traditional remedies 2

There are many everyday ailments which can be treated in the home, without a visit to the doctor, or buying medicine from a chemist.

Can you suggest natural remedies for any of the following?

Birth contractions

Bruises and sprains

Burns

Catarrh

Cold and chills

Constipation

Coughs

Cystitis

Diarrhoea

Indigestion

Insomnia

Menopausal problems

Mouth infections

Muscular aches and pains

Nervous tension

Period pains

Premenstrual tension

Sore throats

Thrush

Toothache

WORKSHEET 10.3
Complementary medicine and the NHS

	Against inclusion	For inclusion
DOCTORS	There are over 100 complementary therapies – how would we select which ones to provide under the NHS?

Is it realistic to think of expanding NHS provision when we are struggling to keep what exists intact?

Orthodox medicine depends largely on medical trials to prove effectiveness of treatment. Complementary therapies often cannot prove effectiveness in the same scientific way. How can we justify allocating scarce resources to treatments where it is difficult to justify effectiveness with trials and statistics? | As a GP I already use homeopathy and acupuncture in my practice. I would like to make this service more widely available.

In England anyone can set her/himself up as a therapist providing s/he doesn't pose as a medical doctor. This leaves the system open to abuse and threatens the reputation of many bona fide practitioners. Bringing practitioners under the umbrella of the NHS would mean greater standardisation of training and registration, and therefore greater protection for the consumer. |
| COMPLEMENTARY PRACTITIONERS | By retaining our independence, we can provide the kind of service we feel is appropriate. We fear the kind of control the orthodox dominated NHS would attempt to impose.

Complementary medicine does not fit into the same framework of science and technology as orthodox medicine does. We cannot test effectiveness in the same way – the body is not a machine made up of parts – it is a complicated combination of lifestyle, physical, emotional and spiritual | If made more widely available through the NHS, complementary therapies could mean substantial savings for the NHS. Orthodox medicine depends largely on the use of drugs, surgery, etc. which are expensive and have side-effects. There are few known side-effects for most complementary therapies. Certain approaches use meditation, relaxation and diet as an integral part of the treatment, which require minimal costs. Complementary therapies use a holistic approach, focusing on prevention and |

△

For inclusion (cont.)

identifying the root of the symptoms. This could lead to savings, particularly for chronic recurring conditions.

Complementary approaches are often expensive and are therefore only available to those who can pay. Provision under the NHS means more people can have access to them.

Many people are interested in complementary treatments but don't know where to find them. If they are under the NHS they will be more accessible.

There is always the fear of going to a quack and hopefully the NHS will help to ensure standards and provide more protection for us.

Against inclusion (cont.)

components, and treatment involves all of these. Also, people are seen as individuals and therefore treatment plans are different for each person. None of the above lend themselves to trials and scientific research. Our independence will enable us to contribute in this way.

As it exists now there are long waiting lists for treatment under the NHS. One rarely has to wait for treatment with most complementary practitioners – inclusion might imply long waiting lists.

We would be worried about losing the individual attention we now receive from complementary practitioners.

PATIENTS

WORKSHEET *10.4*

Food as medicine and as cosmetics

TYPE OF FOOD   MEDICINAL USE

TYPE OF FOOD   COSMETIC USE

RESOURCES

For contact details of distributors and organisations listed here, see the list of organisations in Chapter 11 *General resources*.

Publications

Bauer, Cathryn, *Acupressure for Women* (1987), Women Crossing Press, £6.95.
Acupressure techniques applied to women's problems. A how-to guide.

Campion, Kitty, *A Woman's Herbal* (1992, c1987), Vermillion, £6.99.
Preventive herbal medicine for a range of health problems, body maintenance and beauty.

Curtis, Susan and Fraser, Romy, *Natural Healing for Women: Caring for Yourself with Herbs, Homoeopathy and Essential Oils* (1991), Pandora, £7.99.
Includes a repertory of ailments organised by body systems and areas of health, the material medica, an A–Z of remedies and treatment, and a section on lifestyle.

Gemmell, D, *Everyday Homoeopathy: a Safe Guide for Self-treatment* (1987), Beaconsfield Publishers, £7.95.
How to use homeopathic medicine in the everyday context of your own personal and family health care. The theory of homeopathy is explained, and basic information is given on how to observe symptoms and select the correct dosage of remedy.

Grant, Belinda, *An A–Z of Natural Healthcare* (1992), Optima, £9.99, ISBN 0 356 20560 6.
Provides information on a full range of natural therapies which includes details of how they work, what can be expected of each treatment, what to expect from a practitioner, managing and treating minor ailments and self-healing techniques. The book emphasises self-help and taking responsibility for individual health throughout.

Hall, Nicola, *Thorsons Introductory Guide to Reflexology* (1991), Thorsons, £3.99.
Second revised edition of the guide to reflexology, how it works, treatment and how it is practised.

Hopkins, Cathy, *The Joy of Aromatherapy: Sensual Remedies for Everyday Ailments* (1991), Angus and Robertson, £3.99.
Suggestions for treatment of a range of conditions.

Inglis, Brian and West, Ruth, *The Alternative Health Guide* (1984), Joseph, £10.99.
An introduction to alternative health care.

Marcus, Paul, *Thorsons Introductory Guide to Acupuncture* (1991), Thorsons, £3.99.
Second revised edition of this clear guide to acupuncture.

McIntyre, Anne, *Herbs for Common Ailments* (1992), Gaia, £6.99.
A guide to common problems such as insect bites and stings, bruises, travel sickness and others, and the use of herbs to treat them.

Nagarathna, R, Nagendra, H R, and Monro, Robin, *Yoga for Common Ailments* (1990), Gaia, £6.99.
Illustrated guide includes many women's problems.

Nissim, Rina, *Natural Healing in Gynaecology: a User's Manual* (1986), Pandora, £4.95.
A wide range of women's health concerns dealt with through natural techniques.

Scott, Julian and Scott, Susan, *Natural Medicine for Women: Drug-free Healthcare for Women of all Ages* (1991), Gaia, £8.99.
Natural therapies for a range of women's conditions and ailments.

Shapiro, Debbie, *The Bodymind Workbook: Exploring How the Mind and the Body Work Together* (1990), Element, £7.99.
Spiritual guide to a wide range of health problems.

Sharma, Ursula, *Complementary Medicine Today* (1992), Routledge, £12.99.
Sociological look at the users and practitioners of complementary medicine.

Stevens, Chris, *Alexander Technique* (1990, c1987), Optima, £4.99.
How the Alexander technique can help general health and well-being.

Tisserand, Maggie, *Aromatherapy for Women: Beautifying and Healing Essences from Flowers and Herbs* (1990), Thorsons, £3.99. Looks at children's illnesses, pregnancy, skin care, immune system and massage.

Westcott, Patsy, *Alternative Health Care for Women: a Compendium of Natural Approaches to Women's Health and Wellbeing* (1991), Thorsons, £6.99.
Full range of health problems and how complementary therapies can help.

Wildwood, C, *Aromatherapy – Massage with Essential Oils* (1991), Element Books Ltd, £4.99.
Has a brief history and explains how aromatherapy works. Very useful tips about blending different oils and massage techniques to use for different complaints. Useful reference table of oils and complaints.

Worsley, J R, *Acupuncture: is it for you?* (1988), Element, £6.99.
Guide to different uses of acupuncture.

Organisations

The Institute of Complementary Medicine
Has registers of a wide range of practitioners and their organisations. For other organisations, either ring the number listed or send a large stamped self-addressed envelope for further information.

Alexander Technique Society of Teachers (STAT)

Bach Flower Remedies, Edward Bach Centre

British Acupuncture Association and Register

British Homeopathic Association

British Naturopathic and Osteopathic Association

International Federation of Aromatherapists

International Federation of Reflexologists

Relaxation for Living

School of Phytotherapy (Herbal medicine)

Vaginal health

BACKGROUND INFORMATION

- Women may feel uncomfortable about the genital area, which is often associated with discharges, infections, and embarrassing internal examinations. Doctors may contribute to these feelings by using complicated Latin names, or euphemisms such as 'down there'.

- Women are particularly prone to recurring problems such as thrush and cystitis. They may be caught in a vicious circle, for example cystitis treated with antibiotic, which then causes thrush; or being treated for thrush and reinfected by their partner who does not seek treatment.

- A greater understanding of the vaginal area can help dispel fears and give women the confidence they need to ask doctors the right questions and look towards prevention and promoting their own vaginal health. Understanding what is normal for them, recognising early signals, when to go to the doctor, and simple home remedies can all alleviate the misery these common problems can cause.

- Information Sheets 10.4 *Vaginal health* and 6.3 *Pelvic floor exercises* (see Chapter 6) give practical guidelines for promoting vaginal health.

- For more information about infections see the *Sexually transmitted diseases* section of Chapter 9.

PRACTICAL POINTS

- Women may be embarrassed talking about vaginal health, and sharing experiences. Many women will have had vaginal examinations at some time, and it may be helpful to share experiences about embarrassment and communication difficulties, and ideas about what can help.

- Be familiar with the most common problems. It may be helpful to bring in books and other information for women to look at. Find out where women may get more information if they need it.

- If giving information about self-help remedies, it is important to be clear about their limitations. Point out that self-help remedies may offer relief for some problems, but if there is not a rapid improvement or the condition worsens it is important to see a doctor.

- There is a danger with these sessions of ending on a negative note. Try to focus on the positive things we can do to prevent or deal with the most common problems.

INFORMATION SHEET *10.4*

Vaginal health

If we know more about the vagina and how infections may develop, we can take some preventive measures.

The vagina is self-cleansing. Secretions produced by glands in the walls of the vagina lubricate and cleanse it. The amount, texture and colour of mucus produced will vary between individual women and also during different stages of our reproductive and menstrual cycles. It also changes if you are on the Pill, when you are pregnant and when you get older and your periods stop. For most of the month the liquid looks milky, is fairly thick, and dries on your pants as a white or cream mark. Two weeks before your next period it will be thinner, stretchy and clear. Just before your period it will be creamy and can be thicker. It will have a very faint musky smell that is not unpleasant.

It's a good idea to get into the habit of noticing what your vaginal secretion looks, feels and smells like and how it changes through the month. Then you should be able to tell if something is wrong.

Apart from normal changes, something could be wrong if:

- there is more discharge than you would normally expect;
- it looks different, especially if the colour is unusual;
- it feels different;
- it has a strong, unpleasant or unfamiliar smell; or
- it makes your vagina itch.

Something could also be wrong if you have:

- redness or soreness in and around your vagina;
- pain when you pass water; or
- rashes and tiny cracks in the skin around your vagina.

Many kinds of bacteria live in the healthy vagina (and in the healthy mouth and stomach). Most of these are 'good' bacteria for the vagina, as they fight off possible infections. If we take an antibiotic (for a sore throat, for instance) it can kill off the 'good' bacteria in the vagina leaving us vulnerable to infection. This is why many women develop thrush after taking an antibiotic.

▷

© Health Education Authority, 1993

▷ 10.4 cont.

The natural environment of the vagina is easily disturbed – vaginal deodorants, bubble bath and even soap may affect the balance to make the vagina less acidic, so that infection may develop. This is why natural yoghurt is sometimes recommended as a remedy for thrush. It can help the vagina re-establish its natural acidity and so fight infections. Wearing underwear made of synthetic material, tights or tight trousers creates a warm and moist environment in which infection can flourish. Taking the contraceptive pill produces hormonal changes, which in some women alter the vaginal balance and make them more susceptible to thrush.

Vaginal infections such as thrush and trichomonas are prevented from spreading into the uterus by a barrier of mucus on the cervix. But if you have a contraceptive coil (IUD) fitted, there is a possibility that an infection may travel up the string and into the uterus. So women with a coil have an increased risk of developing a pelvic infection (PID) and should have vaginal infections treated as soon as they develop, and seek medical attention for any abdominal discomfort.

During the menopause some women experience vaginal dryness which increases susceptibility to infection. (For more information, see the section *The menopause* in Chapter 6.)

Action to promote vaginal health and prevent infections

- Be aware of your own body and what is normal for you, then you will be alert to any changes and be able to respond quickly.

- Do not use vaginal deodorants, and if you are prone to vaginal infections, avoid bubble bath or shampooing your hair in the bath.

- Be careful to prevent bacteria from the anus entering the vagina, as they can cause infection. Make sure your sexual partner is aware of this (for example, a hand that has touched the anus should be washed before it touches the vagina). Wipe yourself from front to back to avoid contaminating the vulva with any organisms that may be present around the anus.

- Always wear cotton pants, and if you are especially prone to infections (e.g. at risk from taking antibiotics or the Pill) avoid tight trousers and tights or wear open gusset tights.

- If you have a sexual relationship, make sure your partner washes before sex. Find out about how infections can be passed on to your partner and then back to you. (See the section *Sexually transmitted diseases* in Chapter 9.)

- Exercise your pelvic muscles to maintain elasticity and improve muscle tone. (See Information Sheet 6.3 *Pelvic floor exercises* in Chapter 6.)

▷

▷ 10.4 cont.

- If you are prone to thrush and are particulary at risk because you are taking antibiotics, you may be able to prevent it developing by restoring the vagina to its acidic balance. Try putting *plain live* yoghurt onto the vulva or into the vagina; dip a tampon in yoghurt and then insert it.

ACTIVITY *10.4*

Vaginal infections

Aims

- To share experiences of having vaginal infections, and show how common they are.

- To explore possible remedies.

Materials

A copy of Information Sheet 10.4 *Vaginal health* for each woman; post-its, pens, flipchart paper.

Method

1 Give each woman three or four post-it stickers and ask them to write down any vaginal infection or gynaecological infections they have had. Stress that information will be anonymous.

2 Stick post-its on the flipchart and read them out to the group.

3 Brainstorm possible remedies that women have used for vaginal infections.

4 Discuss, using the information sheet for back-up information.

Discussion points

- How many different types of infection are there?

- Are they very common – have nearly all women had them or not?

- Do women use Latin names or common names? How familiar are women with Latin names when doctors use them?

- Have many women in the group used self-help remedies? Have they worked?

- Do women go to the doctor with vaginal infections or do they ignore them?

*ACTIVITY *10.5*

Common gynaecological problems – sharing experiences

Aims

- To discuss common experiences and difficulties, and positive ways to deal with them.

- To explore feelings women may have about going to a doctor with gynaecological problems.

Materials

A copy of Worksheet 10.5 *Common gynaecological problems – sharing experiences* for each woman; pens.

Method

1 Ask women to read and fill in the worksheet individually.

2 As a whole group, go through each question and share experiences.

Discussion points

- Where do you draw the line between attempting to treat something yourself, ignoring it or seeking medical help?

- How can you ensure that you are getting the information you want from your doctor?

- Why are women sometimes reluctant to go to their doctor?

- What kind of services would women ideally like? What is available locally?

WORKSHEET *10.5*

Common gynaecological problems – sharing experiences

1 If you have a vaginal infection or gynaecological problem do you:

- leave it for weeks and hope it will disappear;
- go straight to the doctor;
- try to treat it yourself and then go to the doctor if there is no improvement; or
- something else?

2 Generally, when you see a doctor about a gynaecological problem do you:

- clearly explain your symptoms (when they appeared, etc);
- mumble in embarrassment that there's something wrong down there, and leave the rest up to her/him;
- find out as much as you can before you go so you can understand more when you see her/him;
- make a list of questions to ask;
- take someone with you to give support and ask questions;
- something else?

3 Generally, when you see a doctor about a gynaecological problem have you found that they:

- write a prescription and tell you you've got '. . .', which you can't pronounce and don't understand what it is or how it's caused;
- explain clearly what it is and how it's cured;
- discuss prevention; or
- something else?

4 When you have an internal examination do you:

- understand what's being done;
- feel relaxed and comfortable;
- feel tense, but cope;

▷

▷ 10.5 cont.

- find it totally traumatic; or

- something else?

5 Have you ever delayed going for treatment because you did not want an internal examination or felt frightened of the doctor or what s/he was going to tell you?

6 Have you had to inform your partner about vaginal infections? Did s/he also need to be treated? Was it easy to talk about?

7 What response did you get?

- understanding and co-operation;

- accusations that you must have caught it from someone else;

- refusal to co-operate; or

- something else?

RESOURCES

For contact details of distributors and organisations listed here, see the list of organisations in Chapter 11 *General resources*.

Publications

Butterworth, Jane, *Thrush: the Yeast Infection you can Beat* (1991), Thorsons, £3.99. Broad coverage of the topic. Covers dealing with stress, complementary treatments, diet, clothing and more.

Chaitow, Leon, *Candida Albicans: Could Yeast be your Problem?* Thorsons, £3.99. Revised edition provides a non-drug approach to the treatment of candida.

Clayton, Caroline, *Coping with Thrush* (c1984, 1989), Sheldon, £2.95. An easy-to-read, thorough introduction.

Gillespie, Larrian and Blakeslee, Sandra, *You Don't Have to Live with Cystitis: How to Avoid it – What to do About it* (1988), Century, £3.95. Covers cystitis in general and as it relates to ageing, pregnancy, the menopause, cancer and heredity.

Hayman, Suzie, *Endometriosis* (1991), Penguin, £5.99. A clear guide to the subject. Includes groups and a book list.

Hawkridge, Caroline, *Understanding Endometriosis* (1989), Optima, £5.99. Clear guide to all issues. Includes resources. Recommended by the National Endometriosis Society.

Jacobs, Gill, *Candida Albicans: Yeast and Your Health* (1990), Optima, £5.99. Candida and ME – case histories and suggestions for self-help.

Kilmartin, Angela, *Understanding Cystitis* (1989), Arrow, £4.99. Clear, thorough guide to all the issues related to cystitis.

Kilmartin, Angela, *Sexual Cystitis* (1988), Arrow, £3.99. Specific attention paid to the sexual causes of cystitis. Covers psychological issues and includes practical suggestions.

Kilmartin, Angela, *Victims of Thrush and Cystitis* (1986), Arrow, £2.95. Accessible, includes information on self-help, alternative treatments and prevention.

McCutcheon, Ralph, *Diets to Help Cystitis* (1988), Thorsons, £2.99. Brief guide to cystitis and its control through diet and other treatments.

Valins, Linda, *Vaginismus: Understanding and Overcoming the Blocks to Intercourse*, (1988), Ashgrove Press, £7.99. Available from Ashgrove Distribution. A practical guide offering an understanding and resolution of vaginismus, and suggestions for confronting and resolving any emotional problem, free from shame and ridicule.

Women's Health leaflets, including: *Fibroids, How to Cope with Thrush, Pelvic Inflammatory Disease* (40p each). For individual orders, please send a stamped s.a.e.

Video

The Gynaecological Examination – What Happens? (1989), 15 minutes, Brook Advisory Centres, £40.00. Available from Healthcare Productions Ltd.
Aims to encourage women to have regular gynaecological check-ups. Women from different cultures discuss their experiences and worries and the full examination and cervical smear test are demonstrated. Available in six languages: English, Hindi, Bengali, Chinese, Turkish and Greek, and features women from these cultures.

Organisations

Endometriosis Society
Provides support and information. Produces publications.

Hysterectomy Support Network
Provides information and support for those planning to or who have had hysterectomies. Helpline.

Pelvic Inflammatory Disease Network
c/o Women's Health. Produces twice yearly newsletter.

Resolve
A vaginismus support group.

Premenstrual syndrome

BACKGROUND INFORMATION

- PMS can be a confusing topic as there are different theories about its cause as well as doubt as to whether it is actually real.

- It is important for women to be aware of and understand their own specific cycles and the accompanying changes.

- Both social attitudes and personal experience affect how women view these changes. Fifty years ago in this country PMS was not heard of. Has the incidence changed since then or has it become visible because women have discussed and validated their experiences, and found common patterns?

- There is a wide range of symptoms of PMS, including: anger, anxiety, headaches, painful or tender breasts, food cravings, forgetfulness and cramps.

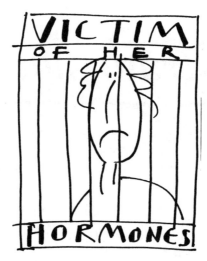

- There are many self-help remedies for PMS, which are often seen as preferable to prescriptions. (See Information Sheet 10.6 *PMS and self-help*.)

PRACTICAL POINTS

- There may be women in the group who do not experience PMS, for example they may have had early hysterectomies.

- The group can be used as a resource for self-help ideas.

- Women may start to compete for who has the worst PMS – this is to be avoided. Small group or paired discussion may help keep a balance between positive and negative aspects to PMS.

- PMS can be a 'catch-all' phrase and there may be other reasons why women feel the way they do.

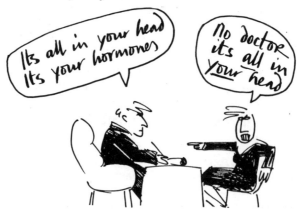

INFORMATION SHEET *10.5*

Premenstrual syndrome (PMS)

Premenstrual syndrome is a term which describes a variety of physical and emotional changes causing problems before a period, but absent during the rest of the cycle. The most commonly experienced feelings are of tension or depression. It is sometimes known as premenstrual tension (PMT).

For many women these changes may be mild and unproblematic; for others, they may lead to discomfort and suffering, frequently affecting relationships with their families, friends, work and other areas of their lives. Some of the more common symptoms include tiredness, irritability, weepiness, clumsiness, sore and swollen breasts, bloatedness, hunger (particularly for sweet things), changes in taste buds and breath, backache.

There are many theories about the causes of PMS. The table that follows shows some of the most common. Each interpretation has specific implications for the way PMS is tackled.

View	Implications
1 It does not exist. This is the view that women are neurotic or more recently that women have these kind of symptoms on and off all the time.	PMS can be dismissed, and women blamed for making such a fuss.
2 PMS is purely psychological and cultural – it is related to our feelings and attitudes towards menstruation.	This implies that a woman's experience of menstruation is culturally defined in any society, and undermines the hormonal basis which can cause physical and psychological changes.
3 PMS is the result of hormonal imbalances and changes. Some go further and claim it is a hormonal disease, to be diagnosed and treated.	If PMS is diagnosed and treated as a hormonal disease, medication, usually hormones, will be given, with little regard to other factors in the woman's life. Often women are presented as being 'ill' every month, and are seen as victims of their hormones.

▷

▷ 10.5 cont.

View	Implications
4 PMS is a result of a nutritional deficiency, making women susceptible to normal, cyclical hormonal changes.	Viewing PMS as a result of nutritional deficiencies implies that a large part of the treatment required is dietary supplements, e.g. vitamin B6 and zinc.
5 Women's cycles put women more closely in touch with their bodies and feelings, and what women experience during PMS are feelings they are unable to express during the rest of the month.	This implies that the *whole* of a woman's life, and her outlets for expressing her feelings and emotions, need to be acknowledged.

PMS may be caused by a combination of the above factors. This is why it is important for women to become more familiar with their own cycles. It is easier then to assess for oneself which symptoms appear to be clustered around the time of our periods and define for ourselves our own experience of PMS. Keeping a menstrual calendar to note changes can be useful in this respect.

There are numerous medical treatments for PMS. These come in the form of hormones, diuretics (water retention tablets) and pain killers. Some women are reluctant to take medication every month, and are also wary of the possible side-effects of certain drugs.

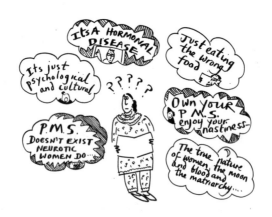

INFORMATION SHEET *10.6*

PMS and self-help

The views expressed here are those of the authors, and do not necessarily reflect the views and policies of the HEA.

Some practitioners identify four different types of premenstrual syndrome. Some women experience changes which don't fit into just one type. But if you do recognise *your* particular 'type' of PMS here, the following self-help ideas could help.

Homeopathic remedies work by giving you a small dose of the symptom you are trying to reduce (a bit like a vaccination). Remedies should match your symptoms, your physical features (colouring, weight etc.) and your personality. It's advisable to talk to a trained homeopath or a doctor who knows about homeopathic medicine before taking homeopathic treatments, because homeopathic medicine is *holistic* and treats you as a whole person, not as a set of symptoms. The following is only a very rough guide.

Type A PMS: Anxiety

Main symptoms: tension, anxiety, mood swings. It commonly begins about one week before bleeding.

Nutrition: basic healthy eating throughout the month. B complex vitamins. Minerals, especially magnesium and zinc. Evening primrose oil.

Other self-help: any form of moderate exercise, relaxation.

Homeopathic remedies: sulphur, nux vomica, aresnicum album. These three remedies are particularly recommended for reducing anxiety.

Type B PMS: Depression

Main symptoms: confusion, depression, possibly suicidal. It often occurs with or after anxiety. It's usually most intense just before your period.

Nutrition: basic healthy eating throughout the month. B complex vitamins. Magnesium, zinc and Optivite. Evening primrose oil.

Other self-help: any form of moderate exercise, relaxation.

Homeopathic remedies: sepia, ignatia. Sepia is also recommended for bringing on a delayed period.

▷

© Health Education Authority, 1993

▷ 10.6 cont.

Type C PMS: Carbohydrate cravings

Main symptoms: appetite increases two weeks before bleeding. Food cravings, especially for sweet foods. Headaches.

Nutrition: It's essential to stabilise the blood sugar. This is done by cutting out sugary foods all month and eating regularly, preferably small amounts every three hours. B complex vitamins. Try to cut out alcohol.

Other self-help: any form of moderate exercise, relaxation.

Homeopathic remedies: calcarea carbonica is recommended for reducing excessive appetite and breast tenderness. Ferrum phosphoricum can also stabilise appetite. Kalium bichromicum is recommended for curing migraine.

Type D PMS: Bloatedness and weight gain

Main symptoms: weight gain, feeling bloated, sore breasts.

Nutrition: basic healthy eating throughout the month. Avoid salt during PMS phase, and reduce saturated fats. B complex vitamins, vitamin E. Magnesium and potassium. Evening primrose oil.

Other self-help: any form of moderate exercise, relaxation.

Homeopathic remedies: calcarea carbonica is recommended for reducing breast tenderness.

Source: adapted from *Female Cycles* (1991), Ealing Health Authority.

ACTIVITY *10.6*

Premenstrual syndrome

Aims

- To explore the range of symptoms which could be included as part of PMS.

- To share the ways women have developed to cope with PMS through their own experiences.

Materials

A copy of Worksheet 10.6 *Premenstrual syndrome* for each woman; flipchart paper, pens, Information Sheet 10.5 *Premenstrual syndrome*.

Method

1 Ask women to fill in the worksheet.

2 Discuss in the large group and flipchart the main points. It may be useful to refer to the information sheet for information.

Discussion points

- There is a lot of overlap between physical and emotional symptoms.

- Some women do not experience any particularly negative symptoms and therefore do not suffer from PMS.

- Women often have the attitude that PMS is something they must grin and bear alone. How useful is it to be more open and share problems and ways of coping together with other women?

ACTIVITY *10.7*

Periods and PMS – sorting out the issues

Aim

- To think about the wider, more controversial issues related to periods and PMS.

Materials

A copy of Worksheet 10.7 *Periods and PMS – sorting out the issues* for each woman; flipchart paper, pens.

Method

1 Divide into small groups and ask each group to select one or more of the case studies on the worksheet, for discussion.

2 In the large group, feed back some of the main issues raised, and discuss.

Discussion points

These are included on the worksheet.

ACTIVITY *10.8*

Logging your PMS

Aim

● To help women develop awareness of their own cycle and the accompanying changes.

Materials

Copies of Worksheet 10.8 *Logging your PMS* and Information Sheet 10.6 *PMS and self-help* for each woman.

Method

1 This activity extends over a six-week period.

2 Explain the worksheet, and identify symbols that they could use to record different aspects of their cycles – it's important to log both good and bad feelings. Give the women copies of the information sheet. Ask them to fill in the chart over a six-week period.

3 After six weeks, women share their charts, noting emerging patterns.

Discussion points

● Did women manage to complete the task?

● Do group patterns emerge as well as personal patterns?

● Can any women identify with the four types of PMS on the information sheet?

● Can the information gained be useful in predicting the onset of PMS?

Source: *Female Cycles* (1991), Ealing Health Authority.

WORKSHEET *10.6*

Premenstrual syndrome

1 How do you feel before your period? (These feelings can be both positive and negative).

	Physical	Emotional
Positive		
Negative		

2 What effect does PMS have on:

your work

relationships with your:

partner

children

friends

others

Have you found any ways of dealing with any of these?

WORKSHEET *10.7*

Periods and PMS — sorting out the issues

CASE STUDY A

Margaret is standing trial for attempted murder of her husband. In her defence she claims she suffers from severe PMS and it was at this time of the month the attack took place.

Brenda appears in court for child battering. She claims that she is fine for most of the month, and it's just before her periods she cannot contain her frustration and lets it out on the kids.

DISCUSSION POINTS

- Statistics show that women are more likely to commit crimes, have accidents, hurt their children, and commit suicide when they have PMS.
- Does this evidence surprise you?
- What are the implications for using PMS as an excuse or defence?
- Does using PMS as an excuse take into account some of the other reasons why Margaret may attack her husband or Brenda batter her children?
- What do you think of the view that some women are victims of their hormones and have little control over what they do when their hormones are imbalanced?

CASE STUDY B

When **Penny** loses her temper the week before her period, her husband will seem very understanding. 'I know you can't help it dear, it's this PMS business'. However, he doesn't take any other feelings seriously during that week. And whenever she's irritable or upset the rest of the month he sighs and asks 'Now when's your period due, dear?'

DISCUSSION POINTS

- How do we get real support for suffering from PMS, without everything being blamed on periods or being a woman?
- What is the best way to get people around us to understand how we feel before/during periods?

▷

▷ 10.7 cont.

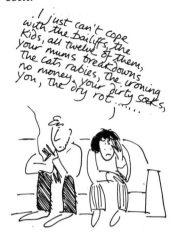

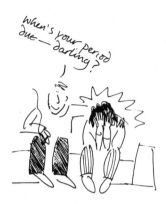

CASE STUDY C

Janet suffers from severe menstrual cramps. She often has to take one or two days off from work each month. Recently her supervisor has started to comment on this.

Sally works in a laboratory. She has noticed that about a week before her period is due she drops slides more frequently and makes more errors. She wants to be out of the lab on these days, possibly to work in the library.

Marlene's child suffers from severe asthma. She frequently has to miss work because of this. She's got a sympathetic woman supervisor, and often uses the excuse that she's got period problems.

DISCUSSION POINTS

- Should 'women's problems' such as PMS and the menopause be placed in the same category as other health and safety issues, e.g. maternity rights and leave, and negotiations made accordingly?
- By highlighting issues such as PMS, do we increase men's awareness of women's health issues, or do we give employers more ammunition to see women as unreliable employees and risk losing gains made in the fight for equal rights at work?
- Do demands that women's specific health needs be taken seriously give fuel to the argument that women are the weaker sex?

WORKSHEET *10.8*

Logging your PMS

	1	2	3	4	5	6	7	8	9	10	11	12	13	14	15	16	17	18	19	20	21	22	23	24	25	26	27	28	29	30	31
Month 1	P	P	P				OK	OK																H				B	I	B	I	I
Month 2	I	P	P	P	P	P																									
Month 3																															
Month 4																															
Month 5																															
Month 6																															

Continue to fill the chart in using symbols. Above, the following have been used:

H = headaches **B** = feeling bloated **I** = feeling irritable **OK** = feeling OK **P** = period, bleeding

©Ealing Health Authority, 1991.

RESOURCES

For contact details of distributors and organisations listed here, see Chapter 11 *General resources*.

Publications

Carpenter, Moira, *Curing PMT the Drug-free Way* (1986), Century, £2.95.
Detailed information on a range of alternative approaches to dealing with PMT including diet, vitamins, homeopathy, herbal remedies and stress reduction.

Dalton, Katherina, *Once a Month* (1991), Fontana, £4.99.
Revised and expanded edition of a guide which covers all aspects of PMS. Favours progesterone therapy.

Dalton, Katherina, *Premenstrual Syndrome Illustrated* (1990), Peter Andrew Publishing Co, £5.95, ISBN 0 946796 41 6.
Draws on the author's 40 years of experience, study and treatment of PMS. The illness and its treatment is explained in an easy-to-follow guide illustrated by a series of cartoons, making it informative and entertaining.

Harrison, Michelle, *Self Help for PMS: Escape from the Prison of Premenstrual Tension* (1987), MacDonald, £7.99.
Covers medical and self-help remedies.

Stewart, Maryon, *Beat PMT Through Diet: the Women's Nutritional Advisory Service Programme Based on Medically Proven Treatment* (1990), Ebury, £6.99.
Very useful, detailed guide. Includes recipes.

Wilson, Robert, *Pre-menstrual Syndrome: Diet Against it: Your Complete Self-help Plan* (1989), Foulsham, £4.99.
Looks at effects of various drugs and harmful additives, gives dietary advice.

Cancer

BACKGROUND INFORMATION

- Women's health courses are an ideal place for talking about cancer. This is especially so once a group is established and has looked at other topics where some of the issues may come up (e.g. self-image, sexual health, food and diet, mental health, older women's health, the NHS, complementary medicine). We can draw once again on the strength of sharing experiences which all women have, whether it is knowing someone who has cancer or having had cancer or fear of cancer oneself.

• While this section looks particularly at screening and early diagnosis, there is scope within the activities for considering wider political issues around cancer, and for acknowledging painful areas like loss, bereavement and our own mortality. Cancer education is a very good focus for exploring feelings of fear, loss and grief.

• The activities facilitate discussion around how much cancer prevention is our responsibility as individuals, and how much it appears to be beyond our immediate control. On the one hand being aware of body changes in general, knowing what to look for, and availing yourself of measures for early detection will enable better treatment choices plus quality of life and survival chances. But within women's groups, stories will be recounted of individuals who took up screening facilities, ate a healthy diet, didn't smoke and didn't drink – yet still got cancer. Women may also feel helpless over the extent to which we as individuals have control over our environment, the food we eat, our working conditions and so on.

• Information on cancers is constantly changing. Medical advancements and opinion move forward. You will need to supplement the information in this section with up-to-date information; the *Resources* at the end of the section will help with this.

PRACTICAL POINTS

• It is important for tutors to think about their own feelings and attitudes to cancer before leading a session. You could look through Worksheet 10.9 *What cancer means to me*, and consider your responses carefully.

• Only deal with the topic of cancer if women in the group have chosen to do it and are prepared for it. Sometimes women who come to every other session on a course do not come to the one on cancer. Tell the group that information will be available for anyone who missed the session.

• Avoid dealing with the topic of cancer early on in a course. Give members of the group a chance to get to know each other so that trust may build up.

• It may be useful to do Activity 10.9 *Feelings about cancer* at the end of the session which comes before the one on cancer. You will then have an idea of the fears of your particular group, and will be better placed to produce a sensitive programme.

• Leading sessions on cancer can be difficult and distressing because of the fears and emotions which can be aroused. Women themselves may have been affected by cancer, or people close to them may have cancer. Some women may want to talk about their experiences, others may not.

- It can be valuable to begin a session by discussing feelings about cancer. This can provide an opening for women who have had a personal experience of cancer to talk about this if they want to. There should be no pressure on any woman to open up.

- Don't assume that women are just at risk of 'women's' cancers such as breast and cervical cancer. Women are also affected by skin, lung, stomach, bowel and other cancers.

- A session on cancer may need a strong information element. Information on cancer is constantly being updated. You may find it helpful to contact your local Health Promotion Unit for the latest information on issues such as cervical cancer screening, breast awareness, and breast screening. Some HPUs have specific Breast Screening Health Promotion Officers who might be available to talk to your group. Many HPUs will have up-to-date leaflets on aspects of cancer even if they do not have a specific person who can help you.

- If appropriate, encourage the group to explore feelings around loss, grief, bereavement and mortality. But it will be better to end a session on a positive note, e.g. by looking at possibilities for prevention and how women can get the quality of services they want to minimise risks.

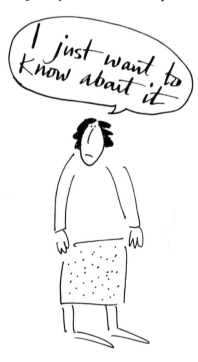

INFORMATION SHEET *10.7*

What is cancer? 1

What is cancer?

Cancer is a general term for more than 200 different types. Cancers occur when there is uncontrolled growth of a group of cells in some part of the body. These new cells don't function properly as part of the organ in which they originate but continue to grow using up oxygen and nutrients and taking up more room. The cells may invade nearby parts of the body, stopping them from functioning properly. Because our bodies are made up of many different types of cells there are many different forms of cancer which grow and spread at different rates. How serious the cancer is depends on the type of cells that are affected, how quickly the abnormal cells are multiplying and how soon the cancer cells spread to other parts of the body.

What causes cancer?

Some substances can be very clearly linked to the development of some cancers, for example 81% of lung cancers are caused by smoking; smoking is also linked to increased risk of cancer of the pancreas, cervix, lip and kidney; some chemical dyes are linked to bladder cancer; and strong sunlight to skin cancer. Such cancer-causing agents are called carcinogens. With the increase in the number of women smokers since the Second World War, the incidence of lung cancer in women is approaching that of men. Other substances may be suspected of causing cancer without any definite evidence being available, for example, some food additives and some hormones. Other factors thought to be involved include diets high in animal fat, exposure to radiation, familial links in some forms of cancer, for example, breast cancer. Comparatively little money is spent on researching environmental causes of cancer and there is much disagreement amongst the 'experts' as to their relative importance. Some forms of cancer are far more common in the UK than others, for example, breast cancer and lung cancer are far more common than leukaemia. The rates of different cancers vary between countries.

Why is cancer dangerous?

Cancer is dangerous when it prevents your body from carrying out essential tasks e.g. lung cancer preventing you from breathing properly, or liver cancer preventing breakdown of waste materials. Tumours may also press against organs

▷

© Health Education Authority, 1993

▷ 10.7 cont.

preventing them from functioning or, as they grow, may erode important blood vessels leading to bleeding. Advanced cancers may divert the body's nutrients away from muscles and organs. Depending on where the cancer is it may or may not be painful, for example, cancer involving the liver is not always painful, whereas cancer involving bones is often very painful.

How does cancer spread?

The initial growth of cancer in the body is called the 'primary' cancer. When cancer spreads to other parts of the body this is known as secondary spread or metastases e.g. primary breast cancer may lead to secondaries in the liver. Spread occurs when some cancer cells break off from the original tumour and travel through the bloodstream to another part of the body. The lymph system, which drains fluid from the tissues, can also carry cancer cells elsewhere.

How is cancer detected?

Cancer is often detected after investigations of persistent symptoms e.g. difficulty in swallowing, a persistent cough, difficulty in passing urine, pain etc. Other cancers may be detected through noticing lumps or swelling e.g. in breast cancer and cancers affecting lymph glands. Changes in the texture or colour of skin may be a sign of cancer. If cancer is suspected, different techniques are used to confirm the diagnosis including X-rays, whole body scans, biopsies (where a small amount of tissue is removed and examined), blood tests and various other medical examinations. Early detection is believed to improve chances of successful treatment in many cases e.g. in cervical cancer. Regular cervical screening, offered to all women of 20-64 years, could significantly reduce deaths from cervical cancer. Early detection of breast cancer can improve the potential for successful treatment. Being 'breast aware' (i.e. knowing what is normal for yourself) and noting any changes and seeking medical advice can only be helpful. The use of mammography (X-rays of the breast) has been shown to be of benefit for women over 50 (but not of benefit, to date, in women under 50).

Can cancer be prevented?

It is currently believed that up to 85% of cancers may be preventable. The prevention of cancer is often confused with early detection of cancer e.g. by cervical screening and breast self-examination, but screening is not prevention. More research needs to be done into environmental causes of cancer such as pollution. Individuals can take steps to reduce their own risks to some extent, for example, by cutting down on tobacco and alcohol and changing their diets. Every possible way should be found to reduce occupational hazards.

▷

▷ 10.7 cont.

Treatment of cancer

Orthodox medicine uses surgery, radiotherapy (X-rays) and chemotherapy (drugs) to treat cancer. A combination of these approaches may be used. These treatments may also be used to control cancer that cannot be successfully treated in order to relieve symptoms.

Complementary approaches to cancer treatment are often aimed at improving the body's own defences and promoting self-healing mechanisms. A holistic approach involves looking at the whole person and may include several approaches e.g. changes in diet, psychotherapy and homeopathy.

INFORMATION SHEET *10.8*

What is cancer? 2

Cancer occurs when some of the cells in our bodies become abnormal and act in an uncontrolled way. To understand how this happens, it helps to know how cells work normally.

Each of us starts life when one cell, the egg cell, or *ovum*, is fertilised by the male sperm and begins to develop in the womb. The ovum then divides millions of times. Soon, groups of cells change their shape and do highly specialised jobs to make bones, muscles, nerves and all the different organs and tissues that make up a human being. After we are born, the cells go on dividing rapidly until we reach our full adult size of at least 10 million million cells. In some parts of the body, such as the brain, the cells then stop dividing altogether. In others this cell division just slows down and replaces any cells that have worn out and died, or that have been damaged in some way.

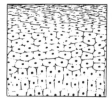

1 Normal cells – there are 10 million in the adult body.

How cells normally work

2 If your cells are damaged for any reason, for example if you cut yourself, it usually isn't long before the cut is completely healed. How does the healing take place?

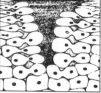

3 Immediately after the skin has been cut and some cells destroyed, the nearby skin cells become very active. Each of these active cells divides into two complete new cells, and these in turn divide and so form new tissue.

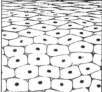

4 Once the cut heals, this process of forming new cells goes back to the steady maintenance routine of replacing the old, dead ones that are constantly being rubbed off the surface of our skin.

When something goes wrong

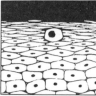

1 Cells are dividing all over the body all the time. They're getting and giving out instructions to carry out normal growth and repair. Usually this system works well. But occasionally the control programme breaks down and something goes wrong in one cell, causing it to get or give the wrong instruction.

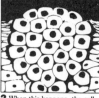

2 When this happens, the cell becomes abnormal, and it starts dividing in an uncontrolled way, forming a group of abnormal cells. These cells don't work properly as part of the organ or tissue where they began. They seem interested only in reproducing themselves, and don't seem to know when to stop. This is called a *primary growth*. As the cells multiply, the growth takes up more and more room. It may invade nearby parts of the body and prevent them from working properly. This is called *local invasion*.

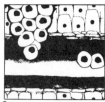

3 Very often, cancer cells will break away and travel, for example through the bloodstream, to *other* parts of the body, where they may settle down and form new colonies of abnormal cells. These colonies are called *secondary growths* or *metastases*. Left unchecked, they too can prevent the organs where they're growing from working properly.

INFORMATION SHEET *10.9*

Reducing risks of cancer

In the UK, one in every three people will develop cancer at some time in their lives. Most of these cases will occur in people over the age of 60. But cancer may take decades to develop, and risks of developing cancer can be reduced by making certain changes in the way we live. Although there is no way of *ensuring* we will not develop cancer, we can *reduce the risk* of developing certain types of cancer.

Smoking

Quit smoking!
- Cigarette smoking causes one third of all cancer deaths.

- Smoking can cause lung cancer (81% of lung cancers are caused by smoking).

- Smoking is also linked to increased risk of cancer of the pancreas, cervix and lip.

Alcohol

Go easy on the alcohol!
- Drinking too much alcohol has been linked to 3% of cancers (of the mouth, larynx, oesophagus and liver).

- If heavy drinkers also smoke, the risk becomes even higher.

Food

Avoid being overweight!

Cut down on fatty foods!

Eat more fibre
- Some cancers are associated with extreme overweight (obesity).

- A diet high in meat, butter and other dairy products may increase the risk of breast cancer, bowel cancer (and coronary heart disease).

- Eating more fruit and vegetables may help reduce the risk of cancer.

- Food containing fibre may actually protect against cancer of the bowel.

▷

▷ 10.9 cont.

Sun

Take care in the sun!

Too much sun may cause skin cancers. Enjoy the sun, but protect your skin, especially during holidays abroad and in hot countries, and avoid burning.

Health and safety at work

Observe health and safety regulations at work!

In the workplace, some 40 chemicals and processes are known to cause cancer. Many have been banned by law. Others are strictly controlled by regulations drawn up by the Health and Safety Executive.

Screening

Have a regular cervical smear test!

- Every 3–5 years for women who are sexually active.

- A smear test can detect abnormal changes in the cells of the cervix (neck of the womb) before cancer has actually developed.

Be breast aware!

- Examine your own breasts regularly and be aware of any changes. Seek medical advice if you notice any changes in your breasts.

- Women aged 50–64 will be invited for screening (mammography) every three years. This X-ray can show up very early changes in breast tissues.

See your doctor if there is any unexplained change in your normal health which lasts for more than two weeks. Most symptoms are unlikely to mean cancer, but see your doctor at once if you notice:

- a lump;

- a change in a skin mole;

- any unusual bleeding;

- a persistent cough;

- a change in bowel habits; or

- unexplained weight loss.

INFORMATION SHEET *10.10*

Cervical cancer screening

Cancer of the cervix can be prevented. The signs that it may develop can be spotted in advance, and it can be stopped before it even gets started. Yet more than 2,000 women in Britain die from cervical cancer every year. Most of these women have never had the simple and quick test that might have saved their lives.

An NHS cervical smear test is now available to all women aged 20–64, at least once every five years.

Pre-cancer signs can develop in women of any age.

- If you have passed the menopause you still need to be tested to check that your cervix is healthy.

- If you have had a hysterectomy or if you have any other doubts about whether you still need to be tested, your doctor will advise you.

- If you are 65 and over you should ask your doctor about how often you need to be screened.

Cervical smear test

This is a test to check the health of your cervix (neck of the womb). For most women it shows that cells are normal and healthy, but for a few women it shows changes in the cells which might develop into cancer if left untreated.

A qualified doctor or nurse will carry out the test. If you prefer a female, ask when you make your appointment. You cannot be tested while you are menstruating, so be sure to get an appointment before or after your period is due. If you use a spermicide or a barrier method of contraception or a lubricant jelly, you should avoid having intercourse for 24 hours before the test as the chemicals may affect the smear.

The test may cause slight discomfort – trying to relax by taking slow, deep breaths, may help. You will be asked to undress from the waist down, and lie on a couch. The doctor or nurse will then gently insert a small instrument called a speculum into your vagina to hold it open. Then a smooth, wooden or plastic spatula will be lightly wiped over the inside to pick up a few cells from your cervix. The cells will then be sent away to be looked at under a microscope.

▷

▷ 10.10 cont.
Results of the test

When you have the test you will be told how, where and approximately when you will get the results. Before you leave the clinic or surgery, make sure that you have been given this information.

If you get asked to come back

- Only very rarely does it mean that you have cancer. It might only be that your sample didn't show up clearly, and another smear is needed.

- It could point to some slight irregularity or an infection that can be treated easily.

- Rarely, it may show abnormal cells which could develop into cancer in the future. In this case, you need further monitoring.

Abnormal cells

Your doctor will explain what needs to be done. You may be asked to come back for more smear tests. If the results still show abnormal cells you may be asked to go into hospital for a closer examination. The treatment of abnormal cells is quite a minor one and if the treatment is done early enough, it almost always leads to a complete cure.

Regular smear tests are important – they pick up the early warning signals that could save your life.

INFORMATION SHEET *10.11*

Cervical screening – terminology

- **Cell**: the smallest unit of the body capable of independent life; hardly ever visible to the naked eye.

- **Cervix**: the neck of the uterus (womb) at the top of your vagina.

- **Os**: entrance to the canal through the cervix, from vagina to uterus.

- **Smear test**: a few flaky cells scraped off the surface of the cervix and examined under the microscope for abnormal changes.

- **Speculum**: a duck-billed instrument to open the vagina and view the cervix.

- **Colposcopy**: examination of the cervix through a colposcope (a specially high powered microscope placed at the entrance to your vagina) which shows up the shape of cells.

- **Dysplasia**: abnormally developing cells.

- **Non-invasive cells**: cancerous cells that have not yet begun to grow inwards.

- **Invasive cells**: cells that are growing inwards, changing normal body tissue into abnormal, cancerous tissue.

- **Pre-cancerous cells**: abnormally shaped cells one stage away from being cancer.

- **CIN**: cervical intraepithelial neoplasia – abnormal cells on or near the cervical canal.

- **Biopsy**: Diagnosis by cutting off a small part of the body that's suspected of being abnormal in some way, and testing it.

- **Punch biopsy**: very small piece of tissue cut out to be tested.

- **Cone biopsy**: removal of part of the cervix (in the shape of a cone) for tests.

- **Laser**: treatment for abnormality using a high-energy beam trained directly onto the abnormal cells to destroy them.

- **Cryocautery**: treatment for abnormality using gas to freeze and destroy tissue.

- **Radiotherapy**: treatment of cancer by X-ray which destroys cancer cells near the surface of the body.

- **Carcinoma**: cancer

- **Carcinoma-in-situ**: cancer which has not yet invaded the underlying tissue.

INFORMATION SHEET *10.12*

NHS breast screening

Why have breast screening?

One in twelve women in the UK develops breast cancer. It is much more common in women over 50. Breast screening can help to find small changes in the breast before there are any other signs or symptoms of cancer. If these changes are found at an early stage, there is a good chance of a successful recovery.

What is breast screening?

Breast screening (mammography) is an X-ray examination of the breasts.

Who is it for?

Free breast screening is being offered by the NHS to all women aged 50 to 64.

If you are under 50, you will not receive an invitation for breast screening. Breast cancer is not so common in your age group, and general screening of women under 50 has not yet proved to be helpful in reducing the number of deaths from cancer. However, if you are ever worried about any breast problem, contact your doctor who will refer you for a specialist opinion if necessary.

If you are 65 or over you will not automatically be invited for screening, but you will be screened if you request it. If you are interested in being screened, talk to your GP or contact your local screening office.

How the service works

All women in the UK aged 50–64 who are registered with a GP receive an invitation to attend a screening centre for a mammography every three years. If you are in this age group, your name will be taken from your GP's list and you will receive an invitation. It is very important that your GP always has your correct name and address. So remember to let your doctor know if you move house.

The breast screening service is being introduced throughout the country. From 1990 all services should have been operational. It will take a full three years to screen all women aged 50–64 for the first time. It may therefore be some time before you get your first invitation. But all women in the age group who are registered with a GP should have received an invitation by the end of 1993.

▷

▷ 10.12 cont.
What happens when you go for breast screening?

The screening centre may be in a hospital or clinic, or it may be a mobile unit. On arrival a nurse or radiographer will explain to you what will happen and will ask you a few questions. Feel free to ask them any questions you may have.

When you are ready and comfortable the radiographer will compress first one and then the other breast between two special plates and take the X-rays. Some women may find the test a bit uncomfortable, but most do not. Try to relax, since the test only lasts a few minutes.

When you have had the mammogram you should be told how and approximately when you will get the results. Make sure you have been given this information before you leave.

After mammography – the results

Most women will receive a normal result and will be automatically recalled in three years' time.

Some women will need to have the test repeated for a technical reason before the results can be given. For example there may have been a problem with the film.

Some women will be called back because the appearance of the X-ray suggests that tissue in the breast needs further investigation. Do not be surprised if you are called back and then told that there's nothing to worry about: most women will be found not to have any problems and will then be recalled in three years' time.

If you are called back, and found to need further specialist treatment, you will be cared for by a team who will be working with you and for you, to ensure that you are given the best care and treatment at all times.

Breast care

You should be alert to any changes in your breast (even if you have had a mammogram), since breast cancer can still develop at any time. If you notice anything which is unusual such as a lump, pain, discharge from the nipple or abnormal appearance or sensation, you should arrange to see your GP as soon as you can.

Further information and support

If you have any questions about the service, ask your GP or contact your local screening office. Your health visitor, district nurse or well-woman clinic should also be able to answer your questions.

INFORMATION SHEET *10.13*

Skin cancer

Too much sun may cause skin cancer (the second most common cancer in the UK). Most skin cancers are completely curable, but some can be fatal. One type of skin cancer is malignant melanoma. Malignant melanoma can show itself by a change in the look of a skin mole.

In the UK melanoma is twice as common in women as men. For women of 15–64 years, it is the fourth most common cancer. The incidence is 10–12 times higher in women with white skin (who have little protective melanin pigment) by comparison with Black women living with the same lifestyle.

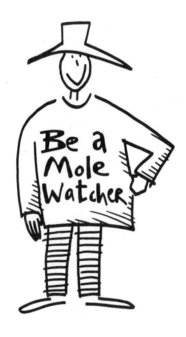

▷

▷ 10.13 cont.

Skin types and sun exposure

Type 1 White skin, never tans, always burns
Type 2 White skin, burns initially, tans with difficulty
Type 3 White skin, tans easily, burns rarely
Type 4 White skin, never burns, always tans, Mediterranean type
Type 5 Brown skin
Type 6 Black skin

Individuals with skin types 1 and 2 are more likely to develop melanoma than those with other skin types.

Melanoma is a prime case for early detection – *"be a mole watcher!"* Most people have some moles on their skin which remain harmless all their lives. However any new, growing or changing moles should be shown to your doctor *straight away*.

If your doctor thinks you have an early malignant melanoma, s/he will refer you to a hospital specialist. At the hospital you will have a careful examination, a photograph and if the specialist thinks it is a possible melanoma, it will be removed by a simple operation carried out under local anaesthetic (often in the outpatients' department). You will be told if further treatment is required.

Protect yourself

- With clothing (wear hats, long-sleeved shirts and skirts/trousers).

- With suncream with the correct sun protection factors (SPF).

*ACTIVITY *10.9*

Feelings about cancer

Aim
- To enable women to share feelings about cancer within a supportive atmosphere.

Materials
Small cards, pens, bag.

Method
1 Give each woman a small card and pen and ask her to write down on the card her biggest fear or other feelings about cancer. Stress that what she writes will be anonymous, though it will be shared among the group.

2 Put the completed cards in bag.

3 Ask women to take a card from bag (replacing it and taking another if she takes her own).

4 Women read out in turn what is on the card.

Discussion points
- Were there similar feelings? Or very different?

- Are there fears for ourselves, as well as fears for those we care about?

- Why do we fear cancer so much?

Note for tutor
This could also be a useful activity for the end of a previous session (where it has been agreed with the group that the next session will be on the subject of cancer). You would not need to discuss there and then the issues that have arisen, but the responses would help you plan a session on cancer based on group needs.

ACTIVITY 10.10

What cancer means to me 1

Aims

- To enable women to begin to share their feelings about and experience of cancer.

- To explore individual responsibility versus factors outside of individual control in relation to cancer prevention.

Materials

A copy of Worksheet 10.9 *What cancer means to me* for each woman; pens, flipchart, markers.

Method

1 Give a copy of worksheet to each woman.

2 Working individually, ask women to underline the statements they agree with (while women are doing this, write the statements on flipchart).

3 Taking each statement, ask women if they agree, and record the number of agreements against each statement.

Discussion points

- Has everyone in the group known someone who has been affected by cancer?

- How many women prefer not to even think about cancer? Why might this be so?

- Why is it so difficult to talk about cancer with someone who has it?

- How much is cancer prevention our individual responsibility, and how much appears beyond our control? What can we do about it?

- What is women's experience of cancer screening?

Note for tutor

Women may wish to share a personal experience of cancer. Question 10 on the worksheet is there so that women feel they may share with the group *if they so wish*. This must be entirely up to individual women.

*ACTIVITY *10.11*

What cancer means to me 2

Aim

- To enable women to begin to share their feelings about and experience of cancer.

Materials

A pile of different kinds of women's magazines, flipchart sheets, glue, scissors, markers.

Method

1 Ask women to spend a minute beginning to think about what cancer means to them. Explain that it might be helpful to portray this in a collage rather than in words.

2 Place the pile of magazines in middle of room and give out flipchart sheets, glue, scissors, markers.

3 Women can work alone, or with others. Ask women to flick through the magazines, cutting out pictures and words which express what they feel about cancer. It may be helpful to do all the cutting out before gluing onto flipchart paper.

4 When women appear to have finished, ask if anyone would like to share what their collage means with the rest of the group.

Discussion points

- Was there a wide range of feelings expressed in different collages?

- Were there similar or very different images portrayed?

- What words had women added to the collage? What did they signify?

Notes for tutor

- Collage can be a powerful medium to work with. Producing a personal collage may bring out intense emotions and feelings, so ensure enough time for the activity to offer women the opportunity to express what they are feeling.

- It may be helpful to participate by making a collage yourself. You can then explain your collage to the group first, if it seems that women are hesitating.

ACTIVITY *10.12*

Knowledge of cancer

Aims
- To find out the group's existing knowledge about cancer generally.
- To promote discussion on the facts about cancer.

Materials
A copy of Worksheet 10.10 *Cancer – true or false?* for each woman; pens.

Method
1 Give a copy of the worksheet to each woman.
2 In pairs, ask women to tick true/false/don't know for each question.

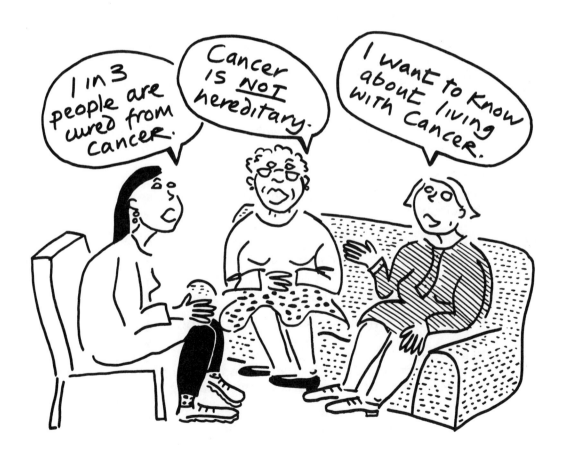

3 In the large group, go through each question and invite responses from the group.

(Tutor: see *'Answers' to* Cancer – true or false? *questionnaire.*)

4 If there are lots of 'don't knows', be prepared to offer information.

Discussion points

- With some questions there is not a straightforward 'true' or 'false' answer. Why might this be so?

- How much of cancer prevention is the individual's responsibility, and how much appears to be outside of our immediate control?

- How can we as individuals act to minimise our risk of cancers?

- Is it possible for us to take on the wider issues? How can we do this?

- What other information do women need?

ACTIVITY *10.13*

Reducing risks of cancer

Aim

- To enable discussion on what women themselves can do to minimise risk of cancer.

Materials

Flipchart and markers; Information Sheet 10.9 *Reducing risks of cancer* for each woman.

Method

1 In the large group, brainstorm all the different ways women can reduce the risk of cancers.

2 Discuss how to go about these.

3 Give out the information sheet and discuss further.

Discussion points

- How can women help each other to stop smoking? Where can they get outside help? What factors affect women smoking?

- Is help available for women to reduce their alcohol intake? What are the wider issues around alcohol consumption?

- What can women do to eat more healthily? What can make healthy eating more difficult?

- What can be done to minimise risk of skin cancer?

- If women are in paid employment outside of the home, are they aware of the health and safety regulations governing their workplace? If women have male sexual partners, do their partners ensure health and safety regulations at work are complied with? What are the implications?

- Do women have regular screening checks? If they do not take up the opportunity, why might this be so?

ACTIVITY *10.14*

Benefits of and barriers to cancer screening

Aims
- To enable discussion on the benefits of, and barriers to, screening for cervical and breast cancer.
- To share ways of overcoming barriers to screening.

Materials
Flipchart and markers.

Method
1 Divide women into small groups, each group with a flipchart with two columns headed 'benefits' and 'barriers'.

2 Ask women to brainstorm all the benefits of screening, and all the barriers.

3 Share responses in the large group.

4 Discuss how to overcome the barriers.

Discussion points
- Benefits of screening could include:

    – prevention of serious disease;
    – saving your life;
    – learning more about your own body;

– helping you feel you are taking more responsibility for your own health;
– helping you feel you are more in control of your life; and
– saving the NHS money.

- Barriers for screening could include fear, lack of time and lack of opportunity:

  – being embarrassed by the test;
  – fear of something being wrong;
  – worry because you haven't been for a while;
  – fear because of lack of information (relevant and in the appropriate language);
  – being unsure if the benefits of screening outweigh the risks of X-ray used in breast screening;
  – fear that you could be judged for being sexually active;
  – the closure of a family planning clinic;
  – no well-woman clinic;
  – an unsympathetic GP;
  – no woman GP available; or
  – facilities not open at a convenient time.

- What can be done to overcome barriers?

- How can we get the kind of screening services that we want at the times that we want?

ACTIVITY *10.15*

Local screening services

Aims

- To share information on local services available for cervical and breast screening.

- To consider the quality of the services offered.

- To look at how services might be improved.

Materials

A copy of Worksheet 10.11 *Local screening services* for each woman; pens, flipchart, markers.

Method

1 Give each woman a copy of worksheet.

2 Individually, or in pairs, women fill in worksheet.

3 In large group, discuss and share experiences and knowledge.

Discussion points

- Have all eligible women had cervical cancer screening? If not, why might this be so?

- Have all eligible women taken up the opportunity for breast screening? If not, why might this be so?

- What did women like about the service offered?

- What didn't women like about the service offered?

- How could services be improved?

- How can women campaign for improved services?

- How can women find out about the range of screening services in their area?

Family Health Service Authority: all GPs now have to produce a practice leaflet which details what services they offer.

District Health Authority: will be able to let you know where screening services are available.

Community Health Council: should have up-to-date information.

Workplace: do facilities exist within the workplace for screening? Would your union help set this up? Can you get time off work for screening?

Other sources of information?

WORKSHEET *10.9*

What cancer means to me

Tick the statements you agree with:

1 I don't even like *thinking* about cancer.

2 I find it difficult to *talk* about cancer with someone who has it.

3 I'd rather not know if I have cancer.

4 It is my responsibility to prevent cancer.

5 Whether or not I get cancer is beyond my control.

6 Screening for breast cancer is a good idea.

7 Screening for cervical cancer is a good idea.

8 I can reduce my risks of getting cancer.

9 Someone I know has been affected by cancer.

10 Personally I have been affected by cancer (tick this only if you feel comfortable about sharing your experience with the rest of the group).

WORKSHEET *10.10*

Cancer – true or false?

1 Cancer is different from all other diseases   TRUE/FALSE/DON'T KNOW

2 The following can increase your risk of cancer:

   – smoking   TRUE/FALSE/DON'T KNOW
   – alcohol   TRUE/FALSE/DON'T KNOW
   – obesity   TRUE/FALSE/DON'T KNOW
   – sun   TRUE/FALSE/DON'T KNOW
   – fatty foods   TRUE/FALSE/DON'T KNOW
   – workplace chemicals   TRUE/FALSE/DON'T KNOW
   – the Pill   TRUE/FALSE/DON'T KNOW
   – some viruses   TRUE/FALSE/DON'T KNOW
   – stress   TRUE/FALSE/DON'T KNOW

3 Cancer is hereditary   TRUE/FALSE/DON'T KNOW

4 Cancer cannot be cured   TRUE/FALSE/DON'T KNOW

5 Cancer is infectious   TRUE/FALSE/DON'T KNOW

6 Cancer can be avoided   TRUE/FALSE/DON'T KNOW

7 Complementary medicine can help
   in the treatment of cancer   TRUE/FALSE/DON'T KNOW

8 Screening can prevent some cancers   TRUE/FALSE/DON'T KNOW

9 85% of cancers may be preventable   TRUE/FALSE/DON'T KNOW

10 25% of all deaths in Britain
    (15–64 years) are from cancer   TRUE/FALSE/DON'T KNOW

11 Approximately 33% of all deaths from
    cancer are caused by smoking   TRUE/FALSE/DON'T KNOW

12 In men aged 15–64, cancer
    accounts for almost 33% of deaths   TRUE/FALSE/DON'T KNOW
    and
    In women aged 15–64, cancer
    accounts for almost 50% of deaths   TRUE/FALSE/DON'T KNOW

'Answers' to Cancer – true or false?

1 Cancer isn't a single disease. It covers a number of different diseases which have different causes, and which can be treated in different ways. Some cancers are incurable at present. Cancer often *feels* different from other diseases. There are now available cures for previously fatal diseases. We are used to modern medicine being able to cure all. Cancer is often perceived to be about suffering and dying. With the advent of AIDS, issues around death are becoming more acceptable to talk about.

2 – Smoking increases your risk of cancer.
  – Too much alcohol appears to increase your risk of cancer.
  – Obesity may increase your risk of cancer.
  – Too much exposure to sunshine may increase your risk of cancer.
  – Fatty foods may increase your risk of cancer.
  – Workplace chemicals may increase your risk of cancer.
  – Taking the contraceptive pill appears to increase your risk of cervical cancer slightly (but other factors such as age of first intercourse, partner's job, use of barrier methods of contraception appear to be more important). But taking the Pill appears to reduce your risk of cancer of the ovaries and womb. It is not clear at present what effect the Pill has on breast cancer.
  – Some viruses appear to increase the risk of cancer. Both the herpes virus (HSP) and the wart virus (WPV) appear to increase the risk of cervical cancer.
  – It has not been proven that stress increases the risk of cancer.

3 Cancer is not hereditary, but some families appear predisposed to certain cancers. There is an increased risk of breast cancer if there is a family history of breast cancer on the maternal side.

4 Over 50% of cancers can be cured.

5 Cancer is not infectious (though in some cases it may be associated with a virus which can be transmitted from one person to another).

6 While it cannot be said that cancer absolutely can be avoided, it is thought that up to 85% of cancers may be preventable, either through individual responsibility or through tackling other causes.

7 Complementary medicine may well have a useful role in the treatment of cancer.

8 Screening cannot *prevent* some cancers. Screening can detect the very early stages of cancer, when quick treatment can lead to complete cure.

9, 10, 11 and 12 – all true.

WORKSHEET *10.11*

Local screening services

Have you had a cervical smear?

- Where did you have it?
- What did you like about the service?
- What didn't you like about the service?

Have you had breast screening?

- Where did you have it?
- What did you like about the service?
- What didn't you like about the service?

What facilities are available locally for cervical screening?

NHS

- GP
- well-women clinic
- family planning clinic
- antenatal clinic
- other

Workplace

Private

What facilities are available locally for breast screening?

NHS

Private

How might you find out about cervical and breast screening facilities in your area?

RESOURCES

For contact details of distributors and organisations listed here, see Chapter 11 *General resources*.

Publications

Butler, Sandra and Rosenblum, Barbara, *Canon in Two Voices* (1991), Spinsters, £9.95.
A collection of essays, journal entries and letters by two women, one of whom has cancer and the other is the partner who survives.

Boston, Sarah, *Disorderly Breasts: a Guide to Breast Cancer, Other Breast Disorders and their Treatments* (1987), Camden, £5.95.
Useful look at a wide range of breast problems, including cancer.

CancerLink, *Complementary Care and Cancer* (1991), free. Available from Cancer-Link.
Aims to help people make choices. Written in question and answer format, the booklet contains a brief outline of the types of complementary care which may be used by people with cancer.

CancerLink, *Directory of Cancer Support and Self Help Groups*, 7th Edition.
Single copies free with large s.a.e., £4.00 for additional copies. Available from CancerLink.

CancerLink, *Life with Cancer* (1990), £2.75. Available from CancerLink.
Deals with the what, how and why of feelings experienced, treatments offered, and physical and psychological changes of cancer. Explains many medical terms in a straightforward way and includes descriptions of radiotherapy and chemo-therapy. Deals with hospitalisation and complementary therapies.

Chomet, Jane and Chomet, Julian, *Smear Tests, Cervical Cancer: its Prevention and Treatment* (1991), Thorsons, £3.99.
A thorough look at abnormal smears and cervical cancer: prevention treatments and control.

Cirket, Cath, *A Woman's Guide to Breast Health* (1989), Thorsons, £4.99, ISBN 0 7225 1790 4.
Aims to empower women with the knowledge and confidence to face the fear and anxiety surrounding breast disease. Explains why and how to look after the breasts, and provides biological and medical information. Argues for a holistic approach and therefore looks at complementary treatments.

Cochrane, John and Szarewski, Anne, *The Breast Book* (1989), Optima, £5.99.
Looks at self-examination, breast-feeding, surgery, the Pill and emotional aspects. FPA approved.

Dawson, Donna, *Women's Cancers: the Treatment Options – Everything you Need to Know* (1990), Piatkus, £8.95.
Looks at main women's cancers and both orthodox and complementary treatment.

Doyal, Lesley et al, *Cancer in Britain: the Politics of Prevention* (1986), Pluto, £8.95.
A study of factors – particularly industrial ones – causing cancer in Britain.

Faulder, Carolyn, *The Women's Cancer Book* (1989), Virago, £5.99.
An excellent general look at the cancers of particular concern to women. Shows how to make informed choices.

Harvey, Judith, Mack, Sue and Woolfson, Julian, *Cervical Cancer and How to Stop Worrying about it* (1988), Faber, £3.95.
A clear guide to abnormal smears and cervical cancer treatment.

Health Education Authority, *Cancer Education* (revised March 1992). Free.
A resource list prepared by the Health Education Authority. Available from the Health Education Authority.

Health Education Authority, *NHS Breast Screening: the Facts* (leaflet), in Bengali, Cantonese, Greek, Gujarati, Punjabi, Hindi, Turkish, Urdu, Vietnamese, English. Available from the Health Education Authority.

Hopkins, L, *I'm Alive* (1991), Changing Places Publications, £5.50, ISBN 0 9517671 0 0.
Lily Hopkins was one of 500 women recalled after a smear test blunder in Liverpool. This is her story of the events of that time, and the consequences for her life, and other women's. A moving account which should be read by all practitioners working with women with abnormal smears.

Kfir, Nira and Slevin, Maurice, *Challenging Cancer: from Chaos to Control* (1991), Routledge, £8.99.
Shows people with cancer how they can stop feeling like victims and regain control over their lives. People with cancer talk.

Kidman, Brenda, *A Gentle Way with Cancer* (1986), Century, £2.95.
Looks at the methods of the Bristol Cancer Help Centre.

Lorde, Audre, *The Cancer Journals* (1985), Sheba, £2.95.
A Black American feminist's response to the loss of her breast. She strongly and movingly challenges both societal and medical thinking and treatment of breast cancer.

Marks, Ronald, *The Sun and your Skin* (1988), MacDonald Optima, £5.99, ISBN 03561 474 01.

Phillips, Angela and Rakusen, Jill (eds), *Our Bodies, Ourselves* (1989), Penguin, £15.99.
Includes very substantial and useful introduction to cancer and women.

Posner, Tina and Vessey, Martin, *Prevention of Cervical Cancer: the Patient's View* (1988), Kings Fund Centre, £6.95.

Based on the first research study to consider the impact on women of positive cervical smears and subsequent investigations.

Quillam, S, *Positive Smear* (1989), Penguin, £3.99.
Expanding on her personal experience, the author details indications of a positive smear, what treatments are available, how you can prevent further positive smears. Emotional issues are also considered.

Shaw, Clare, *Cancer Special Diet Cookbook: Over 100 Recipes to Help Overcome Eating Difficulties and Enjoy a Healthy Diet* (1991), Thorsons, £5.99.

Singer, Froog Albert and Szarewski, Anne, *Cervical Smear Test: What Every Woman Should Know* (1988), Optima, £5.99.
Clear, thorough guide to the topic.

Westgate, Betty, *Coping with Breast Cancer*, Breast Care and Mastectomy Association of Great Britain, £1.25.
Booklet which tells about the association and gives advice, resources and suggestions for exercises.

Womens Nationwide Cancer Control Campaign, *Calling All Women* (leaflet on breast and smear test). Bengali, Cantonese, Hindi, Punjabi, Turkish, Urdu, Vietnamese, English.
Available from Womens Nationwide Cancer Campaign.

Videos and audio tapes

CancerLink – Cancer Information on Cassette, £3. Available from CancerLink.
Raises and answers questions on cancer.

BACUP, *Breaking the Silence on Cancer* (1988), 14 minute video. Available from Concord Films.
Video on how the BACUP information and support service can help people with cancer. Not aimed specifically at women.

Breastscreening Your Questions Answered (in Arabic, Bengali, English (for blind and partially sighted women), Urdu). Price for 1 tape £2.50, bulk buy, price on application. Available from Salford Health Promotion Centre.
These cassettes have been piloted by local women.

The Breast Self-Examination and the Gynaecological Examination (Cantonese with English subtitles), 20 minute video, £35.25 incl VAT and p&p. Available from Health Care Productions Ltd.
Aimed at encouraging Cantonese women of all ages to have cervical smear tests and highlights the importance of breast self-examination.

Cancer – a Patient's View (1985), 21 minute video, Available from Concord Films.
An interview with a young woman doctor who had cancer. She speaks with insight of both the physical and emotional problems.

The Cervical Smear Test (1988), video (Bengali, English, Gujarati, Hindi, Punjabi and Urdu), plus booklet. £20 + VAT. Available from the Leicestershire Health Authority, Health Education Video Unit.
Aimed at Asian women and those health professionals and voluntary workers concerned with improving health care for people from ethnic minorities. It briefly explains what the smear test is and what the results mean. It does not cover causes or prevention.

Down There (1987), 30 minute video, Yorkshire Women video. Purchase £40.00 or hire. Available from Concord Films.
A play about two women who discover they may have cervical cancer.

Looking Good after Breast Surgery (1988), 14 minute video, Breast Care and Mastectomy Association of Great Britain. Available from Concord Films.
Women talk about how they have coped with clothing problems after breast surgery.

Mrs Khan goes for Breastscreening (1992), National Breast screening Programme and Department of Health. (Produced in Urdu and Hindi, dubbed versions in Bengali, English, Gujarati and Punjabi), £35.00 plus VAT. Available from National Breast Screening Programme.
Shows what happens at a breast screening clinic.

Test in Time, 10 minute video, Perspective Photography and Audio Visual, and Women's Nationwide Cancer Control Campaign, £25 plus VAT (or £10 to hire). Available from Women's Nationwide Cancer Control Campaign.
Stresses the importance of cervical smear tests for all women. Shows what happens during the test and if any abnormalities are discovered.

Organisations

Breast Care and Mastectomy Association of Great Britain
For women who have or fear they may have breast cancer, providing emotional support, information and practical advice on prostheses, clothing and swimwear.

Bristol Cancer Help Centre
Complementary holistic approach to cancer, used alongside orthodox medicine. Therapy, support, education, self-help, healing.

British Association of Cancer United Patients (BACUP)
Information service for people with cancer. Newsletter, leaflets, counselling. Helpline.

Cancer Aftercare and Rehabilitation Society (CARE)
National organisation of people with cancer with 47 self-help groups throughout the country. Information, support/counselling, advice.

CancerLink

Information and support for people with cancer, families and professionals. Details of self-help groups nationally. Training, publications.

DES Action

Network of women affected by the drug diethylstilboestrol, given to thousands of pregnant women in Europe and North America between the 1940s and 1960s, causing an increased risk of cervical cancer and other reproductive problems in the offspring of those women.

The Lesbian Network

For lesbians affected by cancer. Support and information for lesbians, their partners, family and friends.

Women's Nationwide Cancer Control Campaign (WNCCC)

Promotes measures for early detection of cancer in women. 24 hour taped phone lines on breast awareness and cervical screening.

Smoking

BACKGROUND INFORMATION

- Some groups may feel that smoking is not an immediate concern for them, or the issue may bring up conflicting feelings for women in the group. They may reject the 'stop smoking' message coming from health professionals, or react with guilt and resentment because of unhelpful stereotypes about what smokers and non-smokers are like as people.

- But some women may welcome the chance to talk about smoking with others, especially if the group is supportive and sympathetic. Tobacco use is an important influence on women's health, both for those who are affected by smoke at home or at work, and for those who themselves smoke. Even if smoking is not discussed as a separate issue, it may be useful to look at tobacco use in the context of other coping strategies which, like drinking too much alcohol, can be harmful.

- Women who are poor or socially isolated are much more likely to smoke, particularly those who are unemployed, or caring for young children on a low income. By 1990, fewer than 3 in 10 adult women were smokers, but women in the poorest social group were twice as likely to smoke as those in the most affluent group. But there is no simple relation between the amount of stress which women describe, and how likely they are to smoke.

- Over the two decades 1972–92 the number of adult women smokers fell by less than half a per cent a year, compared with about one per cent for men. This isn't because women are less successful than men at giving up smoking, but because more young women than young men are taking up smoking.

- Most women who smoke would like to stop, but may feel anxious about how they will cope with their emotions, or that they will put on weight. Women are often denied real power in society, but we are encouraged to put our energy into keeping control over our bodies and feelings. Other influences which may make it difficult to stop smoking include high spending on tobacco promotions, increasingly targeted at women across the world, and low tax increases in some years, so that the price of tobacco falls compared to other items. Smoking in public places has also been largely accepted, although this is now changing rapidly.

PRACTICAL POINTS

- It is helpful for the tutor to acknowledge her own experience of smoking at the start of a general session on smoking, but to emphasise that her role is to encourage sharing of ideas, rather than advise on stopping.

- The word and picture collage Activity 10.16 *Smokers and non-smokers* could be a useful start to the session in breaking down stereotypes.

- Many of the activities in this book could be used for a course to help women stop smoking – particularly those activities focusing on food and healthy eating, self-image, emotional and mental health, dealing with stress, and relaxation and massage. Looking at a range of related issues helps women to understand smoking in context, and acknowledges that women will be at different points in the process of stopping.

INFORMATION SHEET *10.14*

Smoking and health

Cigarette smoke consists of more than 4,000 chemical constituents which may be present as a gas or particle.

The *particles* include nicotine (which causes addiction) and tar (a complex mixture of chemicals, many of which cause cancer).

The *gases* include carbon monoxide, ammonia and acrolein.

Heart disease and stroke

Carbon monoxide and nicotine promote the development of atherosclerosis, or hardening of the arteries. Narrowed arteries may become blocked, leading to:

- difficulty in walking, and possible loss of the limb if the artery is in the leg;
- a heart attack if a coronary artery is blocked; or
- a stroke if the artery is in the brain.

About one in ten deaths from heart disease and stroke among women are related to smoking, more than the number of deaths from smoking-related lung cancer among women. After stopping smoking the level of carbon monoxide in the blood falls to that of non-smokers within a day, and oxygen can be carried more efficiently. Women who stop smoking greatly reduce their risk of heart attack and stroke within a few years. The occurrence of many tiny strokes is related to mental deterioration in old age, so even very elderly women may benefit from stopping smoking.

Use of high-oestrogen contraceptive pills increases the risk of heart disease or stroke in women smokers. None of the contraceptive services recommend pills containing oestrogen for smokers over the age of thirty-five.

Respiratory problems

Irritant and toxic gases in tobacco smoke damage the respiratory system causing:

- destruction of the cilia, the small hairs which sweep debris out of the respiratory system;
- increased production of mucus; and
- damage to the alveoli, the tiny air-sacs which absorb oxygen in the lungs, leading to emphysema.

▷

▷ 10.14 cont.

Eventually the airways become clogged with mucus and debris, oxygen is poorly absorbed, and breathing becomes very difficult. About seven out of ten cases of chronic bronchitis and emphysema among women are caused by smoking. On stopping smoking the cilia usually start to recover within a month or so – many women notice worse coughing for a while when they stop smoking, as the cleaning system starts to work again.

Cancers

The particles of cigarette smoke consist mainly of tar from partly burnt tobacco leaf, which contains many cancer-causing agents such as benzene and nitros-amines. Some of the gases in cigarette smoke and derivatives of nicotine also cause cancer. Chemicals in cigarette smoke damage the immune system too, so that early cancer cells are less likely to be destroyed.

Smoking causes about seven out of ten lung cancers among women. The incidence of lung cancer among women in the UK has increased greatly over the past few decades, particularly for older women, and in some areas has overtaken breast cancer as the most common cancer. Among women, about half of all cancers of the mouth, larynx and oesophagus, and a third of all cancers of the pancreas, bladder and cervix are also related to smoking.

Reproductive health

As well as the link with cervical cancer, smoking affects other parts of the reproductive system. Women smokers may have more difficulty becoming pregnant, and reach menopause two or three years earlier, which increases the risk of osteoporosis. If a pregnant woman smokes, the poisons in cigarette smoke pass through the placenta and affect the baby's heart rate and breathing processes. The baby also grows more slowly, leading to low birth weight and increasing the risk that the baby may die around the time of birth.

Stopping smoking

When a woman stops smoking the level of nicotine in her blood is halved within about a day, although adaptation to being without nicotine goes on for much longer. Some women notice that when they stop smoking their hands and feet are warmer, and their skin feels better as blood flow increases. Many women also feel more relaxed after the first few weeks of stopping.

Although nicotine is called an addictive drug, there is no clear relation between how long or how heavily a woman has smoked and her experience of stopping. For many women, good social support and confidence about stopping may be the best cessation aid.

INFORMATION SHEET *10.15*

Starting and stopping smoking

Why do women start smoking?

- Most women who smoke started before the age of sixteen.

- Smoking is a part of social life for many young people, and may allow young women to feel more confident when forming early sexual relationships.

- Cigarettes may seem to help with frustration or depression, particularly for those who see little chance of a job or further education.

- Young women are very concerned with their weight and appearance, and tend to believe that smoking keeps weight down.

- By 1990, young women from the early teens to the early twenties were slightly more likely to smoke than young men.

Why do women continue to smoke?

- Although smoking can have a very serious effect on a woman's health, having a cigarette can be an understandable response to the pressures of women's lives.

- Women are more likely to be living in poverty through low pay or inadequate benefits, particulary those who are single parents. Cigarettes are often the only item of personal spending.

- Women's roles emphasise caring for others, but smoking is something we feel we can do to fulfil our own needs.

- Many women are isolated by unemployment or lack of affordable childcare and transport. Smoking may feel like a small link with the social world.

- Women usually have little time to themselves, and having a cigarette may be a precious opportunity for a break, even if only a few minutes away from children or a work situation.

- But the relation between smoking and social disadvantage is not simple. Many women who are employers and managers smoke, perhaps because of the pressure of succeeding in largely male occupations.

- African-Caribbean and Asian women often experience the effects of social disadvantage through discrimination and racism, but are less likely to smoke than white women.

$\triangleright$

▷ 10.15 cont.

Stopping smoking

Most women who smoke would like to stop, but may feel anxious about how they will cope with anxiety or depression, or fear that they will become irritable with children or a partner. Like overeating or using tranquillisers, smoking can be used to suppress feelings. Many women also worry about getting fat. Metabolic changes, and perhaps eating more, may result in women putting on weight. This is not a health risk, but worry about weight gain is very discouraging for women smokers who want to stop, in a society obsessed with our shape and size.

Many women find stopping smoking easier than they expected, but some find it a struggle. Most women make several attempts before they stop long-term. Short lasting attempts to stop need not be seen as failures, but as part of a learning process. Stopping smoking may involve learning to relax or socialise without cigarettes, and this takes time. Women often return to smoking because of depression or an emotional crisis – long-term stopping may depend on learning how to cope with these feelings in other ways.

The process of stopping can be seen as a spiral, perhaps going through each stage several times, but with more skills and a better chance of long-term stopping each time.

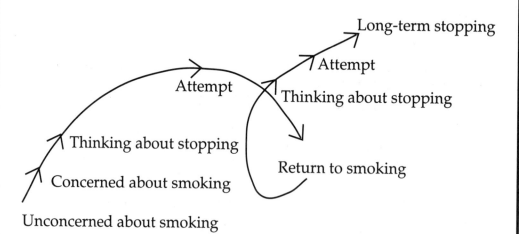

Most women who stop do so without any particular help. The important issues seem to be:

- *Wanting to stop.* Wanting to feel healthier and have more money are important for many women. The great majority of women do feel healthier within a few months of stopping.

▷

▷ 10.15 cont.
- *Planning.* Setting a date for stopping, and thinking about how to cope with difficult times.

- *Getting support.* Most women find it very important to get support from friends, family, a group or a telephone helpline.

Some women have found it useful to see a hypnotist or acupuncturist, although the effect may be short lasting. Nicotine gum, which can now be obtained without prescription, may be helpful for some heavier smokers, especially if social support is also available. New nicotine substitutes are also being developed.

Cutting down rather than giving up is usually difficult, and may have few health benefits, but many women will want to try this as part of the stopping process. The following diagram shows the range of influences on smoking and stopping smoking.

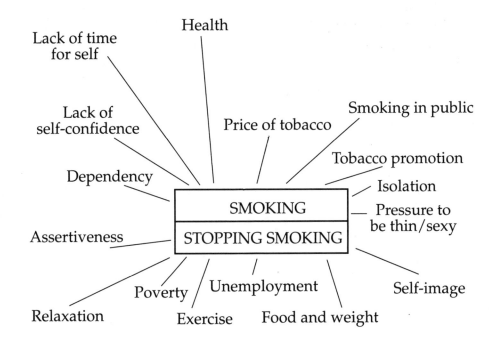

INFORMATION SHEET *10.16*

Other people's smoke

Breathing other people's smoke (passive smoking) can cause a lot of discomfort for non-smokers and sometimes smokers too. A smoky environment can cause headaches, sore throats, nausea, and eye irritation – especially for contact lens users. Passive smoking can bring on symptoms for people with angina and asthma, and regular exposure to tobacco smoke has been linked with serious smoking-related illnesses, such as lung cancer and heart disease, and possibly cervical and other cancers. Passive smoking when a woman is pregnant increases the risk of a low-birth-weight baby, and children growing up in a smoky environment are more likely to get asthma and chest or ear infections.

Over the past few years, many public places and transport services have introduced smoke-free areas. The number of workplaces with a smoking policy also tripled during the 1980s. In the UK the Health and Safety at Work Act 1974 says that it is the duty of employers to do everything that is reasonably practicable to ensure the health, safety and welfare of employees at work. This should include protection from environmental tobacco smoke, but by late 1992 the law had not been fully tested. The article *Smoked out* shows how one health authority dealt with the problem of smoking at work.

▷

▷ 10.16 cont.

Smoked out

Claire Laurent looks at a case arising from Greater Glasgow Health Board's total ban on staff smoking

Health unions have condemned as 'heavy-handed' Greater Glasgow Health Board's ban on staff smoking after a theatre auxiliary claimed it had forced her out of a job.

Mrs Dryden, a smoker for 50 years, who smokes 30 cigarettes a day, handed in her resignation three days after Greater Glasgow Health Board brought in a total staff smoking ban on its premises last July.

She claims that in an eight-hour working day, her half-hour lunch break did not give her sufficient time to change out of her theatre clothes to go outside hospital premises to have a cigarette.

Mrs Dryden, who just lost a claim of constructive dismissal against the health board, explained: 'I wanted to achieve the return to designated areas that smokers could go to. They were only taken away for the staff – patients are still allowed to smoke.'

The RCN spokesperson said that while the college supported no-smoking policies, it felt they should be brought in 'in a supportive way that encourages staff to give up smoking. We do feel that Greater Glasgow Health Board's policy does seem to be severe rather than taking a caring approach.'

NUPE national officer Malcolm Wing said: 'To introduce a ban on smoking and actually drive people out of the hospital or into the toilets to smoke is not the way to deal with a problem. We certainly support the need for designated smoking areas which don't impinge on the rights of non-smokers. We very much support the provision of counselling services for people who smoke and want to give up.'

Mrs Dryden said she had tried hypnosis and acupuncture and had been prescribed Nicorette chewing gum twice in the past to help her give up smoking but had not succeeded.

A spokesman for Greater Glasgow Health Board said that before the ban, introduced in July 1991, there had been designated smoking areas for both staff and patients.

The board decided to introduce a total ban on staff smoking anywhere on its premises because it thought 'it was the correct thing to do' although, he added, 'there were those who thought it was not a good idea.'

Some patients, such as long-stay patients, are still allowed to smoke in designated areas, he said. 'The premise for that was that a long-stay hospital was their home.'

A COHSE spokeswoman said that while the union appreciated the difficulties faced by smokers trying to give up, seeing hospital workers smoking would only encourage patients to do the same.

Nursing Times, February 5, Vol 88, No 6, 1992.
Article reproduced by kind permission of Claire Laurent and *Nursing Times*.

ACTIVITY *10.16*

Smokers and non-smokers

Aims

- To explore ideas about ourselves and other women as smokers and non-smokers.

- To allow feelings about stereotypes to be shared in a safe way.

Materials

A copy of Worksheet 10.12 *Smokers and non-smokers* for each group; flipchart paper, markers, glue, scissors, a selection of magazines, post-its.

Method

1 In small groups, women write words or phrases describing smokers or non-smokers on post-its. Quotes from the worksheet may give some ideas.

2 Using two sheets of flipchart paper, headed 'smokers' and 'non-smokers', the groups draw pictures or symbols, or choose images from the magazines, and make a collage with the words and images.

3 In the large group, allow time to look at the finished collages.

Discussion points

- Are there any ideas which come up on both sheets, for example in relation to confidence or attractiveness?

- How do group members feel about the images and words?

- Where do stereotypes about smokers and non-smokers come from, and does health information create stereotypes too?

ACTIVITY *10.17*

Changing ideas about smoking

Aims

- To look at how social attitudes and smoking habits have changed over time.

- To put personal changes in a social context.

Materials

A copy of Worksheet 10.13 *Changing ideas about smoking* for each woman; post-its, flipchart paper, blutack, pens.

Method

1 Using the worksheet as a prompt, women work in small groups to draw out their own recollections or family stories about smoking in previous times. Do women remember: the first time they saw someone smoking; school lessons on smoking; family smoking habits; the first try of a cigarette; stopping attempts; old cigarette adverts? It's not important to remember exact dates.

2 Write recollections on post-its and stick onto a sheet of flipchart paper in date order, in relation to timing of events on the worksheet.

3 In the large group, share charts. Time and space permitting, the group can make a single line of stickers around the walls of the room to create a group history of smoking.

Discussion points

- What trends have there been? These could relate to social attitudes, advertising methods, smoking in public places, and so on.

- What changes would group members like to see in the next 5, 10 or 20 years? These could be personal changes, or relate to policy or attitudes to smoking.

ACTIVITY *10.18*

Starting and stopping smoking

Aim

- To look at the processes of starting and stopping smoking among women.

Materials

A copy of Information Sheet 10.15 *Starting and stopping smoking* for each group; flipchart, markers.

Method

1 In small groups, read through the information sheet, and discuss the issues raised.

2 Using the diagram at the end of the sheet, try drawing in the way the different factors interconnect, and discuss.

3 In the large group, brainstorm strategies women may use to give up smoking and write these on the flipchart, drawing especially on the experiences of women in the group.

Discussion points

- Why might young women take up smoking?

- Why do women continue to smoke, even when they want to stop?

- How have different women in the group experienced giving up smoking?

- What is the best way to help women stop smoking?

- How does poverty relate to smoking, and is it fair to tax tobacco?

- How do tobacco promotions affect women?

ACTIVITY *10.19*

Other people's smoke

Aim

- To look at the problem of environmental tobacco smoke, and the connection with good working conditions.

Materials

A copy of Information Sheet 10.16 *Other people's smoke* for each woman.

EITHER:

Method

1 Give out the information sheet for women to read.

2 In small groups, discuss smoking in public places and at work.

Discussion points

- What can be done if someone is bothered by smoke at work? What about at home, which is also a workplace for most women?

- Have women ever asked someone not to smoke, or wanted to do so, or have they ever been asked not to smoke? What happened?

- How can smokers/non-smokers reach agreement about smoking in shared spaces?

- In what other ways might smoking affect the environment, locally and across the world?

OR:

Method

1 Give out the information sheet for women to read.

2 Divide into two groups, one a group of smokers, and one non-smokers. Ex-smokers can go in either group, to balance numbers a bit.

3 Ask the 'smokers' group to imagine they are the non-smokers, and 'non-smokers' group to imagine they are smokers. Each group is asked to decide on a fair smoking policy for a hospital (or other workplace if preferred).

4 In the large group, report back on smoking policies developed.

Discussion points

- How might smoke/not being able to smoke affect working life?

- What choices are there for different areas of the hospital (or other workplace)?

- How might the policy affect patients, visitors and staff?

ACTIVITY *10.20*

Making decisions about smoking

Aims

- To look at different women's perspectives on smoking issues.

- To share ideas for resolving problems.

Materials

A copy of Worksheet 10.14 *Decisions about smoking* for each group.

Method

    1 In small groups, choose one or more situations from the worksheet for discussion.

    2 In the large group, report back on the discussion.

Variation: using role-play, one woman takes the main role, and two others present alternative viewpoints, in the role of a friend, colleague or family member. Sometimes it is more interesting for a participant to argue for a point of view opposite to her own.

WORKSHEET *10.12*

Smokers and non-smokers

'Smoking spoils your looks.' (Brooke Shields)

'I'm attracted to the image of a woman with a cigarette. It looks tough and confident.'

'When I've got a difficult meeting the first thing I do is light up.'

'It does not look nice if Bengali women smoke, but if they do that is their decision.'

'A cigarette gives me a ten-minute break.'

'Smokers are more fun, more down to earth.'

'Smokers must be more stressed – when I stopped I was hyper.'

'A lot of the women I know who smoke are rebels. They don't want to be the nice girls they're told to be.'

'I think women smoke to do something with their sense of frustration or fear, to flatten their emotions.'

'Smokers want to be in a gang when you're young, then later you start to enjoy it.'

'When people make a fuss about smoking I think they're drippy.'

'I smoke because I'm addicted. I smoke because I'm a dickhead.'
('Graffiti' from leaflet for young people.)

WORKSHEET *10.13*

Changing ideas about smoking

An occasional history of smoking

1904 New York cop arrests woman for smoking in a car on Fifth Avenue.

1910 President Roosevelt's daughter scolded for smoking in the White House, says she will smoke on the roof.

1928 Amelia Earhart endorses Lucky Strike brand as helping to 'lessen the strain' of her Atlantic flight. (She didn't smoke at all!)

1935 Survey in the USA shows that nearly a third of film heroines smoke, but only one in forty female villains.

1940 Chesterfield Cigarette campaign aimed at women war-workers 'When you're doing a bang-up job, you need a bang-up smoke.'

1950 Sensation throughout the fashion world as Norman Parkinson shows a woman smoking in Vogue magazine.

1955 The woman's cigarette Marlboro ('Mild as May') relaunched as a man's brand.

1962 First major health report *Smoking and Health* from the Royal College of Physicians in the UK.

1976 Virginia Slims brand for women launched onto the British market with the slogan 'We've come a long, long way.'

1980 First major report on smoking and women, *The health consequences of smoking for women: a report of the Surgeon General*, published in the USA.

1981 Prime Minister Margaret Thatcher photographed admiring a John Player Special racing-car.

1982 Martina Navratilova wears the colours of Kim brand for her winning match at Wimbledon.

▷

▷ 10.13 cont.

1986 Health Education Council and ASH launch the campaign booklet *Women and smoking: a handbook for action.*

1988 An American court holds the makers of Chesterfield brand responsible for the death of Rose Cippolone, who died of lung cancer.

1991 Princess Diana, president of the British Lung Foundation, launches No Smoking Day.

1991 Joan Clay, civil servant in the UK, wins a claim for disability benefit, following lung damage caused by others smoking at work.

1992 First International Conference on *Women and Smoking* held in Northern Ireland.

1993 Woman awarded £15,000 damages for ill-health caused by passive smoking at work.

WORKSHEET *10.14*

Decisions about smoking

Choose one or more of the following situations to discuss or role play:

1 An older woman has smoked for a long time and is bothered by chesty colds. Her doctor has suggested attending a stop-smoking group or trying nicotine gum. One of her daughters is pregnant and keen for her mother to stop as soon as possible, but the mother thinks that no group or gum will be much help, and perhaps she's too old for stopping to make any difference.

2 A woman who's newly self-employed has stopped smoking for two weeks, but her period's due, and she's very irritable and shouting at her children. Some of her friends feel it's not a good time for her to stop, but others think her family should give her more support.

3 A young woman who stopped smoking at New Year has put on several pounds and is worrying about how she'll look in summer clothes. Her best friend doesn't know whether to tell her that she's getting fat, but her mother says it doesn't matter what she weighs, as long as she's healthy.

4 A woman who's just started a new job finds that she's smoking more than usual. Some of her non-smoking colleagues want to ask her not to smoke in the office, but others say there's no rule against it, so they're not going to interfere.

5 A woman with two teenage daughters is worried that they're smoking at school, although they say it's only their friends who smoke. Her older daughter feels she hasn't got a problem, as she only smokes a few now and then. Her sister is smoking regularly, and finds she gets breathless at games. She would like to ask for advice.

6 A woman who's unemployed is feeling really fed up with being stuck at home. Her local shop is advertising cheaper cigarettes to 'Beat the budget', and she's thinking about buying in extra. Her partner thinks she's silly because she said she will stop if the price goes up. Her neighbour thinks it's really unfair that poor people get hit hardest by a price rise.

RESOURCES

For contact details of distributors and organisations listed here, see Chapter 11 *General resources*.

Publications

ASH Women and Smoking Group, *Smoke Still Gets in Her Eyes: a Report on Cigarette Advertising in British Women's Magazines* (1990), £1.50 inc. p&p from Action on Smoking and Health (ASH)

ASH Women and Smoking Group, *Teenage Girls and Smoking: a Review of Research and Implications* (1988), £1.50 inc. p&p from Action on Smoking and Health (ASH).

ASH Women and Smoking Group, Reports on *Smoking and Poverty*, and *Smoking in Pregnancy* are due at time of writing, (1992). Enquiries to ASH.

Carr, Allen, *The Easy Way to Stop Smoking* (1987), Penguin, £5.99.
A very popular guide to developing an optimistic attitude to stopping smoking.

Canadian Council on Smoking and Health, *Taking Control: An Action Handbook on Women and Tobacco* (1989), £3. Available from the HEA HELIOS Project, University of the West of England.
A Canadian update of the ASH handbook *Women and Smoking – a Manual for Action*.

Chollat-Traquet, Claire, *Women and Tobacco* (1992) World Health Organisation, Geneva. Available from HMSO.

HEA HELIOS Project, *Smoking Prevention for Minority Ethnic Groups: a Resource Pack* (1992). Funded by the Department of Health and the Health Education Authority. £5 plus postage. Available from HEA Helios Project, University of the West of England.
Presents facts and figures about smoking, and then looks at smoking prevention, giving up smoking, and campaigning. Ideas of possible activities are given, examples of good practice, and information on resources. The pack includes photocopiable handouts in English, Bengali, Gujarati, Chinese, Turkish, Urdu and Punjabi.

Health Education Authority, *Women and Smoking: a Handbook for Action* (1986), £2.00. Available from the Health Education Authority.
Draws together the ideas, experiences and activities of women already involved in action on smoking, and acts as a practical guide for those who wish to become involved.

Jacobson, Bobbie, *Beating the Ladykillers* (1988), Victor Gollancz, £4.95.
A comprehensive discussion of the health and social aspects of smoking for women.

Woodhouse, Kate with Rigg, Elaine, *Quit and Get Fit*, Free. Available from the HEA HELIOS Project, University of the West of England.
Session plans and handouts for a stop-smoking course for women.

Videos

The Ladykillers (1983), 50 minutes, Channel 4. Weekly loan £10; purchase £60 (plus VAT and p&p) from Concord Video and Film Council.
An excellent survey of the pressures on women to smoke at work and at home, and hardly dated. Includes a look at health effects, advertising, and giving up, with a good soundtrack.

Organisations

Action on Smoking and Health (ASH)
A medical charity. Provides an information service, information bulletin, and free packs on smoking in the workplace for employees/employers. ASH has branches throughout England.

HEA HELIOS Project
Aims to support local Health Promotion/Education Units in England in their work against smoking by ensuring a flow of new ideas, and a sharing of good practice. Provides links between national agencies and health workers at a local level. Offers information, advice and resources.

International Network of Women Against Tobacco (INWAT), c/o American Public Health Association.
A group promoting links between women working in smoking control.

QUIT
A charity specialising in smoking cessation. Quitline (071 487 3000), is a national stop-smoking helpline. Usual call charges apply – recorded message outside normal hours.

Drinking

BACKGROUND INFORMATION

- The most commonly used, potentially addictive, substances in Britain are nicotine and alcohol, both of which are legal and socially acceptable drugs. Tranquillisers are more widely used than any other prescribed medicines, and anti-depressants and sleeping pills may also be more often prescribed to women.

- There are many reasons for our use of different substances, some positive and others negative, and often this becomes something we do merely from habit. Terms like dependent or addicted are used to describe people who become either physically or psychologically dependent upon something.

- For many people, their use of tobacco or alcohol is not seen as a problem until or unless they experience obvious health or other difficulties. Sometimes, at this stage, it is difficult for that person to stop smoking or drinking, or to cut down their drinking.

- A common public misconception of drinking is that it is only a problem if you become addicted to it, become an 'alcoholic', which ignores the wide range of social and health problems associated with inappropriate or heavy drinking. To understand why we use certain substances, what risks are associated with their use and what we can do to change this, the following activities take drinking alcohol as an example.

INFORMATION SHEET *10.17*

Women and drinking

Sensible drinking

- There are recommended weekly sensible drinking levels to reduce the risk of harm from drinking alcohol. For women, the recommended limit is up to 14 units of alcohol a week, spread throughout the week, with one or two drink-free days. This limit does not apply to pregnant women.

A unit is:

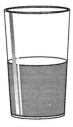   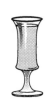 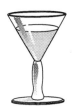

| Half a pint of ordinary beer, lager or cider | A small glass of wine | A measure of spirits | A small glass of sherry | A single measure of aperitif |

- For men, the limit is up to 21 units of alcohol a week.

- The limits are different because women have less body water and are generally smaller than men which means that the alcohol they drink is less diluted in the body. So, drink for drink, women will reach a higher blood alcohol level than men.

- Some alcoholic drinks are extra strong – all bottles and cans now carry % ABV symbol (alcohol by volume) so you can compare the strength. Measures poured at home are usually more generous, so you may be drinking the equivalent of two or three units.

- On average, it takes one hour for the body to get rid of one unit of alcohol.

Effects of alcohol

- Some women find that alcohol affects them differently a few days before their period.

▷

▷ 10.17 cont.

- Alcohol and medicines do not mix – check with your doctor or pharmacist.

- When you drink the alcohol is quickly absorbed into your blood and carried round the body. The health risks from heavy drinking include damage to the liver and brain, stomach disorders, high blood-pressure and strokes. Some cancers, e.g. mouth, throat and liver, are related to heavy drinking.

- Drinking affects your co-ordination and judgement and the risks of having an accident after drinking are high.

- Alcohol is a depressant and can be linked to mental health problems such as anxiety, tension, depression and paranoia.

- The use of alcohol is related to a range of social problems: arguments, the break-up of relationships and families, work difficulties, money problems, child neglect or abuse, vandalism, public disturbance or violence.

Pregnancy

- Alcohol passes from a mother's bloodstream to the baby through the placenta and can affect the baby's development. So cutting down how much you drink before you become pregnant is advisable.

- There is no evidence that light or occasional drinking will affect the baby, so if you limit yourself to one or two drinks once or twice a week there will be little risk. You may choose to stop drinking altogether.

- If you breast-feed, small quantities of alcohol will be passed to the baby in your breast milk. This may affect the baby's feeding, bowels or sleeping. If you have had several drinks it is advisable to allow time for your body to get rid of the alcohol.

Seeking help

- Tips on cutting down: keep one or two drink-free days; choose low alcohol or alcohol-free drinks instead; sip slowly; drink smaller measures; find alternative ways to relax.

- Traditional images of women as carers may conflict with the image of women with drink problems and this can make it harder for some women to seek help.

- Help is available from a range of sources: either ask your GP or look in the telephone book under 'Alcohol'. Alternatively, contact Alcohol Concern or Alcoholics Anonymous (details under *Resources* at the end of this section).

ACTIVITY *10.21*

Why do women drink?

Aim

- To encourage women to look at the way they drink and the many influences on them to drink.

Materials

Flipchart and markers.

Method

1 Introduce the session and its aims. Reassure the group that there is no need for anyone to disclose aspects of their drinking which they do not wish to discuss. Stress that the discussion is confidential.

2 Ask the group to 'brainstorm' reasons why women drink and write on flipchart. A finished list might include –

- Like the taste;
- Because friends drink;
- To relax;
- To quench your thirst;
- To be more confident;
- To help with PMS;
- To help cope with children;
- Because your partner drinks;
- To look sophisticated;
- Because its there, e.g. at parties;
- To celebrate something;
- To 'drown your sorrows';
- To help you to sleep.

3 Try to draw out a balance between 'good' reasons and 'bad' reasons and see if there are any conclusions about the amount drunk, i.e. small quantities of alcohol are most likely to achieve the 'good' effects. Make links with reasons for women's use of other substances such as prescribed or illicit drugs, food, tobacco.

4 Discuss how much women take their own decisions about drinking and how much is determined by other people – for example, women being allocated the 'driver' on occasions when their partners want to drink. How much are women influenced by other people's drinking?

Discussion points

- The excessive use of alcohol can cause more problems than it solves.

- Women's lives are complex and there are many demands made on us but there are *other* ways of coping with these things.

ACTIVITY *10.22*

How much do we drink?

Aim

- To look at how to measure the amount of alcohol in our drinks and to know how much we can drink without risks to our health.

Materials

A copy of Information Sheet 10.17 *Women and drinking* for each woman.

Method

1 Using the information sheet, introduce units of alcohol – stress that the same amount of alcohol is in half-a-pint of ordinary strength beer, a small glass of wine, a glass of sherry or a single spirit (pub measures).

2 Discuss sensible limits and strategies for knowing how much we drink.

Discussion points

- Women are more liable to suffer physical effects from drinking heavily and so limits for women are lower than for men.

- Alcohol can have an increased effect during the premenstrual period for some women and can be dangerous when used in combination with other drugs e.g. tranquillisers and anti-depressants.

- The Pill can slow down the rate at which women absorb alcohol.

- Pregnant women should only drink one or two units of alcohol, once or twice a week or, to be absolutely safe, no alcohol at all.

- Some drinks can have deceptively high alcohol content e.g. strong lager.

ACTIVITY *10.23*

Drinking problems

Aims

- To draw attention to the fact that women are more prone to physical damage from excessive use of alcohol than men.

- To stress that alcohol-related problems may be physical, social or psychological.

Materials

Flipchart paper and markers for each group, copy of Information Sheet 10.17 *Women and drinking* for each woman.

Method

1 Divide into small groups of three or four. Give flipchart paper and pens to each group and ask them to nominate someone to do the drawing/ writing.

2 Ask someone to draw the outline of a body on a piece of flipchart paper.

3 Ask women to make a list – on the paper – of different physical problems relating to different parts of the body, and separate lists for social problems and psychological problems; these can be written around the figure.

4 Report back from each group and make a list on the flipchart. Use the information sheet to check out responses.

Discussion points

- Alcohol problems are not just about physical problems or 'being an alcoholic'; heavy drinking can cause many problems – arguments in the home, links with child abuse, depression etc.

- Even moderate drinking at inappropriate times can lead to problems – drink driving, accidents at work etc.

- You may need to refer to other resources for more details of the effects of alcohol.

ACTIVITY *10.24*

How to cut down

Aims

- To help women decide if they are happy with how much they drink.

- To offer tips and advice for those who would like to cut down.

Materials

A copy of Worksheet 10.15 *Drink diary* for each woman; flipchart, markers.

Method

1 Give a copy of the worksheet to everyone and ask them to fill it in for the last week (this can be given out a week in advance if the group meets regularly). Stress that they do not need to share this information with anyone unless they wish to.

2 When everyone has recorded how much they have drunk in the last week, ask the group to think about ways that they could cut down their drinking if they wanted to. Many women will be happy with their drinking but ask them to put themselves in the place of someone who does want to cut down.

3 Make a list on the flipchart of all the different ways of reducing your drinking.

Discussion points

- It is important to know how much you drink before you can decide whether or not you are risking problems through your drinking.

- There are many different ways to reduce your drinking, depending on your lifestyle and circumstances.

- If someone has a serious drinking problem they may need experienced help. A list of agencies which can offer services is included in the resources at the end of this section.

WORKSHEET *10.15*

Drink diary

	WHAT	WHERE/WHEN/WHO	UNITS	TOTAL
MON				
TUES				
WED				
THURS				
FRI				
SAT				
SUN				
		TOTAL FOR THE WEEK		

RESOURCES

For contact details of distributors and organisations listed below, see the list of organisations in Chapter 11 *General resources.*

Publications

Brown, George W, and Harris, Tirrill, *The Social Origins of Depression: a Study of Psychiatric Disorder in Women* (1990), Routledge, £12.99.
The classic study of depression in women from a sociological perspective.

Camberwell Council on Alcoholism, *Women and Alcohol,* (1980), Tavistock, London.

DAWN, *Women and Drinking* (booklet), £1.00. Available from DAWN.

Health Education Authority, *Women and Drinking* (1992), free.
Booklet providing information on sensible drinking for women.

HMSO, *Women and Alcohol* (1992), £10. Available from HMSO.
Report of a national conference arranged jointly by the Department of Health and the Royal College of General Practitioners.

Kent, Rosemary, *Say When: everything a woman needs to know about alcohol and drinking problems* (1989), Sheldon Press, £4.50. Available from Institute for the Study of Drug Dependence.

McConville, Bridgid, *Women Under the Influence: Alcohol and its Impact* (1991), Grafton, £4.99.

Swallow, Jean (ed), *Out from Under: Sober Dykes and Our Friends* (1983), Spinsters Ink, £7.95. Available from Sisterwrite.
Lesbians and alcoholism; drug dependency; the politics of addiction.

Wilson, Mary, *Living with a Drinker; how to Change Things* (1989), Pandora, £4.99.

Wolfson, Devora and Murray, Jayne (eds), *Women and Dependency: Women's personal accounts of drug and alcohol problems* (1986), £2.50. Available from DAWN.

Videos

Well Being: Name Your Own Poison (1982), 45 minutes, Channel 4.
Looks at a range of addictions.

Women and Alcohol, 35 minutes. Available from Alcohol Counselling Service.

The Mental Health Film Council Information Service produce a catalogue of films. Available from the Mental Health Film Council.

Organisations

Alcoholics Anonymous
Many local groups.

Alcohol Concern
Aims to raise awareness, improve services and promote preventive action at local and national level. Library, leaflets and journal.

Alcohol Counselling and Prevention Services
Offer counselling on a one-to-one basis for problem drinkers, families and friends. Provide a service for lesbian and gay drinkers. Offer a creche service.

DAWN (Drugs, Alcohol, Women Network)
Offers advice and information on drugs and alcohol for women.

GLAAS (Greater London Alcohol Advisory Service)
Provides advice and information on alcohol in the London area.

Institute for the Study of Drug Dependence
Provides advice and information on drugs.

Coronary heart disease

BACKGROUND INFORMATION

- It is a common misconception that heart disease is a man's illness, and many women have got used to thinking that warnings about heart disease do not apply to them. However, figures show that one in four women will die from coronary heart disease (CHD). In 1989 more than 23,000 women died prematurely of heart disease.

- Although CHD is a major killer for women as well as men, the general CHD death rate is actually falling. This is especially true for women aged 35–44. After menopause women lose the protective effects of their hormones and the risk of CHD starts to equal that of men. This is why CHD in women accounts for almost 45% of all CHD deaths.

- There are marked differences in CHD for different groups of people. Asian women have a much higher incidence of CHD than white women; in fact people born in the Indian subcontinent have a 20% higher incidence of CHD than other people. Women born in the Caribbean or African Commonwealth countries have a reduced mortality rate from CHD of 20% to 50% of the rate for women in general.

- Working class people experience a greater incidence of CHD than middle class people. This class difference is greater for women than for men. The British Regional Heart Study found that living in areas of high unemployment, not owning a car and living in council housing were factors closely linked to heart disease. An American study found that women with children, who were doing boring repetitive paid work, as well as unpaid work in the home, were twice as likely to suffer from CHD as women who worked only in their homes.

PRACTICAL POINTS

- If women do not request a specific session on CHD, it can be built in to other topics such as emotional and mental health, stress, or food and healthy eating.

- Tutors may feel they do not have enough medical knowledge to tackle this topic. However, the information sheet provides useful basic information about CHD and ways to help prevent it. The *Resources* suggested offer further sources of information.

INFORMATION SHEET *10.18*

Coronary heart disease

- Coronary heart disease is also known as coronary artery disease and ischaemic heart disease. It is caused by arteries becoming narrowed and roughened by fatty deposits called plaque. These block the flow of blood to the heart and when insufficient blood is reaching the heart, part of the heart dies from lack of oxygen and other nutrients. This is a heart attack.

- There seem to be several individual based risk factors associated with CHD, including:

  - previous family history;
  - gender (men at greater risk than women);
  - age (risk increases with age);
  - smoking;
  - physical inactivity;
  - high blood-pressure;
  - diabetes;
  - excess cholesterol in the blood; and
  - obesity.

- 29% of all deaths in this country are caused by coronary heart disease.

- CHD affects men more than women, because women's hormones may reduce their risk. Levels of these fall after the menopause, so the risk of CHD for women then begins to equal that for men.

- CHD accounts for 1 in 4 deaths for women who are post-menopausal.

- Raised blood-pressure increases the risk of CHD. You may suffer raised blood-pressure without any visible symptoms.

- Blood-pressure usually rises as you get older.

- Although there are things women can do to reduce their risk of CHD, some factors are harder to control – for example home and work environments which may cause stress.

- The Coronary Prevention Group (1986) looked at the very high rates of CHD for Asian people, and concluded that these could not be explained simply by the classic risk factors of smoking, high blood-pressure and high cholesterol. They suggested that poverty, poor working and housing conditions, and unemployment were significant. The extra stress of migration and racism may also be contributory factors. ▷

▷ 10.18 cont.

- If you have had CHD, and have experienced heart attacks, you can still enjoy gentle exercise such as swimming, cycling and walking. It depends how much you feel you can do and what your doctor advises.

Prevention of CHD

Advice about preventing CHD includes: stopping smoking, being more active, changing diet and reducing stress.

Smoking

Smoking increases the pulse rate, raises blood-pressure and cuts down on the amount of oxygen your blood can carry. It also increases the chance of your arteries becoming clogged.

Although fewer women smoke now than in the past, one in five of all deaths from heart disease are thought to be due to smoking – and half of Britain's smokers are women. Girls appear to be smoking more at younger ages than boys. In addition women who smoke and take the Pill have ten times the risk of having a heart attack or stroke than women who do neither of these.

Many women don't want to stop smoking for fear of gaining weight, yet non-smokers weigh only 5lb (2kg) more than smokers, on average. Any large weight gain after stopping smoking is usually only temporary. It has been calculated that on average women need to gain three stone (18kg) in weight before the risk is equivalent to smoking 20 cigarettes a day.

Physical activity

It seems that women, especially younger women, are starting to exercise more. Exercise can help you to relax and helps to prevent CHD by improving circulation, reducing blood-pressure and helping the heart work more effectively. Cycle, swim, jog and dance – do anything you enjoy and that makes you a bit out of breath. Walking is one of the best forms of exercise. Try to exercise two to three times a week for half an hour or more at a time.

Diet

- One in three women in England is thought to be overweight, and at any one time 12% of women are on a slimming diet. The type of diet recommended for prevention of CHD is very similar to slimming diets: less fats, less sugar and salt, and more fibre.

▷

▷ 10.18 cont.

- Weight is related to both diabetes and high blood-pressure which are both risk factors for CHD.

- Cutting down on alcohol can also lower blood-pressure and contribute to weight loss.

Stress

At least two thirds of women in England do paid work, which effectively means that they have two jobs. The growth in smoking, alcohol and tranquilliser use by women points to disturbing levels of anxiety and stress.

For more information about stress and relaxation see Chapter 4 *Mental Health*.

ACTIVITY *10.25*

CHD – true or false?

Aim
- To extend knowledge about coronary heart disease and women.

Materials
Copies of Worksheet 10.16 *CHD – true or false?* and Information Sheet 10.18 *Coronary heart disease* for each woman; pens.

Method
1 In small groups, ask women to go through the worksheet, noting their responses.

2 Give out the information sheet for groups to check up on the facts.

3 In the large group, feed back and discuss.

Discussion points
- How much did women already know?

- Where does most of our information about CHD come from, and how accurate is it?

- How can women find out more?

ACTIVITY *10.26*

CHD – personal action plan

Aim
- To encourage women to consider changes they can make to reduce their risk of CHD.

Materials
A copy of Information Sheet 10.18 *Coronary heart disease* for each woman; pens, flipchart, marker.

Method

1 Give each woman a copy of the information sheet and ask them to think about ideas for preventing CHD.

2 In pairs, women begin to identify small changes they could make to their everyday life to reduce their own risks. Give each other ideas and support, and choose two steps to start with.

3 In the large group, share ideas, flipchart ideas for action, and discuss.

Discussion points

- What do women already do that helps to protect them from CHD?

- How easy is it for women to make the changes they have chosen? What might help them? What may hinder them?

- Could the group offer opportunities or support for women to achieve their first steps?

WORKSHEET *10.16*

CHD – true or false?

- Almost one third of all deaths of people aged under 75 are caused by CHD.

- Heart disease is a man's illness.

- After menopause, women's chances of getting CHD are equal to that of men.

- Once you have had CHD you are an invalid for the rest of your life.

- You can't do anything about high blood-pressure.

- Responsibility for prevention of CHD lies with the individual.

- Exercise is only good for you if it hurts.

- If you are over 35 and smoke it is not advisable to use the Pill.

- Smoking is one of the main factors which can cause CHD.

- Blood-pressure usually rises as you get older.

- The CHD-related death rate for Asian women is 30% higher than the UK average.

RESOURCES

Good Housekeeping with Coronary Prevention Group, *Eating for a Healthy Heart*, (1988), Ebury Press, £8.95.

Health Education Authority, *Health Update 1 – Coronary Heart Disease* (1990), Free. Available from the Health Education Authority.
Reviews the prevalence and distribution of coronary heart disease in England and the risk factors which give rise to it.

Health Education Authority Look After Your Heart Programme, *Workplace Action Plans*, £2.95 plus p&p. Available from the Health Education Authority.
A set of action plans for employers to improve the health of their employees. Topics covered include smoking, stress, sensible drinking, healthy eating, cancer, physical activity and women's health.

Kowalski, Robert E, *Cholesterol and Children: the parent's guide to giving children a future free of heart disease* (1989), Thorsons, £8.95, ISBN 0 7225 214 5.

Lynch, Barry, *The BBC Diet: the Easy Healthy Diet* (1989), BBC, £2.95, ISBN 0 56320 689 6.
Includes diet plans from Heartbeat Wales.

Mervyn, Leonard, *New Self Help Heart Disease: a practical guide to all aspects of heart disease and its prevention* (1990), Thorsons, £1.99. ISBN 0 72252 256 8.

Mulcahy, Risteard, *Beat Heart Disease! How to help your heart and lead a happier, healthier life* (1990), Optima, £5.99, ISBN 0 35619 670 4.

Patel, Chandra, *Fighting Heart Disease: a practical self help guide to prevention and treatment* (1987), Dorling Kindersley/British Holistic Medical Association, £6.99.

Shreeve, Caroline, *Lower your Blood Pressure in Four Easy Stages* (1989), Thorsons, £3.99. ISBN 0 72251 635 5.

Videos

Amar Dil, (in English, Gujarati, Punjabi, Hindi, and Bengali), Leicestershire Health Authority. Compilation of 50 minutes (10 minutes in each language). Available from Leicestershire Health Authority, Health Education Video Unit.
Aimed at the general public looking at contributory factors to coronary heart disease, with accompanying leaflets.

Prevention of Coronary Heart Disease (1990), (in Hindu, Urdu, Bengali, Gujarati, Punjabi and English). Available from Concord Films.
Alerts Asian people and health workers to the risk factors of CHD. Through the story of a man who has a mild heart attack, the film shows how this encourages the whole family to change its lifestyle. Accompanying book.

Organisations

Coronary Prevention Group
Carry out research into issues surrounding coronary heart disease. Provide information and publications.

LAYH: LAY Project Centre
A national project which promotes the benefits of a healthy lifestyle through exhibitions, classes and seminars, in community settings and workplaces. The project provides training and an extensive range of publications and display materials.

The Stroke Association
Work in the field of stroke prevention, research and rehabilitation, advice and welfare. Produce many publications.

11 General resources

For resources on specific topics, see the list at the end of each section or chapter.

Publications

Ammer, Christiner, *The New A to Z of Women's Health* (1989), Facts-on-File, £16.99. Easy to read but detailed encyclopedic guide to women's health topics.

Bolton Health Authority, *Health Information for Women* (booklet), (Urdu, Gujarati, English). Available from Bolton Health Authority. 10 copies price £8 inclusive.
Covers: pre-menstrual syndrome, thrush, cystitis, menstruation, breast care, family planning, and the cervical smear test, safer sex and HIV/AIDS and the menopause.

Bradford, Nikki, *The Well Woman's Self-help Directory* (1990), Sidgewick and Jackson, £12.99.
Includes details of many conditions, how to do self-help, information on complementary medicine and lists of self-help groups.

Bryan, B, Dadzie, S, and Scarfe, S, *The Heart of the Race . . . Black Women's Lives in Britain* (1985), Virago, £5.50. Due for reprint 1992.

Butler, Sandra and Wintram, Clare, *Feminist Group Work* (1991), Sage, £10.95.
Looks at the purposes, practice and effectiveness of group work with women. Speaks in favour of liberating consequences of group work.

Cabot, Sandra, *Women's Health* (1990), Pan, £6.99.
General guide which covers PMS, contraception, sexuality, and a range of topics with both conventional and alternative treatment discussed. Australian.

Carers National Association, *Starting a Carers Group* (1991), Free to carers, £2 to organisations. Available from Carers National Association.
An information pack with contact and book lists. Practical details and ideas, resources needed, suggestions for speakers.

Centre for Contemporary Cultural Studies, *The Empire Strikes Back* (1982), Hutchinson London.
Includes Hazel Carby's article *White women listen! Black feminism and the boundaries of sisterhood*, and P. Parmar's article, *Gender, race and class: Asian women in resistance*.

Community Education Training Unit, *Training and How to Enjoy it* (1988), £6.70. Available from Community Education Development Centre.
Devised especially for community and voluntary groups, this book provides creative ways of helping groups and trainers to develop new skills, knowledge and awareness. It uses techniques such as brainstorming and role play and covers such themes as groups and meetings, equal opportunities, planning and problem solving.

Community Links, *Ideas Annual* (yearly), £5. Available from Community Links, Training and Development Unit.
Over 100 ideas from community groups from all over the country, including setting up a telephone translating service, a lunchtime women's health course and diet group, and a school-age mothers' counselling and support group.
Chapters on participation and representation, ideas for exploiting local resources, ways and means of working, and getting messages across.

Community Projects Foundation/Health Education Authority/Scottish Health Education Group, *Action for Health: Initiatives in Local Communities* (1988), £3.75 (voluntary/community groups), £4.50 (statutory bodies). Available from National Community Health Resource.
Explains the growth of the community health movement, the key issues it has taken up and its potential significance, using detailed examples from 25 projects.

D-Ashur, Shamis, *Silent Tears* (1989), £5.95, ISBN 0 951 4858 0 6. Available from London Black Women's Health Action Group.
Using interviews this booklet brings together firsthand experiences of women living in Britain who are affected by female genital mutilation. Highlights the complex issues surrounding this practice and supports the case for eradication, within the overall context of Black women's health in the UK.

The Diagram Group, *The Modern Woman's Body* (1990), Sidgwick and Jackson, £9.99.
An illustrated guide to a wide range of health topics as they relate to women. Wider than 'women's health' including for example, dentistry, social health, fitness.

Disability Alliance, *Disability Rights Handbook*, £6.95. Available from Disability Alliance.

Doyal, Lesley and Pennell, I, *The Political Economy of Health* (1989, c1979), Pluto, £7.50.
A classic discussion and sociological overview of health, illness and medicine and their relationship to the economy in both British and international contexts. Special emphasis on the oppression of women.

Everywoman, *The Everywoman Directory 1991–1992: Handbook of the Women's Movement* (1991), £5.95.
A directory of women's businesses, networks and campaigns, including health, therapy and others.

Gillinder, Cathy, Hanby, Gill and Wells, Christina, *A Woman's View – Living in a Rural Area* (1991), Huntingdon Health Authority/National Community Health Resource/West Huntingdon Rural Development Project, £3.50 (voluntary/community groups), £4.50 (statutory/professional bodies). Available from National Community Health Resource.
Report of a one-day conference for women living and working in rural areas which provides an account of the major issues affecting them. Useful for anyone working in a rural area as it describes the planning process and highlights examples of good practice.

Graham, Hilary, *Women, Health and the Family* (1984), Wheatsheaf, £12.99.
A sociological examination of women as providers of health care in the family.

Efua Graham, Stella, *Female Circumcision: Information for Health Professionals*, Foundation for Women's Health Research and Development. Available from FORWARD.
This pamphlet is part of a pack aimed at raising the awareness of UK health professionals to the subject of female genital mutilation.

Grant, Jane, *Sisters Across the Atlantic: A Guide to Networking in the USA* (1988), National Council for Voluntary Organisations, £4.95, ISBN 07 199 12261. Available from NCVO.
How and why American women organise; the imaginative fund-raising strategies they have developed; and how these can be adapted to the UK situation. Demonstrates that women in the UK can learn from the American experience, and lists more than 90 key organisations in the USA to enable women to extend their networks across the Atlantic.

Hayman, Suzie, *The Well Woman Handbook: a Guide for Women Throughout their Lives* (1989), Penguin, £3.99.
A clear guide to general women's health concerns.

Health Education Authority, *Women Together: a Health Education Training Handbook for Ourselves and Others* (1992), £12.95. Available from the Health Education Authority.
Provides information and practical suggestions on how to plan, organise and facilitate women's health education, and how to identify new opportunities for health promotion initiatives. The information will help women who are running health sessions themselves or are training others to do so. For all those workers and managers in health and local authorities, adult education, voluntary and community settings who are seeking to promote women's health.

Hepburn, Cuca, *Alive and Well: Lesbian Health Guide* (1989), Crossing Press (Airlift), £7.95.

Krzowski, Sue and Land, Pat (eds), *In our Experience: Workshops at the Women's Therapy Centre* (1988), Women's Press, £6.95.
Articles by many authors cover a range of workshop topics from lesbians to working class to Black women, body work and others.

Last, Pat and Rushton, Ann, *Women's Health Questions Answered: a Guide to Over 500 Common Health Problems* (1990), Thorsons, £5.99.
Answers a wide range of practical questions from a woman's perspective.

Laws, Sophie, *Down There: an Illustrated Guide to Self Examination* (booklet) (1981), Onlywomen, £1.50. Available from Women's Health.

Lothian Health Board, *Women and Wellbeing: a Resource Pack* (1987), £3.50.
Aimed at women interested in or already working with women's health groups. Guidance on setting up groups, approaches to use and resources. Includes ten workshops on specific issues.

Lonsdale, S, *Women and Disability: the Experience of Physical Disability among Women* (1990), Macmillan, £8.99.
Describes the experience of physical disability through detailed interviews with women of different ages, races and socio-economic background, and explores the impact of gender on the process of being or becoming disabled. Considers impact on sexuality, relationships, marriage and childrearing.

Macdonald, Fiona, *The Women's Directory* (1991), Bedford Square Press, £6.95.
Lists a wide range of women's organisations nationwide.

Miles, Agnes, *Women, Health and Medicine* (1991), Open University, £11.99.
Sociological view of women as recipients and providers of health care.

Morris, Jenny, *Pride Against Prejudice: Transforming Attitudes to Disability* (1991), Women's Press, £6.95. Confronts the nature of prejudice against disabled people.

NCHR, *Guide to Community Health Projects* (1987), £3.00 (voluntary/community groups), £5.00 (statutory bodies). Available from National Community Health Resource.
A guide to more than 30 local community health projects in Britain. Contains useful guidelines for those wishing to set up a project, including activities, funding, management and evaluation.

NCHR, *Funding for Women's Health Groups* (1992), £4.00. Available from National Community Health Resource.

NCHR, *Selected References on Black and Minority Ethnic Health Issues: Bibliography No. 1* (1990), £3.00. Available from National Community Health Resource.
Provides more than 70 key references on health issues and Black and minority ethnic groups. It also covers provision of health services and employment of Black and minority ethnic workers in health care services.

National Self-Help Support Centre, *Self-Help Groups: A Way to Health* (1991), £4.00. Available from National Self Help Centre, NCVO.
A report based on a one-day seminar looking at developing partnerships between self-help groups and health promoters. It focuses on the roles health promoters and group members can take in the life of a self-help group, the value of developing networking and partnerships in order to support groups and the implications for policy and practice.

Orr, Jean (ed), *Women's Health in the Community* (1987), Wiley, £8.50.
A collection of articles on women's health topics from economics to hysterectomy, childbirth and mental health from a feminist perspective.

O'Sullivan, Sue, *Women's Health: a Spare Rib Reader* (1987), Pandora, £5.95.
Covers a wide range of women's health topics. Taken from articles published in Spare Rib.

Oxford, *The A-Z of Women's Health* (1990), Oxford, £5.99.
Dictionary approach to a wide range of women's health topics. Second edition.

Pattenson, Lesley and Burns, Jan, *Women, Assertiveness and Health* (1990), Health Education Authority, £5.95. Available from the Health Education Authority.
A rationale for the use of assertiveness in women's health education and promotion.

Pearse, M, and Smith, J, *Community Groups Handbook* (1990), Pluto Press, £5.95, ISBN 1 85172 037 5.
A useful and practical guide on how to make your community group effective. It explains how groups are organised, how they relate to public authorities and reviews tactics for taking action. Particularly valuable for its coverage of topics such as pressure groups and communicating with the neighbourhood.

Phillips, Angela and Rakusen, Jill (eds), *Our Bodies, Ourselves: a Health Book by and for Women* (1989), Penguin, £15.99.
Updated British edition of the classic Boston Women's Health Book Collective comprehensive guide to women's health.

Roberts, Helen (ed), *Women's Health Counts* (1990), Routledge, £10.99.
Covers a number of women's health issues (including hysterectomy, women's mortality differences, research practice) from a sociological perspective.

Roberts, Helen (ed), *Women's Health Matters* (1992), Routledge, £10.99.
Sociological essays on a range of topics including multiple birth, midwifery, birth and violence, nutrition. Includes Jenny Douglas' article, *Black women's health matters*, an excellent appraisal of the complex inter-relationships between race, class and gender in Black women's lives in England.

Rodda, A, *Women and the Environment* (1991), Zed Books Ltd, £9.95.
Looks at the deterioration of the earth's environment in terms of its significance for women, especially in terms of their health and basic needs. Reveals how women can be a major force for environmental change. Good diagrams, well set out.

Rodmell, S, and Watts, A (eds), *Politics of Health Education* (1986), Routledge and Kegan Paul.
Includes M Pearson's article *Racist notions of ethnicity and culture in health education*.

Saxton, Marsha and Howe, Florence, *With Wings: an Anthology of Literature by Women with Disabilities* (1988), Virago, £4.95.

Many different women – young, old, rich, poor, heterosexual, lesbian, Black and white – write about their feelings about disability.

Sapin, Kate and Watters, Geraldine, *Learning from Each Other* (1990), William Temple Foundation, £14.95. Available from Community Education Development Centre.
A handbook for participative learning and community work programmes, useful for those involved in adult learning or work with community groups.

Slavin, Hazel (ed), *Organising Health Events for Women* (1991), Health Education Authority, £2.95. Available from the Health Education Authority.
A guide to planning, organising, running and evaluating women's health conferences and workshops. Aimed at anybody needing to organise such events for women.

Smyre, P, *Women and Health* (1991), Zed Books Ltd, £9.95.
This comprehensive book looks at the position of women worldwide, and asks why so many women in all parts of the world fail to get the health care and health information they need. It examines key health problems for women workers, refugee and migrant women, young girls and older women. Very well laid out.

Szirom, Tricia and Dyson, Sue, *Greater Expectations: a Source Book for Working with Girls and Young Women* (1990, second edition), Learning Development Aids, £12.95. Available from Healthwise, Family Planning Association.
A resource for those who are concerned to raise the awareness and self-esteem of the girls and young women with whom they work. It offers a compendium of activities and strategies to help groups and individuals understand the nature of women's role in society.

Townsend, Davidson and Whitehead, *Inequalities in Health* (1990), Penguin, £6.99. Contains both the Black Report and the Health Divide.

White, Evelyn C, *The Black Women's Health Book: Speaking for Ourselves* (1990), Seal, £10.95.
A collection of essays on subjects ranging from midwifery to child sexual abuse, Black women physicians, teenage pregnancy, hypertension and others. American perspective.

Videos, films and audio tapes

From Boredom to Boardroom: Helping Ourselves to Health: the Wirral Women's Experience (1991), video, £9.95. Available from the Health Education Authority.
Records the way in which community involvement and participation can lead to improved health education policy, planning and provision in both the statutory and voluntary sectors.

Leeds Animation Workshop, *Give us a Smile* (1983), 13 minute video. Available from Leeds Animation Workshop.

A witty and provoking look at the constant harassment which women suffer – institutional, verbal and physical – and ways in which they are fighting back.

Open University, *Health Choices* (undated), video resource pack, study pack £26.00, video £47.00, assessment pack £15.00, course £38.
Deals with a wide range of health, fitness and stress topics.

Leeds Animation Workshop, *Out to Lunch* (1989), 12 minute video. Available from Leeds Animation Workshop.
Covers issues of sexuality and sexism.

Sporting Health, video £35, hire fee £15. Available from Cinema of Women.
Made in Hounslow, London, showing a pilot initiative of health and fitness courses for women including weight training for pensioners, fencing, trampolining and martial arts as well as the more traditional swimming, relaxation, healthy eating and reflexology.

Women Feeling Good, exhibition on women's health with text in six languages. Available from Sandwell Health Promotion Unit.
Aims to reflect women's everyday experience of what health means.

Women's Film List (1989), BFI Publications, £7.75. Available from BFI Publications.
Provides comprehensive details of films directed by women and/or dealing with important aspects of women's lives, such as health and sexuality. All the material listed is currently available for hire in the UK.

Organisations

Feminist Audio Books
Provides materials on tape for women who are blind, partially sighted or who have trouble with the printed word.

Health Education Authority
Publishes an extensive range of health education materials.

Health Search Scotland
A free information service on self-help and voluntary groups throughout Scotland, with an extensive collection of self-help leaflets and booklets.

Help for Health Trust
Produces leaflets on a wide range of topics. Produces a newsletter with details of self-help groups, publications, videos, etc. Has a database of self-help groups throughout Britain.

Liverpool Central and South Community Health Council
Produces a set of 30 regularly updated leaflets written by Dr Katy Gardner in conjunction with the Liverpool & Neighbourhood Health Project. No copyright on the leaflets.

London Black Women's Health Action Project
Works primarily with the Somali community in London, especially with women and young people.

London Interpreting Project
A London-wide organisation committed to facilitating access to public services for all linguistic minorities by providing information, training and support for all those involved in community interpreting initiatives.

National Alliance of Women's Organisations
Umbrella organisation with more than 185 member organisations.

National Community Health Resource
Membership organisation providing information about women's and Black and minority ethnic health groups and community health projects around the UK, community health and women's health issues. Enquiry service, information centre, publications and networking for voluntary and statutory sectors. Bi-monthly newsletter.

National Self-Help Support Centre.
Supports networks for self-help support workers, local workers, Black workers and for specialist organisations. Produces reports and organises seminars.

Open University
Has 13 regional centres. Produces educational materials in health. Open University Department of Health and Social Welfare Newspaper gives news of developments in OU programmes and publications in health.

Repetitive Strain Injury Association
National information body for sufferers of repetitive strain injury.

Well-woman clinics/centres
Ask at your GP surgery if they have a well-woman clinic or contact Women's Health (see below) or your local Community Health Council for local well-woman clinics which will provide a number of services.

Women and Diabetes Network
A national self-help network open to any woman with insulin dependent or non-insulin dependent diabetes. For information, please send large s.a.e.

Women and Theatre
Provides witty, entertaining and provocative theatre on a wide variety of issues such as tranquillisers, HIV, weight, alcohol and PMS. Also offers workshops, training packages and conference presentations which combine drama, group work and role play techniques and structured, reflective discussion.

Women's Environmental Network
Runs seminars, workshops and public meetings, produces action packs and leaflets.

Women's Health
Formerly Women's Health and Reproductive Rights Information Centre (WHR-RIC). Provides enquiry service by visit (phone to make an appointment), phone or letter. Extensive resource centre covers all women's health topics. Send stamped s.a.e. for publication list of over 40 leaflets. Reductions on bulk orders. Leaflets on tape.

Women's Health Information Resource Collective, Australia
Has an impressive collection of resources, leaflets and reports on many women's health topics many of which are translated into languages other than English (mostly Greek and Italian, but also Arabic, Serbo-Croatian, Spanish, Turkish and Vietnamese). May be used, adapted or reproduced as needed.

Women's Health Network
A project of National Community Health Resource. Develops links between women's health initiatives in the community. Produces a bimonthly newsletter. Subscriptions £5 for unfunded groups and unwaged individuals, £12 for waged individuals and voluntary organisations and £20 for statutory bodies.

Bookshops

Healthwise/Family Planning Association
Carries a large range of health topics, with particular emphasis on sexuality, pregnancy, birth control and a number of women's health topics. Mail order service available.

Silver Moon
Women's bookshop carrying a wide range of women's health materials. Will order books not in stock. Mail order available.

Sisterwrite
Has a large stock of women's health materials, will do mail order and will order books not held in stock.

West and Wilde
Will do orders worldwide. Has a range of women's health materials.

Film and video distributors

Academy Television
Handles programmes from Tyne Tees, WTN, HTV, Scottish TV, Thames, Channel 4 and Yorkshire.

Broadcasting Support Services
Support materials on a range of topics. Contact them for titles currently available.

Concord Video and Film Council
A range of films on women's health and related issues.

Organisations: contact details

This list includes details of all organisations listed in *Resources* sections throughout the book.

Academy Television, 104 Kirkstall Road, Leeds, LS3 1JS, Tel: 0532 461528

Action on Smoking and Health (ASH), 109 Gloucester Place, London W1H 3PH, Tel: 071 935 3519

Age Concern England, Astral House, 1268 London Road, London SW16 4ER, Tel: 081 679 8000

AIDS Awareness/Sex Education Project, Harperbury Hospital, Harper Lane, Radlett, Herts WD7 9HQ, Tel: 0923 854861 Ext 4420

Aidsline Health Promotion Services, Enfield Health Authority, Pavilion 1, Highlands Hospital, Winchmore Hill, London N21 1PN, Tel: 081 366 9187

Albany Video Distribution, Battersea Studios, Television Centre, Thackeray Road, London SW8 3TW, Tel: 071 498 6811

Alcoholics Anonymous, PO Box 1, Stonebow House, Stonebow, York, YO1 2NJ, Tel: 0904 644026

Alcohol Concern, 305 Grays Inn Road, London WC1X 8QF, Tel: 071 833 3471

Alcohol Counselling and Prevention Services, 34 Electric Lane, London SW9 8JT, Tel: 071 737 3579

Alexander Technique, Society of Teachers (STAT), 20 London House, 266 Fulham Road, London SW10 9EL, Tel: 071 351 0828

Arrowhead Productions, 51 Thames Village, Hartington Road, London W4 3UF, Tel: 081 994 0896

Ashgrove Distribution, 4 Brassmill Centre, Brassmill Lane, Bath BA1 3JN

Association of Community Health Councils for England and Wales, 30 Drayton Park, London N5 1PB, Tel: 071 609 8405

Association of Community Interpreters and Translators, Advocates and Link-workers (ACITAL), c/o London Interpreting Project, 20 Compton Terrace, London N1 2UN, Tel: 071 359 6798

AWAAZ, Manchester Council for Community Relations (MCCR), Elliot House, 3 Jackson Row, Deansgate, Manchester, M2 5WD

Bach Flower Remedies, Edward Bach Centre, Mount Vernon, Sotwell, Wallingford, Oxon, OX10 OPZ, Tel: 0491 34678

Bailey Distribution Ltd, Department KFP, Learoyd Road, Mountfield Industrial Estate, New Romney, Kent, TN28 8XU

Barony Film and TV Productions Ltd, 4 Picardy Place, Edinburgh, EH1 3JT, Tel: 031 558 3275

Berkshire Education Department, Education for Racial Equality, 41 Stanhope Road, Reading, Berkshire, RG2 7HW, Tel: 0734 311625

Beth Johnson Foundation, Parkfield House, 64 Princes Road, Hartshill, Stoke-on-Trent, ST4 7JL

BFI Publications, 29 Rathbone Street, London W1P 1AG, Tel: 071 636 3289

Birth Control Trust, 27-35 Mortimer Street, London W1N 7RJ, Tel: 071 580 9360

Birthright, 27 Sussex Place, Regent's Park, London NW1 4SP, Tel: 071 262 5337

Black HIV/AIDS Network (BHAN), 111 Devonport Road, London W12 8PB, Tel: 081 749 2828. Helpline: 081 742 9223

Blackfriars Photography Project, Blackfriars Settlement, 44 Nelson Square, London SE1 OQA, Tel: 071 928 9521

Bolton Health Authority, Bolton Centre for Health Promotion, 3 Chorley New Road, Bolton, BL1 4QR, Tel: 0204 320891

Breast Care and Mastectomy Association of Great Britain, 15 Britten Street, London SW3 3TZ, Helpline: 071 867 1103, Tel: 071 867 8275; Suite 2/8, 65 Bath Street, Glasgow, G2 2BX, Tel: 041 353 1050

Bristol Cancer Help Centre, Grove House, Cornwallis Grove, Clifton, Bristol, BS8 4PG, Tel: 0272 743216

British Acupuncture Association and Register, 34 Alderney Street, London SW1V 4EU, Tel: 071 834 1012

British Agencies for Adoption and Fostering, 11 Southwark Street, London SE1 1RQ, Tel: 071 407 8800

British Association of Cancer United Patients (BACUP), 121 Charterhouse Street, London EC1M 6AA, Information: 071 608 1661, Counselling: 071 608 1038, Freephone for outside London: 0800 181199, Admin: 071 608 1785

British Association of Counselling, 1 Regent Place, Rugby, Warwickshire, CV21 2PJ, Tel: 0788 578328

British Homeopathic Association, 27A Devonshire Street, London W1N 1RJ, Tel: 071 935 2163

British Naturopathic and Osteopathic Association, Frazer House, 6 Netherhall Gardens, London NW3 5RR, Tel: 071 435 8728

British Pregnancy Advisory Service, Austy Manor, Wootten Wawen, Solihull, B95 6BX, Tel: 0564 793225

Broadcasting Support Services, PO Box 7, London W3 6XJ

Brook Advisory Centres, Central Office, 153a East Street, London SE17 2SD, Tel: 071 708 1234

Brook Advisory Centres, Education and Publications Unit, 24 Albert Street, Birmingham, B4 7UD, Tel: 021 643 1554

Cancer Aftercare and Rehabilitation Society (CARE), 21 Zetland Road, Redland, Bristol, BS6 7AH, Tel: 0272 427419

CancerLink, 17 Britannia Street, London WC1X 9JN, Tel: 071 833 2451, Edinburgh Information Service: 031 228 5557

Carers National Association, 29 Chilworth Mews, London W2 3RG, Tel: 071 724 7776

Central Council for Education and Training in Social Work (CCETSW), Derbyshire House, St Chad's Street, London WC1H 8AD, Tel: 071 278 2455

Centre for Health and Retirement Education, Department of Educational Studies, Nodus Buildings, University of Surrey, Guildford, GU2 5XH, Tel: 0483 39390

Centre Prise Trust Ltd, 136 Kingsland High Street, Hackney, London E8

CFL Vision, PO Box 35, Wetherby, West Yorkshire, LS23 7EX, Tel: 0937 541010

Child Abuse Studies Unit, The Polytechnic of North London, Ladbroke House, 62-66 Highbury Grove, London N5 2AD, Tel: 071 607 2789 Ext 5014

Child Poverty Action Group, 1-5 Bath Street, London EC1V 9PY, Tel: 071 253 3406

Cinema of Women, 27 Clerkenwell Close, London EC1R 0AT, Tel: 071 251 4978

College of Health, St Margaret's House, 21 Old Ford Road, London E2 9PL, Tel: 081 981 1225, National Waiting List Helpline: 081 983 1133

Community Education Development Centre, Lyng Hall, Blackberry Lane, Coventry, CV2 3JS, Tel: 0203 638670

Community Links, Training and Development Unit, Aizlewood's Mill, Nursery Street, Sheffield, S3 8GG, Tel: 0742 823163

Concord Video and Film Council, 201 Felixstowe Road, Ipswich, Suffolk, IP3 9BJ, Tel: 0473 715754

Confederation of Indian Organisations, 5 Westminster Bridge Road, London SE1 7XW, Tel: 071 928 9889

Coronary Prevention Group, 102 Gloucester Place, London W1H 3DA, Tel: 071 935 2889

Cruse Bereavement Care, 126 Sheen Road, Richmond, London TW9 1UR, Tel: 081 940 4818

DAWN (Drugs, Alcohol, Women Network), c/o 30-31 Great Sutton Street, London EC1V 0DK, Tel: 071 253 6221

Department of Health, Health Publications Unit, Eileen House, 80–94 Newington Causeway, London SE1 6EF, Tel: 071 972 2000

Derbyshire FHSA, Derwent Court, Stuart Street, Derby, SE1 2FZ

DES Action, c/o Women's Health, 52 Featherstone Street, London EC1Y 8RT

Directory of Social Change, Radius Works, Back Lane, London NW3 1HL, Tel: 071 431 1817

Disability Alliance, Universal House, 88-94 Wentworth Street, London E1 7SA, Tel: 071 247 8776

Discern, 34 Heathcoat Street, Nottingham NG1 3AA

Dramatic Distribution Ltd, 41 Stanhope Road, Reading, Berks, RG2 7HW, Tel: 0734 311625

Eating Disorders Association, Sackville Place, 44 Magdalen Street, Norwich, NR3 1JE, Tel: (9:00–4:00) 0603 621414; 11 Priory Road, High Wycombe, Buckinghamshire, HP13 6SL, Tel: (11:30–2:30) 0494 521431

Educational Media International, 235 Imperial Drive, Rayners Lane, Harrow, Middlesex, HA2 7HE, Tel: 081 868 1908

Endometriosis Society, 35 Belgrave Square, London SW1X 8QB, Tel: 071 737 0380

Exploring Parenthood, Latimer Education Centre, 194 Freston Road, London W10 6TT, Tel: 081 960 1678

Family Health and Nutrition Information Group, PO Box 38, Crowborough, East Sussex, TN6 2YP

Family Planning Association, 27-35 Mortimer Street, London W1N 7RJ, Tel: 071 636 7866

Feminist Audio Books, 52 Featherstone Street, London EC1Y 8RT, Tel: 071 251 2908

Health Board, Glenrothes House, North Street, Glenrothes, Fife, KY7 5PB, Tel: 0592 754355

The Food Commission, 5–11 Worship Street, London EC2A 2BH, Tel: 071 628 7774

Food Safety Advisory Centre, 14 Soho Square, London W1V 5FB

FORWARD, 38 King Street, London WC2E 8JT, Tel: 071 379 6889

General Council and Register of Osteopaths, 56 London Street, Reading, RG1 4SQ

Gingerbread, 35 Wellington Street, London WC2E 7BN, Tel: 071 240 0953

GLAAS, 30–31 Great Sutton Street, London EC1 0DX, Tel: 071 253 6221

Good Practices in Mental Health, 380-384 Harrow Road, London W9 2HU, Tel: 071 289 2034/3060

Greater London Association of Community Health Councils, 100 Park Village East, London NW1 3SR, Tel: 071 387 2171

Health Care Productions Ltd, 116 Cleveland Street, London W1P 5DN, Tel: 071 267 8757

Health Education Authority, Hamilton House, Mabledon Place, London WC1H 9TX, Tel: 071 383 3833

Health Education Authority, HELIOS Project, University of the West of England, Redland Hill, Bristol, BS6 6UZ, Tel: 0272 238317

Health Education Authority Primary Health Care Unit, The Churchill Hospital, Headington, Oxford, OX3 7LJ, Tel: 0865 226061

Health Rights, Unit 405, Small Business Centre, 444 Brixton Road, London SW9 8EJ, Tel: 071 274 4000 Ext 326

Health Search Scotland, Woodburn House, Canaan Lane, Edinburgh, EH10 4SG, Tel: 031 452 8666

Healthwise, Family Planning Association, 27 Mortimer Street, London W1N 7RJ, Tel: 071 636 7866

Healthwise Productions, 9 Batley Enterprise Centre, 513 Bradford Road, Batley, West Yorks, WF17 8JY, Tel: 0924 474374

Help the Aged, St James's Walk, London EC1R 0BE, Seniorline: 0800 289404, Admin: 071 253 0253

Help for Health Trust, Highcroft Cottage, Romsey Road, Winchester, S022 5DH, Tel: 0962 849100

Herpes Association, 41 North Road, London N7 9DP, Tel: 071 609 9061, Helpline: 071 607 9661

HMSO Bookshops, 49 High Holborn, London WC1V 6HB, Tel: 071 873 0011 (counter service only); PO Box 276, London SW8 5DT, Tel: 071 873 9090 (telephone orders)

Hysterectomy Support Network, 3 Lynne Close, Green Street, Orpington, Kent, BR6 6BS

Immunity Publications, 260A Kilburn Lane, London W10 4BA, Tel: 081 968 8909

Institute of Complementary Medicine, PO Box 194, London SE16 1QZ

Institute for the Study of Drug Dependence (ISDD), 1 Hatton Place, London EC1N 8ND, Tel: 071 430 1991

International Federation of Aromatherapists, Department of Continuing Education, Royal Masonic Hospital, Raven's Court Park, London W6 0TN, Tel: 081 846 8066

International Federation of Reflexologists, 78 Edridge Road, Croydon, Surrey, CRO 1EF

International Network of Women Against Tobacco (INWAT), c/o American Publication Health Association, 1015 Fifteenth Street, NW, Washington, DC 20005, USA

International Planned Parenthood Federation (IPPF), Regents College, Inner Circle, London NW1 4NS, Tel: 071 486 0741

International Stress and Tension Control Society, 25 Sutherland Avenue, Roundhay, Leeds, LS8 1BY, Tel: 0532 664260

Jensen E A, Attree Drive, Queen's Park, Brighton, Sussex, BN2 2HN, Tel: 0273 605293

Kings Fund Centre, 126 Albert Street, London NW1 7NE, Tel: 071 267 6111

Lancashire FHSA, Caxton Road, Fulwood, Preston, PR2 4ZZ, Tel: 0772 704141

LAYH:LAY Project Centre, Christ Church College, Canterbury, Kent, CT1 1QU, Tel: 0227 455564

Leeds Animation Workshop, 45 Bayswater Road, Leeds, West Yorkshire, L88 5LF, Tel: 0532 484997

Leicestershire Health Authority, Health Education Video Unit, Clinical Sciences Building, Leicester Royal Infirmary, PO Box 55, Leicester, LE2 7LX, Tel: 0533 550461

Lesbian Line, BM Box 1514, London WC1N 3XX, Tel: 071 251 6911

The Lesbian Network, c/o CancerLink (see above)

Liverpool Central and South Community Health Council, 57 Whitechapel, Liverpool, L1 6DX, Tel: 051 236 1176

Liverpool Health Promotion Unit, Sefton General Hospital, Smithdown Road, Liverpool, L15 2HE, Tel: 051 733 4020

Liverpool Institute of Higher Education, Stand Park Road, Liverpool, L16 9JD, Tel: 051 722 7179

London Black Women's Health Action Project, Cornwall Ave Community Centre, 1 Cornwall Avenue, London E1 0HN, Tel: 081 980 3503

London Interpreting Project, 20 Compton Terrace, London N1 2UN, Tel: 071 359 6798

London Rape Crisis, PO Box 69, London WC1X 9NJ, Tel: 071 837 1600

London Voluntary Service Council, 68 Chalton Street, London NW1 1JR, Tel: 071 388 0241

Maternity Alliance, 15 Britannia Street, London WC1X 9JP, Tel: 071 837 1265

M E Action Campaign, PO Box 1126, London W3 0RY

Meet-A-Mum Association (MAMA), 58 Malden Avenue, London SE25 4HS, Tel: 081 656 7318

Menopause Society, 83 High Street, Marlow, Buckinghamshire, SL7 1AB, Tel: 0628 890199

Mental Health Film Council, 22 Harley Street, London W1N 2ED

Mental Health Media Council, 380 Harrow Road, London W9, Tel: 071 286 2346

The Mental Health Shop, 40 Chandos Street, Leicester, LE2 1BC, Tel: 0533 471525

Metro Pictures, 79 Wardour Street, London W1V 3TH, Tel: 071 734 8508

MIND (National Association for Mental Health), 22 Harley Street, London W1N 2ED, Tel: 071 637 0741

Miscarriage Association, PO Box 24, Ossett, West Yorkshire, WF4 4TP, Tel: 0924 830515 (recorded message)

N. Films, 78 Holyhead Road, Birmingham, B21 0LH, Tel: 021 507 0341

National AIDS Helpline: 0800 567 123 (24 hours), Cantonese: Tues 6–10pm 0800 282 446, Bengali, Gujarati, Hindi, Urdu, Punjabi: Wed 6–10pm 0800 282 445, Minicom: 10am–10pm 0800 521 361, Arabic: Wed 6–10 pm 0800 282 447

National Alliance of Women's Organisations, 122 Whitechapel High Street, London E1 7PT, Tel: 071 247 7052

National Association for Maternal and Child Welfare, 1 South Audley Street, London W1X 6J

National Association for Patient Participation (NAPP), 50 Wallasey Village, Wallasey, L45 3NL, Tel: 051 677 9616

National Association for Premenstrual Syndrome, PO Box 72, Sevenoaks, Kent, TN13 1QX

National Association of Natural Family Planning Teachers, 24 Selly Wick Drive, Selly Park, Birmingham, B29 7JH, Tel: 021 472 3806

National Breast Screening Programme, Trent Regional Health Authority, Fulwood House, Old Fulwood Road, Sheffield, S10 3TH, Tel: 0742 630300

National Childbirth Trust (NCT), Alexandra House, Oldham Terrace, London W3 6NH, Tel: 081 992 8637

National Childcare Campaign, 4 Wild Court, London WC2B 5AU, Tel: 071 405 5617

National Children's Bureau, 8 Wakley Street, London EC1V 7QE, Tel: 071 278 9441

National Community Health Resource, 57 Chalton Street, London NW1 1HU, Tel: 071 383 3841

National Consumer Council, 20 Grosvenor Gardens, London SW1W 0DH, Tel: 071 730 3469

National Council of One Parent Families, 255 Kentish Town Road, London NW5 2LX, Tel: 071 267 1361

National Council for Voluntary Organisations, Regents Wharf, 8 All Saints Street, London N1 9RL, Tel: 071 713 6161

National Extension College, 18 Brooklands Avenue, Cambridge, CB2 2HN, Tel: 0233 316644

National HIV Prevention Information Service, 82-86 Seymour Place, London W1H 5DB, Tel: 071 724 7993

National Osteoporosis Society, PO Box 10, Radstock, Bath, BA3 3YB, Tel: 0761 432472

National Self Help Centre, NVCO, Regent's Wharf, 8 All Saints Street, London N1 9RL, Tel: 071 713 6161

National Society for Research into Allergy, PO Box 45, Hinckley, Leicester, LE10 1JY

Network of Voluntary Organisations in AIDS/HIV (NOVOAH), PO Box 5000, Glasgow, G12 9BL

North East Thames RHA, 40 Eastbourne Terrace, London W2 3QR, Tel: 071 262 8011 Ext 2276

North Manchester Health Promotion Unit, Beech Mount, Harpurhey, Manchester, M9 1XS, Tel: 061 203 4101

Nottingham Community Unit, Memorial House, Standard Hill, Nottingham, NG1 6FX

Oasis AIDS Resource Project, Beechwood Centre, Elmete Lane, Leeds, LS8 2LQ, Tel: 0532 736765

Older Feminists Network, c/o Astra, 54 Gordon Road, London N3 1EP, Tel: 081 346 1900

Older Lesbian Network, BMOLN, London WC1N 3XX, Tel: 071 251 6911

Older Women's Project, Manor Garden Centre, 6 Manor Gardens, London N7 6LA, Tel: 071 281 3485

One-to-One, 404 Camden Road, Islington, London N7 0SJ, Tel: 071 700 5574

Open University, Community Education, Walton Hall, Milton Keynes, MK7 6AA, Tel: 0908 652170. Sales Office, PO Box 188, Milton Keynes, MK7 6DH, Tel: 0908 653140

Parentline – Organisation for Parents Under Stress, Westbury House, 57 Hart Road, Thundersley, Essex, SS7 EPD, Tel: 0268 757077

Parent Network, 44-46 Caversham Road, London NW5 2DS, Tel: 071 485 8535

Parents for Safe Food, 3rd Floor, 5-11 Worship Street, London EC2A 2BH

Pelvic Inflammatory Disease Network, c/o Women's Health, 52 Featherstone Street, London EC1Y 8RT

Pensioners Link, 405–407 Holloway Road, London N7 6HJ, Tel: 071 700 4070

Personal Hygiene Supplies (for re-usable sanitary protection), Ganniull Ltd, 38/40 Market Street, Bridgwater, Somerset, TA6 3EP, Tel: 0278 423037

Picture Talk Films, 61 Cromwell Avenue, London N6 5HP

Plymbridge Distributors Ltd, Plymbridge House, Estover Road, Plymouth, PL6 7PZ, Tel: 0752 695745

Positively Women, 5 Sebastian Street, London EC1V 0HE, Tel: 071 490 5515 (answerphone outside office hours)

The Premenstrual Society (PREMSOC), PO Box 429, Addlestone, Surrey, KT15 1DZ

Pre-School Playgroup Association, 61–63 Kings Cross Road, London WC1X 9LL, Tel: 071 833 0991

QUIT, 102 Gloucester Place, London W1H 3DA, Tel: 071 487 2858

QUITLINE: 071 487 3000 (the national stop-smoking helpline). Usual call charges apply, recorded message outside normal hours

Rainer Foundation, 89 Blackheath Hill, London SE10 8TJ, Tel: 081 694 9497

Relaxation for Living, 29 Burwood Park Road, Walton on Thames, Surrey, KT12 5LH

Repetitive Strain Injury Association, Chapel House, 152–156 High Street, Yiewsley, West Drayton, Middlesex, UB7 7BD, Tel: 0895 431134

Resolve, PO Box 820, London N10 3AW

Rights of Women, 52 Featherstone Street, London EC1Y 8RT, Tel: 071 251 6577; 071 251 6576 (lesbian custody enquiries)

Royal National Institute for the Blind, 224 Great Portland Street, London W1N 6AA, Tel: 071 388 1266

Safe Childbirth for Travellers, c/o London Gypsy Traveller Unit, 205–211 Kentish Town Road, London NW5 2JU, Tel: 071 267 6723

St. Vincent's Centre, Talma Road, Brixton, London SW2 1AS, Tel: 071 737 4255

Salford Health Promotion Centre, Third Floor, Peel House, Albert Street, Eccles, Salford, M30 0NJ, Tel: 061 787 0024

Sandwell Health Promotion Unit, 8 Grange Road, West Bromwich, West Midlands, B70 8PD, Tel: 021 525 5363

School of Phytotherapy (Herbal Medicine), Bucksteep Manor, Bodle Street Green, Hailsham, East Sussex, BN27 4RJ, Tel: 0323 833812

Second Sight Productions, Zair Works, 111 Bishop Street, Birmingham, B5 6JL, Tel: 021 622 4223

The Self-Help Team, 20 Pelham Road, Sherwood Rise, Nottingham, NG5 1AP, Tel: 0602 691212

SHANTI Asian Women and Stress Project, Health Promotion Unit, Coventry and Warwickshire Hospital, Stoney Stanton Road, Coventry, CV1 4FH, Tel: 0203 844178

Silver Moon, 64–68 Charing Cross Road, London WC2H 0BB, Tel: 071 836 7906

Single Parent Network, 14 Robertson Road, Eastville, Bristol, BS5 6JY, Tel: 0272 514231

Sisterwrite Bookshop, 190 Upper Street, London N1 1RQ, Tel: 071 226 9782

Standing Conference of Ethnic Minority Senior Citizens (SCEMSC), 5–5A Westminster Bridge Road, London SE1 7XW, Tel: 071 928 0095

Strathclyde Regional Council Women's Unit, Chief Executive's Department, 314 St. Vincent Street, Glasgow, G2 4PF, Tel: 041 227 2856

Support after Termination for Abnormality (SATFA), 29/30 Soho Square, London W1V 6JB, Tel: 071 439 6124

Survivors Speak Out, 33 Lichfield Road, London NW2 2RG

Telltale International, 12 Parkgrove Drive, Barnton, Edinburgh, EH4 7Q, Tel: 031 336 2512

The Terence Higgins Trust, 52 Grays Inn Road, London WC1X 8JU, Helpline: 071 242 1010, Tel: 071 831 1045

Under Fives Project, Mencap London Division, 115 Golden Lane, London EC1Y 0TJ, Tel: 071 454 0454

Vegetarian Society, Parkdale, Dunham Road, Altrincham, Cheshire, WA14 4QG, Tel: 061 928 0793

Videos in Pilton, 30–35 Ferry Road Avenue, West Pilton, Edinburgh, EH4 4BA, Tel: 031 343 1151

Video Production Unit, Tower Hamlets Health Promotion Service, Tredegar House, 97/99 Bow Road, London E3 2AN, Tel: 071 377 7932

VOLCOF, 77 Holloway Road, London N7 8SZ, Tel: 071 607 9573

Voluntary Action Leicester, 32 de Montfort Street, Leicester, LE1 7GD

Well-Woman Clinics/Centres. Ask at your GP surgery if they have a well-woman clinic or contact Women's Health (see below) or your local Community Health Council for local well-woman clinics which will provide a number of services

WellWomen Information, 24 St Thomas Street, Redcliffe, Bristol, BS1 6JL, Tel: 0272 413311

Welsh Office, S2 Division, Cathays Park, Cardiff, CF1 3NQ

West Birmingham Health Education Unit, Carnegie Centre, Hunters Road, Hockley, Birmingham, B19 1DR, Tel: 021 554 3899

West and Wilde, 25a Dundas Street, Edinburgh, EH3 6QQ, Tel: 031 556 0079

West London Health Promotion Agency, St Bernard's Wing, Ealing Hospital, Uxbridge Road, Southall, Middlesex, UB1 3EU

Women and Diabetes Network, 5 Brundretts Road, Manchester, M21 1DA

Women and HIV and AIDS Network, c/o SOLAS, 2 Abbeymount, Edinburgh, EH8 8EJ

Women and Theatre, 220 Moseley Road, Highgate, Birmingham, B12 0DG, Tel: 021 440 4203

Women's Action on AIDS, c/o AIDS Advice, AIDS Information and Counselling Service, 50 Call Lane, Leeds, LS1 6DT, Tel: 0532 423204

Women's Aid, London office, 52 Featherstone Street, London EC1, Tel: 071 251 6537

Women's Aid Federation England, National Coordination Office, PO Box 391, Bristol, BS99 7WS, Tel: 0272 633494

Women's Environmental Network, Aberdeen Studios, 22 Highbury Grove, London N5 2EA, Tel: 071 354 8823

Women's Health, 52 Featherstone Street, London EC1Y 8RT, Health enquiries: 071 251 6580. Administration: 071 251 6333. (Formerly Women's Health and Reproductive Rights Information Centre (WHRRIC))

Women's Health Concern, 83 Earls Court Road, London W8 6EF, Tel: 071 938 3932

Women's Health Information Mobile, 23 Mill Street, Ashwell, Baldock, Hertfordshire, SG7 5LY

Women's Health Information Resource Collective, 653 Nicholson Street, Carlton North, Victoria 3054, Australia, Tel: 03 3878702

Women's Health Network, National Community Health Resource, 57 Chalton Street, London NW1 1HU, Tel: 071 383 3841

Women's Nationwide Cancer Control Campaign (WNCCC), Suma House, 128 Curtain Road, London EC2A 3AR, Helpline: 071 729 2229, Admin: 071 729 4688 (24 hour taped phone lines), breast awareness: 071 729 4915, cervical screening: 071 729 5061

Women's Nutritional Advisory Service, PO Box 268, Hove, East Sussex, BN3 1RW

Women's Therapy Centre, 6 Manor Gardens, London N7 6LA, Tel: 071 263 6200

Index to activities, information sheets and worksheets